Mosby's textbook for the

HOME

CARE

AIDE

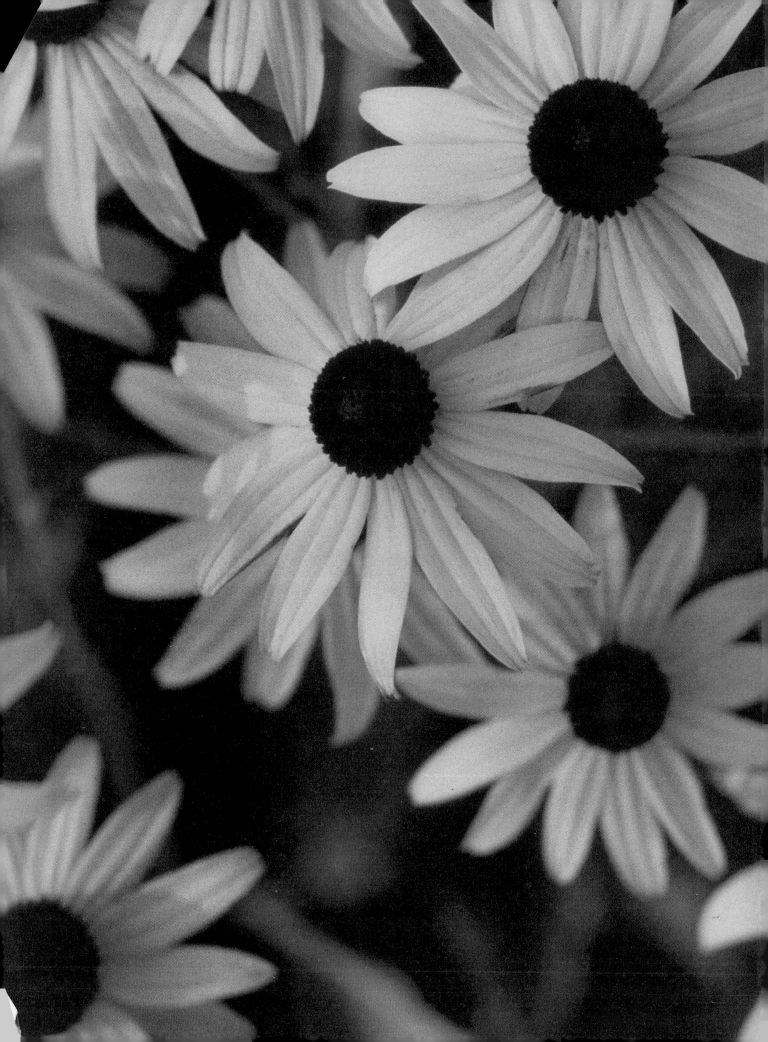

Mosby's textbook for the

HOME

Joan Birchenall

CARE

Eileen Streight

AIDE

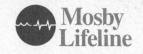

Mosby Lifeline

An Imprint of Elsevier Science

St. Louis   London   Philadelphia   Sydney   Toronto

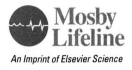

Mosby Lifeline

An Imprint of Elsevier Science

First Edition
Copyright © 1997 by Mosby, Inc.
A Mosby Lifeline imprint of Mosby, Inc.

Printed in the United States of America
Original art by Robin Offenbacher

Mosby, Inc.
11830 Westline Industrial Drive
St. Louis, MO 63146

ISBN: 0-8151-0726-9

02 03 04 05 / 9 8 7 6 5

Dedication

In memory of my mother,
Margaret B. Birchenall,
whose enthusiastic support,
constant encouragement,
keen interest and unwavering love
were her special gifts freely given
during the preparation
of this manuscript in spite of
declining health and energy.

Joan M. Birchenall

To the members of my family—
for their patience, sacrifice,
understanding, and support.

Mary Eileen Streight

To home care aides—
who provide selfless care
for their clients.

Preface

Congratulations on your decision to work in a health occupation. As a student in a program for home care aides, you will learn the skills and knowledge to begin your career in home health care.

Training Program

Most training programs are 75 hours in length. The course takes place in two areas—the classroom and care (clinical) setting.

The classroom portion is 60 hours, and you will learn the knowledge and skills necessary to care for clients. Many topics will be covered, for example: basic human needs, communications, normal growth and development, the aging process, and working with ill persons. Nutrition, special diets, and home management are also included.

Classes are usually taught by a registered nurse instructor and other specialists in home care. They will demonstrate and explain the procedures you need to know to give personal care in a client's home. Your learning will be evaluated through written tests and return demonstrations.

You will spend 15 hours in a clinical experience. This is a supervised field practice in clients' homes where you use the skills learned in the classroom. You will be evaluated on how well you perform the skills learned in this program.

Suggestions for Success

Attend every class. Arrive on time, ask questions, and pay attention to your teachers. Watch all demonstrations carefully. These are important ways to learn as much as you can.

Read all the assigned material in the books and handouts before and after class. When using this book, begin your reading with the chapter objectives. Then read the chapter and the Key Terms found in the margins. When you have finished the chapter, return to the objectives. Ask yourself, "Can I do what the objectives say I should be able to do?" If your answer is "yes"—test yourself by answering the questions at the end of the chapter. If your answer is "no"—read the chapter again and continue with the objectives and this "test yourself process." The list below gives suggestions for study.

PQRST Way to Study

Preview—flip through the chapter, pay attention to headings and bold print.
Question—read the objectives. Ask—"What am I supposed to learn?"
Read—sit in a comfortable, well lighted, and quiet place.
Study—review important points in the chapter.
Test—answer questions at the end of the chapter.

Asking Questions

Have you heard the saying, "The only dumb question is the one that is not asked"? This is very true. Your instructor wants you to ask if you do not understand. Do not be shy or afraid. Remember, there is usually at least one other classmate who did not understand either. Be sure to ask right away. Do not wait and ask classmates to explain it to you after class. They may not know what is correct. Your instructor wants you to succeed and to learn the right information the first time. Asking questions helps you to learn.

Completing Assignments

Your instructor will give assignments to be completed on your own time or during class. These assignments may require that you:

- read pages of your textbook.
- complete workbook questions.
- report to class on a special topic.
- perform a task related to the topic.
- answer questions given by your instructor.

An assignment is given to help you learn more about the topic you are studying. Or it may be given to help you prepare for a new topic to be covered next time. It is important that these assignments are completed with care. Your instructor may give a test to find out whether your assignment was completed properly. Your final grade for the program will include how well you completed your assignments. Set aside a period of time each day or evening when you will study and do your assignments for the next class.

Working with Classmates

You and your classmates make up another "family"—a family of persons who are preparing for a career in home care. You have chosen this career because you like people and want to give the best care to your clients. It is important that you show the same caring concern for your classmates as well. Respecting other persons' points of view and listening to what they have to say are important qualities of a home care aide. You can practice improving these attitudes with your classmates.

Perhaps your instructor will ask two or more of you to work together on an activity. The way you work with others shows your instructor how well you will cooperate with members of the home care team. Team work is very important in this profession. Classroom activities will help you improve your communication skills, listening skills, and cooperation skills.

Taking Tests

Tests are given to show how well you know the subject matter or how well you perform a set of tasks or procedures. They are guideposts that show you and your instructor what you have learned and what areas need improvement. During the program, oral quizzes may be given. These are brief tests where students answer the instructor's questions in class. Sometimes, your instructor will ask you to take the test at home. Directions for completing the test will be given. If the test is "on your honor," it means that your instructor is relying on your honesty to complete the test without any assistance.

During the program, you will have a lot of practice taking tests. Your workbook has sample test questions to help you in the process of learning.

Here are some tips to help you take tests:

- Relax—Take a few deep breaths before you begin.
- Read each question carefully.
- Read the question again.
- Watch for words "all, always, never, and none" in the statement. The statement is <u>usually</u> wrong.
- Do not read into the question something that is not there.
- If you do not know the answer, do not spend a lot of time on it. Go to the next question.
- Return to the unanswered question after you complete the test.

For multiple choice questions:

- Read all the answers carefully.
- Select the one <u>best</u> answer.
- There may be two or more answers that are partly correct, but choose the one that most closely fits the answer you would give.

Evaluation

The process of judging how well you have learned the information and skills required to be a home care aide is called **evaluation**. There are two types of evaluation—classroom and clinical.

The person responsible for evaluating your performance in both areas is your instructor. Other people may have a role in this process, such as part-time classroom instructors. The client and family also may be asked to give information for the clinical evaluation. But the final evaluation is your instructor's job.

Classroom Evaluation

Answers to the following questions are included in the instructor's evaluation of your performance in class.

How well do you:

- participate in classroom discussions?
- contribute your knowledge and experience to topics?
- cooperate with classmates in activities assigned?
- complete assignments in and out of class?
- pass written and oral tests?
- perform the skills needed to be a home care aide?
- listen, cooperate with others, show respect, handle difficult classroom situations?
- come to class on time?

Clinical Evaluation

Clinical evaluation shows how well you perform your duties as a home care aide in the client's home. The questions listed below are answered by your instructor with help from the client and family.

How well do you:

- perform correctly the tasks assigned?
- give safe, considerate care?
- report back to your supervisor?
- record your activities according to agency policy?
- respect the culture of your client and family?
- communicate with your client and family?
- know the policies of your agency and act according to them?

Your instructor will explain how often these evaluations will occur. The instructor will meet with you to review the results. This is the time for you to discuss the evaluation and to ask questions. You can then work on any areas needing improvement.

Certification

State Certification

When you successfully complete the program, your agency or school will send this information to the state agency responsible for certifying home care aides. You will receive a certificate which permits you to practice as a home care aide.

National Certification

Some agencies require that you pass a national test to determine that you have the skills and knowledge needed for the job. Your instructor will give you information about applying to take the test. You must complete an approved program before taking this national exam.

Welcome to the home care training program!

Acknowledgments

We are grateful to many people who gave invaluable assistance during the preparation of the manuscript. They include:

Sandy Robbins, Ambest Surgical Supply Company, Trenton, New Jersey

Melvin S. Babad, DMD, Trenton, New Jersey

Paul Guarner, Massapequa, New York

Ulla Loeffler, OTR, Administrator; Pam Ramus, Exercise Physiologist; Sally Diffley, RN; and Connie McChesney, OTR from Back Rehab Institute, Hamilton, New Jersey

The reviewers of the manuscript, during its development, provided advice and suggestions, and we incorporated much of it into the final text. These additions helped to strengthen the material. We appreciated their careful and conscientious reviews.

A special expression of thanks goes to Gerald K. White, Newtown, Pennsylvania, who assisted with the technical aspects of manuscript preparation. His computer skills were outstanding and his attention to detail and accuracy was flawless.

Thanks to Olsten Kimberly QualityCare, Melville, N.Y., for providing professionals and forms used for illustrations. Also, Marsa Crane, Kathryn Scott, and Donna Vogelsang of Rantoul, Illinois, for the use of their homes, which provided excellent settings for the cover and chapter opener photography, and Doris Ellis of St. Louis, Missouri, for the use of her family portrait as the Chapter 18 opener photo.

Christi Mangold, Project Manager, Mosby Lifeline, guided us through the development and preparation stages of the manuscript offering suggestions and encouragement along the way. We appreciate her tireless efforts.

Finally, our thanks to Doris Smith, Managing Editor, Mosby Lifeline, for her advice and counsel during the initial stages of this project.

Contents

PART 1 Orientation to Home Care

PART 2 Managing the Home Environment

PART 3 Home Care Procedures

PART 5 Professional Skills

Procedures

1 The Home Care Industry

Objectives

After you read this chapter, you will be able to:

1. Explain the importance of home care.

2. Discuss the types of clients requiring care.

3. Identify two types of home care agencies and two sources of income.

4. Describe five members of the home care agency team and a function of each.

5. Identify resources in the community that assist the client at home.

6. Discuss the qualities necessary to be a member of the team.

7. Explain the role of the home care aide as a part of the team.

Home care agencies have been in existence for many years. In the 1880s, visiting nurse societies were established to provide home health services to immigrants in cities, the rural poor, and others in need. Over the years, home care agencies have expanded staff and services to meet the growing needs of society.

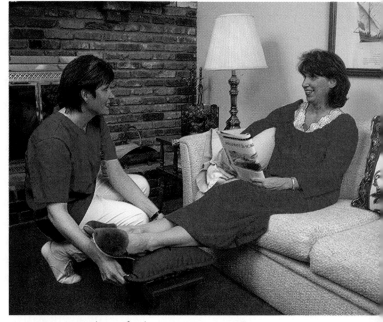

1-1 Most people prefer home care.

Growth of the Industry

There are several factors that influenced the growth of the home health care industry. One major influence came in 1965 when the U.S. Congress passed the **Medicare** laws that allowed funds for home health services for older adults. These new laws caused the number of home care agencies to increase from approximately 1,000 in 1963 to 14,000 by 1993. More than 6,000 of these agencies provide services to Medicare participants.

Another influence on the industry's growth was the 1983 passage of federal legislation that created **diagnostic related groups (DRGs).** A DRG is a list of specific diagnoses used to determine the typical length of stay and the cost of treatment allowed for that particular group of illnesses. The hospital receives only the dollar amount specified in the DRG for Medicare and **Medicaid** patients. If the patient leaves the hospital in less time than specified in the DRG, the hospital gets to keep the excess funds. If the patient stays longer than the time allowed, the hospital loses money. This is one reason that patients are sent home from the hospital as quickly as possible. Other reasons for early hospital discharge include:

1. *Lower costs.* Home care is less expensive. Many times, home care costs about half that of hospital care. Technical improvements in equipment and supplies make it possible to do many of the same things at home as in the hospital.

2. *Greater comfort.* Most people prefer to recuperate in the familiar surroundings of home. Children and older adults often feel more at ease—more comfortable—at home with their family and friends (Fig. 1-1). They can follow their own schedules for eating and sleeping. Many people say they get better faster at home than in the hospital.

3. *Lower risk.* The risk of hospital-acquired infection is reduced because patients' exposure to others who may carry infection— hospital staff, other patients, and visitors—is reduced.

When people come home sooner, they may also come home more sick. An estimated ten million Americans will need ongoing specialized care each year. Home care agencies in the United States provide care on a short-term, long-term or live-in basis to more than six million people. Home care is the fastest growing part of the nation's health care budget.

Medicare
a federal program of hospitalization and health care insurance for persons over 65. Participation is voluntary.

DRG (diagnostic related group)
a listing of diagnoses used in establishing reimbursement by Medicare and Medicaid for hospitalization and medical care.

Medicaid
a state and federal program of hospitalization and health care for low-income persons of all ages.

Home Care Agencies

Home care agencies are as varied as the clients who use them. Each is uniquely organized to best serve the needs of the clients in the community.

Organization and Regulation

Home care agencies are organized and administered in many ways. They may be classified as:

1. *Governmental or official*—sponsored by local or state government. Supported by tax monies, usually a part of the Department of Health.
2. *Voluntary, non-profit*—governed by a volunteer board of directors. Financed through tax-deductible contributions and/or fees for service. For example: visiting nurse associations, church-sponsored home care agencies.
3. *Private, for-profit*—operated by individuals through a franchise or as part of a local or national company. For example: Interim Health Care.

The agency director is responsible for the day-to-day operations of the entire organization. Office staff provide clerical and bookkeeping services. Other staff members responsible for client care are discussed later in this chapter.

The activities of home care agencies may be regulated by state or local authorities. Licensure as a home care agency may be required. These regulations vary in each community. Those agencies that participate in the care of Medicare clients must also meet specific governmental **standards.** The state Department of Health or other designated organization conducts regular inspections to make sure that the agency complies with Medicare regulations.

Sources of Clients

Home care agency clients come from many sources. They include:

1. *Hospitals.* When care needs to be continued at home, but not at the level provided by the hospital, the **hospital discharge planner** arranges transfer of information and doctor's orders to the home care agency.
2. *Rehabilitation Centers.* When a person has reached the highest level of ability following injury or accident but still needs assistance with routine care and therapy in the home environment.
3. *Hospice.* When a terminally ill person wishes to be cared for at home.
4. *Personal referral.* When a family member finds that caring for an ill or disabled relative is too much to handle alone.

Types of Clients

Just as there are many sources of clients, there are many types of clients. A large number are older adults, recently discharged from the hospital after an **acute illness.** Other examples of clients include:

- New mothers and their babies
- Persons with **chronic illnesses**

standard
a gauge that is used as a basis for judgment.

hospital discharge planner
person who arranges for the care of a patient upon release from the hospital. May be a professional nurse or social worker.

acute illness
an illness with a rapid onset, severe symptoms, and of short length.

chronic illness
a disease showing little change, slow progress, and of long duration; not an acute illness.

hospice
a program of care that assists the dying client to stay at home and maintain a satisfactory lifestyle during the end stage of an illness.

reimbursement
to make payment for expense incurred.

- Sick children
- Persons who have had recent surgery
- Persons with fractures
- Persons with amputations
- **Hospice** clients
- Frail older adults
- Persons with disabilities

Payment For Services

Services provided by home care agencies cost about half that of similar care offered by hospitals. But who pays for it? Agencies can turn to several sources for **reimbursement**—or payment—for their services:

1. *Out of pocket.* The client or client's family may be responsible for paying a deductible and/or specific percentage of the cost of care, depending upon the type of health insurance the client has. Sometimes a client must pay "out of pocket" for all care because he/she has no insurance, has exhausted the insurance coverage, or the client's insurance does not pay for home care.

2. *Health care insurance/health maintenance organizations.* An individual or group insurance plan that pays a part—or all—of the cost of medical care and services. The services and payment for them vary depending on the insurance company and the client's type of insurance.

3. *Medicare.* Federal health insurance program for older adults and individuals with disabilities.

4. *Medicaid.* Federal- and state-supported program that provides health care for people with limited income, including children and pregnant women.

5. *Other state and federal programs.* Services are available to eligible clients through special programs for the elderly and disabled.

6. *United Way and other charitable programs.* Provide grants to certain agencies for client services.

The type of care and service provided is limited by the provisions of the programs listed above. Accurate record keeping is essential to show exactly what care was given. If care is not properly recorded, the agency may not receive prompt reimbursement. Most agencies expect you to submit a daily report that lists the exact services performed and the hours worked. This report is signed by the client and is used to complete your payroll record so you can be paid. The report is also necessary to bill the client and/or insurance company for reimbursement.

The Home Care Team

A team is a group of people who work together to accomplish a common goal. Each team member has a special job. The home care team is made up of many members, and they must work together very well to meet the client's special goals (Fig. 1-2).

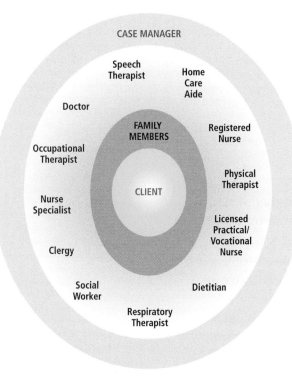

1-2 The circle of home care.

Team Members

Listed below are the types of professionals, in addition to the doctor, who may be included on the home care team. Some typical functions for each member are also included.

Case Manager

- **Assesses** the client's physical, emotional, social, and environmental needs
- Develops a plan to meet these needs
- Recommends services of other professionals
- Reviews or reassesses client's progress and adjusts plan as needed

Registered Nurse (RN)

- Assesses, plans, and implements nursing care required
- Carries out doctor's orders
- Teaches client and family members about care techniques and procedures
- Supervises care given by home care aide and licensed practical/vocational nurse

Nurse Specialist (RN)

- Gives complex nursing care to clients with special needs: cancer care, care of children, care of infants
- Teaches other nursing staff about new procedures
- Acts as an advisor to other agency members about clients with special needs

Licensed Practical/Vocational Nurse (LPN/LVN)

- Gives nursing care under the supervision of an RN
- Cares for clients whose conditions are stable and do not require complex nursing care

Home Care Aide

- Provides personal care according to the client's care plan
- Performs required housekeeping services
- Works under supervision of an RN, therapist
- Reports activities performed according to agency **policy**

Physical Therapist (RPT)

- Assesses the client's muscle strength, balance, and movement of joints
- Plans and implements the physical therapy program
- Teaches the client and family exercises to strengthen muscles and improve movement
- Supervises care given by home care aide

Occupational Therapist (OTR)

- Assesses movement of arms, hands, and fingers
- Determines how well client is able to perform activities of daily living (ADL), such as eating, bathing, dressing
- Supervises care given by home care aide

assess
to determine the client's needs for home care services.

policy, policies
a set of rules and regulations.

Respiratory Therapist (RRT)
- Assesses client's ability to breathe with ease
- Plans and implements the respiratory therapy program
- Explains proper use of breathing equipment
- Checks equipment for proper functioning
- Supervises care given by home care aide

Social Worker
- Determines the need for financial help
- Assesses the need for community services
- Arranges for these services to be provided
- Sees that the client and family receive the needed help

Speech Therapist (Speech Pathologist)
- Assesses the client's speech and language
- Plans and implements program to help client communicate
- Teaches exercises for tongue, mouth, and face
- Teaches family how to help the client who has difficulty speaking and swallowing

Dietitian
- Teaches the client and family about the types of food needed to maintain or improve health
- Teaches proper menu selection and preparation according to diet ordered by doctor

Others
Clergy:
- Provides spiritual help to client and family

Volunteer:
- Gives service to the agency or the client without being paid
- Performs tasks that do not require complex skills
- Supervision is provided by the agency

Forming the Team

The kinds of team members selected will vary according to the needs of each client and family. First, the case manager meets with the client and family to assess the types of services needed. Information received from the hospital's discharge planner (mentioned earlier) is also considered. Next, the case manager determines the type and amount of services needed. The following information is used:

- the client's health and physical condition
- treatments ordered by the doctor
- family members or others able and willing to give care
- the family as a social group—strengths and problems
- reactions of family members to the need for help
- home environment needs—housekeeping required
- other services needed, such as Meals On Wheels, special equipment, transportation
- financial resources of client to obtain services needed
- length of service needed and expected results

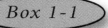

Box 1-1

Plan of Care for Mrs. Stevens

Goal	Mrs. Stevens will gain 1/2 lb. a week until she reaches normal weight (134 lbs.)
Activities	Weigh her once a week
	Mrs. Johnson, home care aide, to visit on Fridays at 10:00 a.m.
Other Agencies Providing Services	Meals On Wheels to give noon meal Monday through Friday
	Local church to provide noon meal on Saturday and Sunday

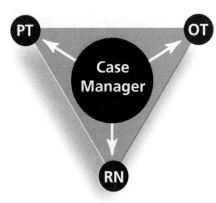

1-3 The case manager coordinates services of team members.

As an example, the client who must receive medications by injection and requires oxygen therapy to help breathe more easily may have a team that includes a registered nurse and a respiratory therapist.

The Care Plan
Establishing the Goal

The case manager develops the goal to be met by the team according to the needs of the client and family. For the client who is disabled, the goal may be to help restore as much function as possible. The goal for a mother and her newborn baby may be to help her gain independence in caring for herself and the baby. For the client who is dying, the goal will be to give the physical care and emotional support needed so that death can occur with dignity. The plan may also include support for the family.

Developing the Plan

The plan of care to meet the goal is based on the information obtained by the case manager while assessing the types of services needed. The plan includes:

- the activities to be performed, who will perform them, and how often
- other agencies performing activities (See Box 1-1).

Several health professionals may be required to give service to the client, such as a physical therapist, respiratory therapist, and registered nurse. Each will develop a plan of care, implement the plan, and evaluate the client's progress. However, the case manager coordinates the total plan of care (Fig. 1-3).

Using Community Resources

The case manager may recommend that resources in the community be used to assist clients and their families with various tasks. Perhaps the client is not able to prepare meals or perform housekeeping duties. Other family members may be at work and unable to help. Community agencies and organizations offer services that may help the client to remain at home rather than to be placed in an institution (Fig. 1-4).

Table 1-1 gives examples of community programs that provide valuable help to both the client and the family.

You, an Essential Part of the Team

The duties you perform as a home care aide are a vital part of your client's care. In some cases, you will be the person who has the most contact each week with the client and family. Information you share with other members of the team is very important. The team relies on your valuable contributions so that the proper care and treatment can be given.

Table 1-1

Examples of Community Programs

Type of Service	Program	Service Provided
Nutrition Services	Home-Delivered Meals (Meals On Wheels) *Sponsor:* State, county, or local community agencies; civic organizations	Provides one or more meals a day, at least five days a week. Food is delivered by a volunteer. A hot meal arrives, ready to be eaten. A cold meal—usually a sandwich, fruit, and milk—may be eaten later.
Social Services	Volunteer Friendly Visitor Program *Sponsor:* Local community agencies; senior citizens' clubs; civic organizations	Offers chance for the homebound person to socialize with mature men and women on a regular basis. The volunteer makes weekly home visits. Activities include writing letters, reading aloud, playing cards, or just talking about topics of interest to the client.
	Telephone Reassurance *Sponsor:* Civic organizations; senior citizens' clubs; police departments; nursing home residents	A volunteer calls the client at a pre-arranged time each day. The conversation with the volunteer may be the only contact with another human being for the entire day.
	Religious Activities *Sponsor:* Church/temple/ synagogue activities	Religious groups provide a variety of services. Visits by clergy and members link the client to the life of the congregation.
Household Services	Volunteer Services *Sponsor:* Local community	Volunteers run errands, do routine home repairs, or perform light housekeeping tasks.
	Housecleaning Services *Sponsor:* Local community businesses	For a fee, the service provides all types of housecleaning tasks according to the needs of the client.

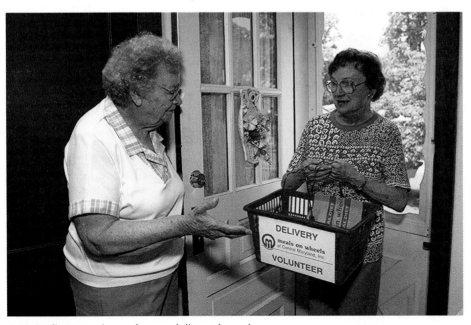

1-4 A client receives a home-delivered meal.

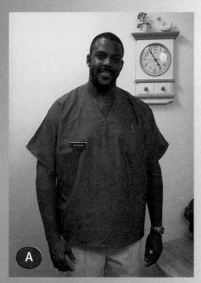

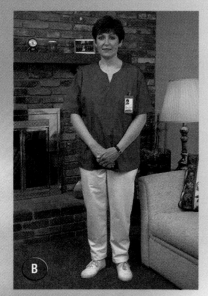

1-5 Good grooming is an important requirement for the home care aide. **A,** A properly groomed male home care aide. **B,** A properly groomed female home care aide.

You will be expected to:

1. LOOK AND ACT PROFESSIONAL.
2. PERFORM YOUR DUTIES PROPERLY.
3. WORK AS PART OF THE TEAM.

Looking and Acting Professional

Looking Professional Your appearance says a lot about the way you will perform your duties. A neat, clean, and properly dressed person conveys an image of one who is ready to perform tasks properly (Fig. 1-5). Your appearance says, "I am proud to be a home care employee." Remember, first impressions are usually lasting ones. Clients and families will appreciate your professional look. Your employer has policies about proper dress and appearance that you will need to follow.

The tips given in the Appearance Checklist will help you present a professional appearance.

Appearance Checklist

Clothing

- Wear a clean uniform each day with undergarments that fit properly and do not show through the uniform
- Iron and repair clothes as needed
- Wear name pin and agency badge at all times

Shoes, Stockings, or Socks

- Wear comfortable, low-heeled shoes with non-skid soles and heels to help prevent accidents
- Polish shoes daily
- Keep shoe laces clean
- Buy the best shoes you can
- Keep shoes in good repair
- Wear clean, properly fitting stockings or socks each day

Jewelry, Cosmetics, Hair, and Nails

- Wear only wedding rings
- Wear watch with sweep second hand
- Do not wear dangle earrings, bracelets, or pendants
- Do not wear a lot of makeup
- Do not wear perfumes, colognes, or after-shave lotions
- Maintain a neat hair style that is easy to manage
- Keep hair clean, free of heavy hairspray

  For men:

  - Keep beard and/or mustache, if worn, trimmed and clean
  - Shave daily
- Keep fingernails short
- Wear nail polish according to your agency's policy
- Do not wear artificial nails

Daily Hygiene

- Bathe each day
- Apply underarm deodorant or anti-perspirant immediately after bathing

- Brush teeth before coming to work and, if possible, after each meal
- Use mouthwash as directed by your dentist
- Avoid foods that produce bad breath—garlic, onions, etc.
- Keep teeth in good repair; see your dentist regularly

Acting Professional   Healthy habits and a positive attitude are keys to acting in a professional manner. As a member of the home care team, you show that you have good personal habits and a positive attitude about yourself and others. The client and family will look to you as an example of the right kind of personal health care practices. You are a role model.

Maintaining healthy habits   The proper balance of food, exercise, and rest are important factors in keeping healthy.

Food. Eating the right kinds of food in the right amounts gives the body the energy needed to function well. Without proper nutrition, you will not have the energy or stamina to correctly perform your duties. Information about daily food requirements is discussed in Chapter 8.

Exercise. Your job will require lifting and moving clients. It is important that your muscles and joints are in good working order. Your doctor is the best person to offer advice about a daily exercise program. Almost everyone can benefit from rapid walking three times a week for 20 minutes. This exercises the long muscles, stimulates the heart and lungs, and promotes restful sleep.

Rest. The body needs rest in order to work efficiently. Make sure you get enough sleep.

Hazards to health   Listed below are three habits that are bad for your body and promote illness:

Smoking. There is nothing positive that can be said about the use of tobacco in any form. Smoking or chewing tobacco—or inhaling snuff—is very harmful to the body's tissues. It can cause cancer of the lung, lip, tongue, mouth, and throat. Secondhand smoke causes the same effects in the nonsmoker. Your agency prohibits smoking while on duty. If you smoke on your off-duty hours, others can smell the odor of smoke. It gets into your hair and clothing. It is often offensive to nonsmokers. For the sake of yourself and others, DO NOT USE TOBACCO.

Alcohol. Alcohol is the most popular and most often abused drug. Even a little alcohol—one drink—can dull the senses. It can reduce judgment and limit the ability to function efficiently. Reporting to work under the influence of alcohol or drinking on the job are causes for immediate dismissal. DO NOT RISK YOUR CAREER AND YOUR LIFE BY ABUSING ALCOHOL.

Drug or Substance Abuse. Drug abuse is a serious medical and social problem. Many people are destroyed by abusing legal and illegal drugs. As a home care aide, you may be caring for a client who is taking drugs prescribed by the doctor. These drugs are for the client's use ONLY. You must never take a drug that has not been prescribed for you. Do not share your prescription drugs with another person. More information about drugs is found in Chapter 17.

Confident

Dependable

Cheerful

Knows Limitations

Skillfull/Competent

Enthusiastic

Well Groomed

Cooperative

Follows Agency Rules

Respectful

Courteous

Honest

1-6 Qualities of a successful home care aide.

Having a Positive Attitude In your experiences of life, you have met people who are friendly, willing to help, and genuinely concerned about you. Their behavior shows that they are worthy of your trust. They demonstrate positive attitudes about themselves and others. You have also met those who do not have these qualities. These people have negative attitudes that show, by their behaviors, that they are not friendly, caring, or concerned about you. Actions do speak louder than words!

As a home care aide, your positive attitude will show in the following behaviors (Fig. 1-6):

- Arriving on time, ready to work
- Being cheerful—smiling
- Being aware of your client's and family's needs, likes, and dislikes
- Willing to adjust your routine to meet their needs
- Being able to understand another point of view
- Being able to accept others' behaviors that may not be familiar to you

Other important rules are:

- Call your agency if you will be late or absent.
- Do not make personal phone calls from your client's home.
- Do not give your home phone number to clients.
- Leave your personal problems at home.
- Refer questions about the tasks you perform to your supervisor.
- Do not make private arrangements with your client for service.
- Respect the privacy of your client and the family members.
- Keep information you receive about client and family matters confidential.
- Do not encourage familiarity with your client or family members.
- Do not get personally involved with your client, the family, or neighbors.
- Do not drive the client in any car—yours or theirs—without agency permission.
- Keep yourself busy elsewhere in the home when visitors arrive.
- Do not expect or accept tips.
- Do not lend or borrow money.
- Treat others as you would want them to treat you.
- Remember, you are a guest in your client's home.

Performing Your Duties Properly

Your training program will prepare you to give safe, competent care to your clients. As a home care aide, you will perform activities under the direction of a nurse supervisor. Your responsibilities will involve care of your client and the home environment. Do not perform any procedures that you have not been taught. Do not perform any duties that your supervisor has not listed in the Care Plan.

The following are examples of some of the duties you will learn to perform.

Care of Client	*Care of Client's Home Environment*
Assist with bathing	Clean equipment
Assist with personal grooming	Purchase food
Assist with dressing	Assist with meal preparation
Help with feeding	Prepare meals
Assist with walking	Launder client's clothes
Collect specimens	Maintain a clean home
Record and report information	Perform light housekeeping tasks

Working as Part of the Team

The team is only as good as each of its members. Most of the time, you will be working alone in the client's home. Therefore, you are the team's representative. How you work with the client and family will tell them how well the team functions. Your attitude and behavior are very important in giving a positive impression of the health care team. Remember, you play a vital role on the team.

CHAPTER SUMMARY

- Home care is a rapidly growing industry.
- Many types of clients are served, from the very young to the very old.
- Most people prefer to be cared for in their own homes.
- Home care is less expensive than hospital care.
- Several types of agencies provide home care; these services are paid through state and federal programs, private insurance, and clients and their families.
- The case manager of the agency coordinates the services and activities of the home care team.
- You, the home care aide, are an important member of the team.
- The agency, your client, and family members expect you to look and act professional. They expect you to perform your duties properly and work as part of the team.

STUDY QUESTIONS

1. List three benefits of home care.
2. Describe four types of clients who receive care at home.
3. How do clients pay for home care?
4. List five duties and responsibilities of a home care aide.
5. Describe three services that are available in your community to assist clients at home.
6. Identify the home care team member who performs the following activities:
   a. teaches crutch walking.
   b. gives breathing treatments.
   c. coordinates the activities of the home care team.
   d. provides spiritual consolation.
   e. helps family with finances.
7. List six qualities you must have to be a good team member and a successful home care aide.

2 Developing Effective Communication Skills

Objectives

After you read this chapter, you will be able to:

1. Define communication.

2. Explain the importance of clear communication in home care.

3. Describe the types of communication.

4. Identify three barriers to effective communication.

5. List five ways to improve listening skills.

6. Use guidelines for good communication with others.

7. Explain the rights and responsibilities of both client and agency.

8. Demonstrate three methods for effective communication with visually-impaired and hearing-impaired clients.

9. Describe the role ethics plays in communicating with the home care team, your client, and the family.

Communication is the sharing of thoughts, information, and opinions with others. This may be done from one person to another on a face-to-face basis, or it may be done in a group setting, such as a teacher and a class of students. Other times, communication occurs through books, newspapers, television, radio, telephone, music, movies, art, sign language, and computer. All around us there is a constant demand for our attention, a constant wish to communicate with us.

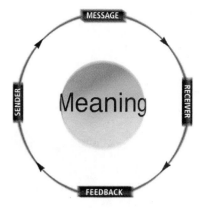

2-1 Four parts of communication.

Communication Process

The process of communication involves four parts: a sender and a receiver, the message, and feedback (Fig. 2-1). The sender is the person who begins the communication—the first speaker. The receiver is the person to whom the message is sent. The message is the actual expression of the thought, information, or opinion. Feedback is the return of information from the receiver to the sender. Feedback is used to tell whether or not the communication was successful.

EXAMPLE

a. Sender:	Home care aide
b. Receiver:	Client
c. Message:	"Goodbye, I'll be back tomorrow at the same time. Please sign my time card."
Meaning:	The home care aide is finished working for the day and will return tomorrow at the agreed upon time.
d. Feedback:	Client says, "Thank you. I'll see you tomorrow," and signs the aide's time card.

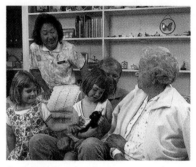

2-2 Talking (verbal communication) and touch (nonverbal communication) are part of this family visit.

Importance

In home care, communication is the link between you, the client, and the agency. You have to be certain that your message has been received and understood exactly as you meant it to be received. That is why feedback is an important part of the process. We must be able to say what we mean clearly and without confusion. By sharing accurate information and observations with the home care team, the aide helps the client receive better care.

Types of Communication

There are many methods of communication, for example, radio, TV, telephone, books, and many others. But all of these can be placed into one of two classifications—verbal or nonverbal communication (Fig. 2-2).

Verbal Communication

Communication using the spoken or written word is known as **verbal communication.** We are most familiar with speaking; we do it all the time. Communicating with clients is not the same as a casual conversation with friends. It is an important part of health care. Use simple words and speak clearly and a little more slowly than in everyday conversation. Remember that the tone of your voice and your expression

communication
sharing of thoughts, information, and opinions with others.

verbal communication
communication using the spoken or written word.

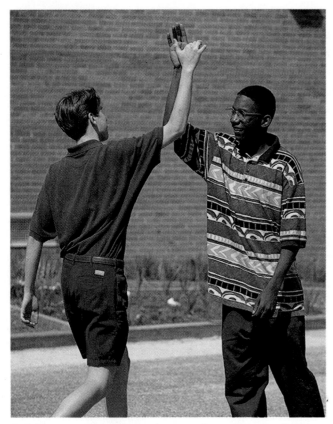

2-3 Young people know the meaning without using words.

can affect the meaning of the message. The words "good morning" don't change when you say them, but their meaning may change, depending on how you use your voice to say those words.

Written communication is usually considered a part of verbal communication because words are included. Written communication is discussed in Chapter 10. A few general rules apply to written messages. They must be legible, spelling must be correct, and the information must be accurate.

Nonverbal Communication

Nonverbal communication is the exchange of information without words (Fig. 2-3). Both positive and negative messages may be sent even when nothing is said. In fact, sometimes saying nothing (silence) can become the message. Silence can be positive—as a hug—or it can be negative—as when angry people do not speak to each other.

Other examples of nonverbal communication include appearance, facial expression, gestures, posture, types of food we eat, and the way we eat our meals. All these combine to send powerful messages to others. Also, many of these are determined by cultural background—our own and our client's.

When verbal and nonverbal communication are combined, the sender can emphasize a point and make the message clearer. For example, the aide holds the time sheet and a pen while asking the client to sign it. Sometimes, combining verbal and nonverbal communication can be confusing when the words tell you one thing but the actions tell you another. For example, it's hard to believe a client who tells you that everything is "OK" and is sobbing into a tissue at the same time. Two different messages are being sent. It's up to you to find out which is correct.

Barriers to Communication

Barriers or blocks to communication occur when something acts as a wall between one or more of the four parts of communication. Then the message just cannot get through. There are many barriers to communication. The more common ones are discussed in this section.

Bias, Prejudice

Preconceived ideas, **biases, prejudice,** "mind already made up," "only one way to do it"—these are clearly barriers to communication. When all we see is a person's color, age, sex, or **disability,** we are unable to accept that person's ideas, opinions, or thoughts. Sex bias is often a problem. Male home care aides may be asked why they are doing a "woman's job." Clients sometimes wonder out loud how "such a tiny little girl" is going to be able to get grandpa out of bed. You can remind people that, in health care, there are no jobs reserved for men or

nonverbal communication
communication without the use of words.

bias(es)
to like or dislike someone or something without a good reason; prejudice.

prejudice
having or forming a preconceived judgment or opinion without fair reasons.

disability
physical, mental, or emotional handicap that interferes with abilities to carry out activities of daily living.

women. Also, you can let your client's family know (in a respectful manner) that you have learned the skills of the job. Once the client and family get to know you as a competent, caring aide, they will come to rely on your assistance and forget their initial preconceived ideas. We have closed the door to communication when we fail to see each person as an individual of worth.

We all have some preconceived ideas, biases, prejudices, but we must do our very best to put these aside to give client care. When clients request and receive care from an agency, they also agree to put aside bias and prejudice in order to receive the care they need at home.

Language, Culture, and Ethnic Diversity

The population of the United States is made up of people from all over the world. You may work in homes where the culture is quite different from yours. The approach to sickness, healing, death, dying, and religious consolation may be unfamiliar to you. Perhaps no one in the household speaks English or any other language that you know. The ideal situation would be to have a home care aide of the same culture in the home, but this is not always possible. The next best thing to do is to find a person who can help you. Discuss the situation with your supervisor, who can assist you to find a neighbor, friend, or another relative who will act as an interpreter. Also, try to learn as much about that culture as possible; it will enrich your life and help you become a more sensitive caregiver (Fig. 2-4).

Sexual Harassment

Unfortunately, you may work in a home where the client or family member may constantly demand sexual favors from you. Even though you perform your duties in a professional manner and in no way indi-

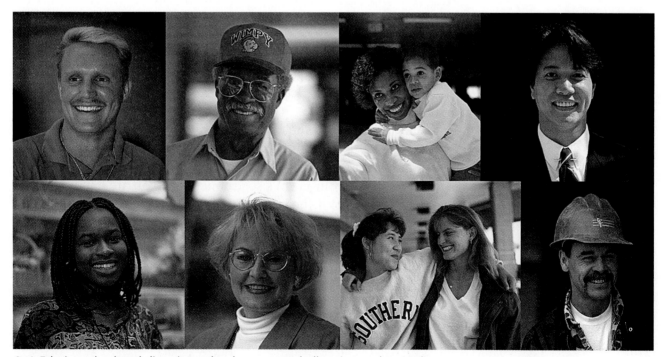

2-4 Ethnic and cultural diversity makes home care challenging and rewarding.

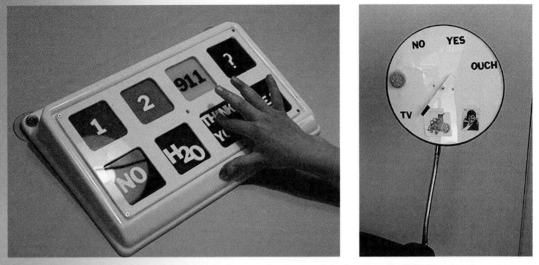

2-5 Communication devices make it possible for the disabled to reach out to those around them. *(Courtesy of Enabling Devices/Toys for Special Children, Hastings, NY.)*

cate any romantic interest in this person, the harasser will not stop bothering you and may become sexually aggressive. This is a situation where no effective communication is occurring, and it is a situation that is unsafe for you. No employer expects you to work under these conditions. Report the situation to your supervisor immediately.

Illness, Pain, and Medications

It is hard to communicate clearly when one is sick. All your client's energy and attention may be focused on the illness and getting well. Sometimes clients are too weak or too sick to talk. Quiet, nonverbal communication and asking questions that can be answered with one word may be appropriate. Some illnesses cause an inability to speak, hear, or comprehend on a temporary or permanent basis. See Chapters 5 and 21 for details on working with ill persons.

Disabilities

Certain disabilities can create barriers to communication. Some examples include blindness, deafness, aphasia (the inability to speak), and brain damage. Please see Chapter 5 for more detail on disabilities. Individuals with disabilities may communicate by using hand signals and eye movements. Sometimes clients use special devices, such as computers, pointers, and speaking tubes, to communicate (Fig. 2-5). You will need to adjust to your client's special needs. If you are having trouble communicating, see if the family can help you. Discuss any communication problems with your supervisor.

Communicating With Agency Personnel

As the eyes and ears of the team, you will be expected to report any problems or changes to your supervisor. You are to report what you observe with your senses:

- Eyes—what you see
- Nose—what you smell
- Ears—what you hear
- Touch—what you feel

Box 2-1

Report to Your Supervisor

Some things to report to your supervisor:

- a change in the physical condition of your client
- a change in the client's emotional or mental condition
- signs of injury, neglect, or abuse (See Chapters 18, 19, and 20.)
- a change in the home environment that may be hazardous for client and family
- you do not understand a procedure or task
- problems with medications
- you are unsure of how to proceed with your assignment
- if the client/family asks you to do something that is not your responsibility
- if you feel unsafe in the client's home

Do not report what you think happened or you thought you saw. Be objective. Give your supervisor the facts—not your opinions. (See Box 2-1.)

Communicating With Your Client and Family Members

Respect for Client and Family

Effective communication starts with the following basic principle— respect for the client and family as human beings. Each person—the sender of the message and the receiver—brings with him/her characteristics that are unique. Physical, emotional, mental, social, and spiritual aspects make up who we are. Try to accept each individual as a person of worth. Listen to what they have to say. Be respectful. Do not "write off" what another person has to say as meaningless and not worth listening to.

Listening

Listening is an essential part of the communication process. The message being sent is much like a football that must be caught for a pass to be completed. So, too, the message must be caught (received) and understood for effective communication to take place. Good listening is essential to receiving and understanding the message being sent.

Good listening involves the use of eyes, ears, and feelings. It takes energy, concentration, and effort to be a good listener. The first step in developing and/or improving listening skills is to decide that you want to become a better listener. This means that you will devote your full attention to the other person (the speaker; the sender). It is difficult to be a listener. Some suggestions to improve listening skills are:

1. Be quiet. Pay attention to what the other person is saying.
2. Stop all other activities. Focus on the speaker.
3. Listen to the entire message.
4. Do not interrupt the speaker. Let the speaker finish, even if it takes a long time.
5. Do not try to think of a response while another is speaking.
6. Keep confidences. Keep private matters private unless the information shared is essential for client care, health, or well-being.
7. Practice listening skills. (See Box 2-2.)

A Learned Skill

Communication is a skill that improves with practice. As your skill increases, you will be able to speak more clearly and send and receive more accurate messages. You will also be more sensitive to the nonverbal messages you are sending and receiving from your client and family. While there are many verbal communication techniques, you will find that a few will be used more often than others. Five examples follow.

1. Use open-ended questions that may be answered with an explanation, instead of closed questions that can only be answered by a "yes" or "no" response. Example:

   Closed question:

   Aide: "Did you eat all of your breakfast?"
   Client: "No."

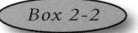

Box 2-2

Listening Skills

- Concentrate—LISTENING is HARD WORK.
- Take time to listen.
- Be patient—let the sender complete the message, even if it takes a lot of time.
- Do not interrupt—let the speaker finish.
- Get feedback—give feedback.
- If you don't understand, do not let the person continue; say, "Would you please tell me again? I do not understand what you just said."
- Observe body language and facial expression.
- Listen to the tone of the sender's voice.
- Do not think about how you will respond before the person has finished talking; use quiet time to mentally summarize main ideas.
- Focus your attention on what is being said, not on what you will say later.

- Show interest, use nonverbal communication to demonstrate your interest.
- Give speaker your full attention.
- Listen for feelings.
- Ask questions that will encourage the speaker to continue.
- Do not be afraid of silence; observe, ask the client to tell you more, and ask them how they feel about what they are discussing.
- Do not finish sentences that the speaker begins.
- Do not jump to conclusions by assuming that you know exactly what your client means.
- Be aware of your own feelings and point of view.
- Listen with an open mind; try to hear everything, not just what you want to hear; avoid selective hearing.

Open-ended question:

Aide:	"What did you eat for breakfast?"
Client:	"Nothing. I was too sick to eat."

2. Restate the message to let the client know you heard what is being said. This encourages further communication. For example:

Aide:	"You were sick this morning and didn't eat any breakfast."
Client:	"That's right. After I took my pain pill, I felt like I was going to throw up, so I didn't have anything to eat."

3. Ask for clarification so the message may be clearly understood.

Aide:	"I am not sure I understand. You say that after you took your pain medicine you were too sick to eat breakfast and you felt like you were going to throw up."
Client:	"Yes. Every time I take that darned medicine it makes me feel like throwing up. That's why I hate to take it, even though it eases the pain."

4. Summarize what you have been hearing.

Aide:	"This sounds like a problem to me."
Client:	"It sure is. I've been putting up with this for a few weeks."

5. Share information with the client.

Aide:	"I'm going to call my supervisor about this. Maybe there is something that can be done to take care of this problem. What do you think about that?"
Client:	"Sounds good to me. I hope I don't have to put up with this much longer."

Practice these techniques with your friends and family. Box 2-3 contains a list of guidelines to enhance communications.

Communicating With the Hearing Impaired

In addition to their illnesses, many of your clients or family members experience difficulty in hearing. Some wear hearing aids; others do not. Communicating with the hearing impaired is a challenge for members of the home care team. The client's record should show what methods team members use to communicate successfully. If you find a technique that works for you, record it so that others can use it, too. In addition to the guidelines outlined in Box 2-3, the following are suggestions for communicating with the hearing impaired:

- Reduce background noise of household appliances (fans, dishwasher, etc.).
- Be sure your face is clearly visible; this will help those who lip-read.
- Lower the tone of your voice.
- Do not exaggerate your speech by mouthing the words.
- Introduce the topic and use a visual aid, if possible.
- Use short, simple sentences.

surrogate
one who is appointed to act for another.

ethics
code of behavior or conduct.

- Rephrase the sentence if it is not understood.
- Pause before changing the topic.
- Keep a pad and pencil ready so that the person can communicate in writing, if possible.
- Try to speak to the side where better hearing occurs, if known.
- Be patient; show by your body language that you are supportive.

Communicating With the Visually Impaired

If your client is visually impaired, the following tips will help you to communicate more effectively:

- Provide adequate light.
- Check glasses, if worn, to be sure they are clean, in good repair, and fit properly.
- Reduce glare from exposed light bulbs, waxed floors.
- Provide aids to communication, such as magnifying glasses.

Box 2-3

Communication Guidelines

- Introduce yourself on the first visit to the client's home.
- Find out the name your client prefers to be called.
- Reduce the amount of background noise (turn off the TV, radio), if possible.
- Get client's attention, face the client, have eye contact (unless this is culturally inappropriate).
- Think about what you will say—organize your thoughts.
- Show interest.
- Explain procedures.
- Use nonverbal communication—a touch on the shoulder, a smile, or hold the client's hand.
- Be polite, courteous, respectful, and considerate.
- Don't talk down to the client.
- Avoid words that may have another meaning.
- Don't use slang, obscene words or gestures.
- Learn the meaning of new words you hear and that the client may use.
- Let the client finish what is being said.
- Be a good listener.

- Say what you mean.
- Use family and/or friends to translate when necessary.
- Use a normal tone of voice—DO NOT SHOUT.
- Speak slowly.
- Speak clearly and distinctly.
- Use words that both you and your client or family member understand.
- Avoid the use of technical or medical terms.
- Use as few words as necessary to convey the message—BE CONCISE.
- Do not mumble or whisper.
- Listen to the client's feedback; ask them to repeat what you said, so you can determine the effectiveness of the communication.
- If you do not understand what your client has said, say so; do not be afraid to say, "I don't understand what you are telling me." Or restate, "Are you telling me...?"
- Smile; use your sense of humor.
- Practice—practice—practice using these guidelines

  with your family.
  with your friends.
  with your classmates.

- Stand directly in front of the client when communicating; side vision may be poor.
- Say the person's name before you start the conversation.
- Speak in a normal tone of voice.
- Touch the client on the hand or shoulder to get and keep attention.

The Client's Bill of Rights

This document explains the rights and responsibilities of the client. (See Table 2-1.) If the client cannot understand the information, a representative (family member or **surrogate**) acts for the client.

There are two parts: (1) What the client has a right to expect from the agency and its members; and (2) What action the client agrees to take.

A copy of the document is given to the client and family by the agency. It is reviewed with them and questions about the statements are explained.

Code of Behavior

Each profession has a code of behavior to follow. This code of behavior is called **ethics.** Ethics are standards to follow in your behavior toward others. The way you act and react to others also has an effect on you.

Table 2-1

The Client's Bill of Rights

CLIENT'S RIGHTS	CLIENT'S RESPONSIBILITIES
Agency Staff	
Receive care without regard to race, color, national origin, religion, age, or disability.	Accept agency staff without regard to race, color, national origin, religion, age, or disability.
Be treated with respect and dignity by agency staff.	Be considerate and respectful of agency staff.
Receive information about the types of team members who will provide care and the number of visits to be made.	Notify the agency when an appointment cannot be kept.
Obtain the name of the supervisor and the agency phone number.	Notify the agency of any problems or dissatisfaction with care.
Request a change in staff to provide home care.	Notify, in advance, of intention to terminate the agency's services.
Receive advance notice of transfer or discharge.	
Client's Property	
Have property treated with respect and consideration.	Store valuables in a safe place. Provide a safe home environment where care can be given.

Continued.

Table 2-1—cont'd.

The Client's Bill of Rights

CLIENT'S RIGHTS

Carrying Out the Plan of Care

Be fully informed, in writing and in advance, about the care and treatment to be given. This includes any changes in care or treatment.

Participate in developing and revising the plan of care or service.

Be fully informed about the expected plan of care or service.

Refuse treatment, medication, or other services.

Be fully informed about the expected outcomes of refusing treatment, medications, or other services.

Accept the results that come from refusing treatment, medication, or other services.

Be informed about completing an **advance directive.**

Payment for Services

Know, ahead of time, charges for services and payment policies, if responsible for payment.
Be informed, in advance, about any changes in service charges or payment policies.

Other

Receive a copy of the agency's policies and procedures.

Be informed about the agency's procedure to voice **grievances** about care or lack of respect, without fear of harmful results.

Confidentiality of all records and information related to care, including financial records.

Be informed about the name, address, and phone number of the state agency that regulates home care.

CLIENT'S RESPONSIBILITIES

Remain under a doctor's care while receiving services of the agency.
Provide the agency with an accurate and complete health history.
Sign required release and consent forms.

Participate in developing and revising the plan of care or service.

Cooperate with your doctor and agency staff.

Provide a copy of the advance directive, if it exists.

Provide agency with all requested financial and insurance records.
Pay for services according to plan for payment.

Follow the procedures outlined.

Follow the grievance procedure in a timely manner.

File a complaint with the state agency, if necessary.

You have chosen to be a home care aide because you like people and want to give them the kind of care you would want to receive. By setting high standards of conduct for yourself, you are contributing to quality home care services for clients.

Home care agencies have policy and procedure manuals that include the code of behavior expected for each employee in performing day-to-day activities on the job. Your agency also has a Client's Bill of Rights similar to the one shown in Table 2-1. It contains standards of behavior for the home care team to follow.

During your orientation to the agency, supervisory staff will discuss the ethical behavior expected of all its employees. Some important behaviors include confidentiality and honesty. Behaviors to avoid will also be discussed.

Confidentiality

As a home care professional, you will receive information about the client and family that is to be treated as private or confidential. You will also observe situations in the home that must only be shared with your supervisor or during meetings of the home care team. You show your respect for the client and family by not discussing any information related to the work assignment with your own family, friends, or other clients. Information you obtain by reading the client's care record must also be kept confidential.

Honesty

You will experience situations in the home where the client or family member may ask you to give them information about the client's condition that you know you are not allowed to give. Be honest. Do not lie by saying, "I don't know." This may give the impression that you do not know what you are doing. Tell the truth. Say, "I really can't answer that question, but I'll ask my supervisor to contact you." Be honest with your client and family at all times. If you do not know the answer to a question, say so. Remember, you are not expected to know all the answers all of the time. Your response may be, "I don't know, but I'll discuss it with my supervisor and get back to you." If you say this, make sure to do what you said you would do. By your actions, you are telling others that you are honest and reliable.

Behaviors to Avoid

Six behaviors to avoid when communicating with your client and family are:

1. Avoid giving advice.
2. Avoid making judgments.
3. Avoid giving false reassurances about your client's physical or emotional condition.
4. Avoid focusing on yourself.
5. Avoid discussing your own problems and concerns.
6. Avoid discussing topics that are controversial, such as religion and politics.

advance directive
documents that indicate a client's wishes about health care.

grievances
a wrong, considered as grounds for a complaint.

confidentiality
something spoken or written in confidence, in secret.

CHAPTER SUMMARY

- Communication is an important skill for the home care aide to develop.

- Clear, accurate communication is necessary so that you can share information and ideas with the client, the family, and your agency.

- There are four parts to the communication process: the sender, the receiver, the message, and feedback.

- Many barriers interfere with clear communication, and there are special techniques to encourage effective communication with clients.

- Guides to ethical behavior are found in your agency's policies and procedures manual and the Client's Bill of Rights.

STUDY QUESTIONS

1. Define communication.
2. Draw and label a diagram showing the parts of the communication process.
3. List three reasons for clear communication.
4. Give three examples of verbal and nonverbal communication.
5. List three barriers to communication.
6. Demonstrate three ways to communicate with
   a. hearing impaired persons.
   b. visually-impaired persons.
7. What would you do in the following situations?
   a. You meet several other home care aides at the local restaurant for lunch. They ask how your client is doing.
   b. Your client says that money is missing from her purse.
   c. The client asks you if he is going to die.
   d. You are caring for two senior citizens in the same apartment building. One client asks you what is wrong with her neighbor.
   e. Your client has several friends who visit regularly. They go into his room, lock the door, and stay for about an hour. You suspect that they are using illegal drugs.
8. Read your agency's Client's Bill of Rights. Identify the rights of the client and the rights of the agency. Identify the responsibilities of the client and the agency. Explain these in your own words.

Understanding Your Client's Needs

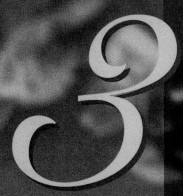

Objectives

After you read this chapter, you will be able to:

1. Discuss basic human needs.

2. Describe three types of families.

3. Explain the importance of the family in society.

4. Discuss the role of the home care aide in helping clients meet their needs.

5. List three principles of growth and development.

6. Discuss each stage of development and identify three characteristics of each.

7. Identify three ways of meeting the client's needs in each developmental stage.

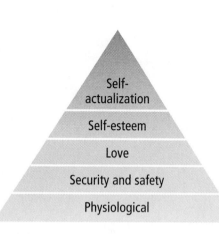

3-1 Basic needs as described by Maslow.

NEED—how often do we use that word? How many times have we said:

"What do we need from the market?"
"I need a new shirt."
"I need a car."
"I need a dress to wear to the wedding."

Over and over, we use the word NEED. Most often, when we say *need*, we are talking about what we want, rather than what we need.

Basic Human Needs

Just what, then, is meant by the term *need?* Need is defined as a requirement for survival. The psychologist, Abraham Maslow, described the basic human needs and used a pyramid shape to illustrate them (Fig. 3-1). At the base of the pyramid is listed **physiological** (or physical) needs. These needs must be met <u>first</u> before any of the others.

Physiological Needs

Physiological needs include:

1. Breathing/Oxygen
2. Food/Nutrition/Water
3. Activity/Rest/Sleep
4. Elimination of body waste
5. Avoidance of pain
6. Personal hygiene
7. Sexuality

It is important to be aware of these needs because they must be taken care of before any others. A person cannot feel loved or give love if he or she is starving. If the most important need is food, then that need takes priority over all the others. Only after that physical need is met can other needs be met. When people cannot take care of their own basic needs for survival, others must help. For children, it is the **primary caregiver**—mother, father, grandparent—who meets their basic needs. For sick persons, the family may provide for the basic needs. Many times, it is the home care aide who will care for basic physical needs.

Safety and Security

Safety and security include:

1. Accident prevention
2. Safe surroundings
3. Religion

Safety is a common concern for most people. "Is my neighborhood a safe place?" "How can fire be prevented?" "Is my seat belt buckled?" All of these questions concern safety. You, the home care aide, are responsible for the safety and security of the client, the client's belongings, and <u>yourself</u>. You will find that safety and accident prevention are stressed throughout the text.

Religion is a very personal set of beliefs, special to the client. As a part of the client's Bill of Rights, religious beliefs are respected. The aide's personal beliefs are just that—personal. What you believe is meaningful to you may not be helpful to clients in meeting their own needs.

need
requirement for survival.

physiological
pertaining to the normal functioning of the body.

primary caregiver
a person who provides most of the care early in one's life.

self-esteem
thinking and feeling good about yourself.

self-actualization
state of reaching one's full potential and being able to cope with problems.

If necessary, your agency and/or the client's family may contact the appropriate clergy to assist your client.

Love

Love includes:

1. Communication
2. Affection
3. Social relationships/friends/companions
4. Identity
5. Belonging and being cared for

We all need to feel loved, wanted, and cared for. We all need some relationship with others—even if it is only with one other person. For many lonely clients, the home care aide fulfills the client's need for love and belonging.

Self-Esteem

Self-esteem includes thinking and feeling good about yourself. It also includes the feeling that others, too, think well of you.

Self-Actualization

Maslow's fifth level of basic human needs is **self-actualization.** This is defined as the state of reaching your full potential and being able to cope with problems. Not everyone achieves self-actualization because the other needs, lower on the pyramid, have not been met.

How well needs are met affects our sense of well-being and our mental health. Most healthy adults are able to meet their own needs—along with the help of their family and friends.

The Family

In the past, the United States was primarily a farming society. Many people lived in rural areas, and the family took care of all its own needs. Family members worked side by side to ensure their survival. Today, few American families live on farms or in rural areas. Most people are employed outside of the home, and, with the exception of family-owned businesses, family members usually do not work side by side.

The Changing Family

As society changed, families changed, too; but some things have remained constant. For example, most of us belong to a nuclear family—that family into which we were born or adopted. We also may belong to a family of procreation: the family we have started.

The word *family* has many meanings. Some are:

- a group of people who are related and may or may not live under the same roof
- a group of people living in the same home
- a circle of friends and relatives who love you
- a group of people living together who share a past and a future

In addition to many definitions of the word *family,* there are also several types of family structures. When you think of the word *family,*

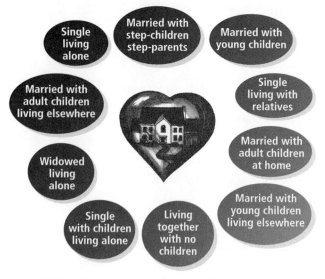

3-2 The changing American family.

a certain image may come to mind. Do you visualize a mother, father, and two children? This is often thought of as the typical American family, the "intact family." But you may have had a different image come to mind—perhaps a widowed grandmother who is raising two young grandchildren. This, too, is an example of a family. In fact, there is <u>NO</u> typical family. There are so many varieties that it is hard to put them into categories. Some examples of family patterns are found in Fig. 3-2.

Families today are more mobile than in the past. Families who have lived in the same home in the same community for generations are the exception. Today, families may move "up" from a starter home or "down" into a retirement home. Some families are homeless, moving from shelter to shelter. Gone are the days when three generations routinely lived under one roof. The extended family (grandparents, aunts, uncles, cousins) is scattered all over the country, perhaps even all over the world.

Importance in Society

The family is the most important structure in society. Within this unit, children are born and reared. Here we learn to love, play, and express our feelings. Our culture and traditions are passed on from generation to generation. Families teach about manners, morals, religion, beliefs, prejudices, hates, and fears. Sometimes family members have so much anger and hate that they may abuse themselves or others in the home. Further information about abuse is found in Chapters 18, 19, and 20.

Psychologists say that one person affects the lives of at least eight others for better or worse, and each one of them will affect the lives of eight more. In other words, the family has a tremendous influence on its members and on society.

Helping Clients to Meet Their Needs

Families still continue to meet many of their own needs, but some organizations and agencies have been created to help when needed. For example, day care centers meet the needs of young children when their parents are at work or school. Home health agencies provide home care when families require help to care for sick members. Meals On Wheels programs help homebound persons to have daily hot meals and good nutrition.

As the home care aide, you will follow the care plan established by the home care team to meet your client's individual needs. When working with a client, you may discover that he or she has additional unmet needs. Notify your supervisor when you identify unmet client needs. For example, your client tells you that she has not been able to sleep ever since she was discharged from the hospital 10 days ago. She is very tired and does not want to get out of bed. The care plan may be changed to meet the client's physiological need for rest and sleep.

role
usual function of a person or object.

The family will also have needs, and, of course, you, too, have personal needs. However, your **role** is to care for the client. That is why you are in the home. The client's needs come first. Sometimes family members will ask you to take care of their needs, such as baby-sitting a grandchild at the same time you are supposed to be caring for the grandfather. If your responsibility is to assist the client with personal care, bathing, grooming, and dressing, how can you also supervise an active two year old? Tell the family politely that the care of the sick person comes first. Also, report the situation to your supervisor, who can explain your role and responsibilities to the family members. If the family requires additional help, such as child day care, the agency may assist by making a referral.

When a person's needs are unmet, many difficult emotions arise, including anger, frustration, fear, and stress. Your client may have these feelings, which are quite common during illness (see Chapter 5). You may experience these feelings, too.

Your Needs vs. the Needs of Your Client

As a home care aide, you will be prepared to recognize and meet the needs of your client. Your needs are important, too—and you must remember to take care of them. However, when you are at work, take great care to see that your needs do not become more important than those of your client. Of course, there may be times when personal problems may make it difficult for you to give proper client care. If this happens, discuss the situation with your supervisor. Perhaps you need a day off or another assignment.

If your own needs are not being met, you will not be able to care for someone else. Sometimes a client may make you feel angry, frustrated, or resentful, but we all get those feelings from time to time. However, you must not forget the client's needs and focus on your own. Consider the following situations:

- Is it quicker, easier, and less messy to feed the client instead of letting him feed himself and gain some independence? Whose need is being met?

- It is a beautiful spring day and you decide to take your client outside in the wheelchair. You really want her to go outside but she doesn't want to go. She refuses to get into the wheelchair and is angry with you. Whose needs are being met? Are you angry and frustrated? Do you feel useless?

- Your client refuses to eat, saying, "Why should I eat; I'm going to die anyway." You become frustrated, angry, and feel guilty. Whose need is being met?

In each case, the need of the home care aide has become more important than the client's need. This can cause unpleasant emotions for you and the client. It is important to recognize these feelings and discuss them with your supervisor.

How We Grow and Develop

Just as a knowledge of basic needs is important, so, too, is an understanding about how people grow and develop. Knowing what is normal for the various stages of development will help you understand how disease and illness are affecting your client. It will also help you modify your care based on the client's stage in the life cycle.

The five principles of growth and development are:

Principle 1

There are many factors that influence the way we grow and develop.

Genes Our physical appearance is determined by genes, which are a part of our body cells. These genes, from mother and father, contain codes that determine bone structure, facial features, and color of eyes, hair, and skin. The statement, "You look just like your Grandma Burns," is true because of the physical characteristics inherited from the family. Genes also contain codes that transmit inherited (hereditary) diseases.

The Primary Caregiver The person who assumes the major responsibility for care early in our lives plays a very important role in how we grow and develop. This person is called the primary caregiver. This is the one who provides for our basic human needs by bathing and feeding us, kissing and hugging us, and talking and playing with us.

In the nuclear family structure, the mother usually assumes the role of primary caregiver. In other families, the biological mother may give up the infant for adoption or get a job shortly after the infant's birth. In these situations, the primary caregiver may be the adoptive parent or the infant's father, grandmother, aunt, other relative, or guardian. Sometimes, the family will hire a person to act as the substitute mother or "nanny." In other situations, the "family" consists of the staff of the institution caring for an abandoned child.

There is no "typical caregiver" in today's society. The primary caregiver may be male or female, married or single, gay or lesbian, older or younger. He or she provides the physical, emotional, and social needs of the infant and child. How successful the caregiver is in meeting these needs has a profound effect on the child's future. As we grow older, **peers,** teachers, other relatives, and friends contribute to our development. But it is the primary caregiver, early in our lives, who plays the critical role.

Nutrition The quantity and quality of the food we eat certainly influences our growth and development. Even before birth, what the mother eats, drinks, and smokes has an effect upon the unborn child. Poorly nourished infants and children are likely to grow and develop more slowly, be prone to illness, and have more infectious diseases.

The Environment Where we live, and with whom; what we receive and how we receive it—all these affect our growth and development. The ideal environment:

- provides for basic human needs of the person
- reflects a loving and caring relationship among all members of the family

peers
persons who are one's equal.

sibling
a brother or sister.

- allows each member to make mistakes, to be corrected or disciplined with love, and to learn from mistakes
- permits each person to grow and develop as a unique human being
- shows that members are accepted for who they are rather than what they can do for others

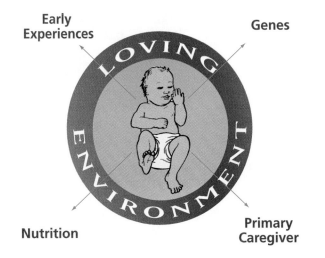

3-3 A loving environment is essential for all of us to grow.

Principle 2

What we experience early in life provides the basis for our growth and development in later years.

A well-nourished infant who receives love and affection in a caring environment has an excellent foundation for the next stage of growth and development. If, however, the infant is poorly nourished, physical growth will be seriously affected. If emotional nourishment—love and affection in a caring atmosphere—is absent or severely lacking, emotional and social growth and development will also be severely affected. A child who is loved learns to love and accept oneself and others, too (Fig. 3-3).

Principle 3

Growth occurs in a logical pattern.

Physical growth and development starts at the head and progresses to the feet. For example, an infant is first able to raise its head before learning to control the shoulders; he/she learns first to crawl, then to walk. This is called the "Head to Toe Principle." Growth is also symmetrical, meaning that the right side of the body grows at the same time the left side grows. Even though the stages of growth and development are the same for everyone, each person grows at his/her own pace. For example, some infants are able to walk when they are nine months old while others may not be walking until they are 14 months old. Children will grow at different paces, even those in the same family. As an example, one child might be outgoing and talkative, whereas his/her **sibling** at the same age was quiet and subdued. In a large family, the youngest child may not begin to talk as early as the older children because needs are being met without having to speak. The rate at which a person grows and develops depends a great deal on the environment and the life experiences of that individual.

Principle 4

We must complete one stage of growth and development before going on to the next.

As we grow and develop, we must first learn how to perform simple tasks before we can learn more difficult tasks. For example, Tommy must learn to walk before he can learn to run. Tamika must first learn how to hold a pencil before she can learn how to write. Because each stage of growth and development builds on the skills learned in earlier stages, no

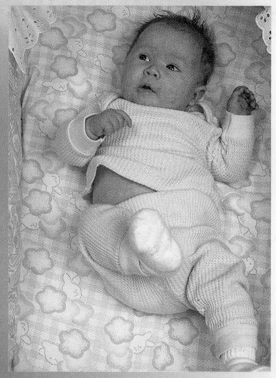

3-4 Infancy is a time of great growth and change.

stage can be skipped. For example, it is impossible for a child to skip the adolescent stage and go right to adulthood.

Principle 5

Physical growth is usually completed around age 21. But we continue to grow emotionally, socially, and intellectually throughout our lives.

Bone growth stops around age 21, but our hair and nails continue to grow. New blood cells are produced as the old ones are destroyed. When injury occurs, new cells and tissues are produced so that healing can take place.

In each stage of growth and development listed below, there are tasks to be accomplished that help to make life meaningful and worthwhile. The experiences of life and how we respond to them influence the way we grow emotionally, socially, and intellectually. While formal education in school may end at a certain time, we continue to expand our knowledge by communicating with others, reading, and learning from other experiences of everyday life. Growing socially, emotionally, and intellectually is a lifetime process.

Stages of Normal Growth and Development

Listed below are the seven major stages of human growth and development, key characteristics of each stage, and some guides for meeting your client's needs during each stage. Additional information is found in Chapters 5, 8, 18, 19, and 21.

Stage 1: Infancy (Total Dependency—Learning to Trust)

Age: Birth to one year

Characteristics Infant learns to survive outside the mother's uterus. A time of tremendous physical growth; birth weight triples. Learns to control head, sits, and grasps objects. Learns to coordinate arms and legs by crawling; takes first step or even walks. From the first cry, develops ability to speak first word and talk. Infancy is the period of the greatest growth and development of all the stages (Fig. 3-4).

Meeting the infant's needs All the infant's needs are provided by the caregiver. Provide a safe environment to prevent injury. Meet needs for food, sleep, warmth. Hold, cuddle, talk to infant. Provide a "world" that is dependable, loving, comfortable, and consistent. Infants develop a sense of trust when this kind of environment exists.

Stage 2: Toddler (Beginning to Exert Independence—"Mine")

Age: One to three

Characteristics This is a period of endless activity—getting into everything. More coordinated—walking, reaching, eating. Develops new skills—climbing, mastering basics of toilet training. Unable to understand danger. Accident prone due to curiosity. Seeks attention and approval. Temper tantrums as a reaction to discipline and developing self-will. Plays alone, then plays alongside other children. Begins to tolerate separation from primary caregiver (Fig. 3-5).

Meeting the toddler's needs Maintain a safe environment by eliminating hazards. Praise to reinforce safe behavior. Be consistent in enforcing rules. Sit down, if possible, when talking to the toddler. Reinforce toilet training techniques provided by primary caregiver. Handling temper tantrums is discussed in Chapter 19.

Stage 3: Preschool (Energetic and Curious—"Why?")

Age: Three to five

Characteristics Better control of complex muscular movements—running, jumping, climbing. A period of almost endless energy. Eager to learn—always asking, "Why?" Imitates adults and older children. May have imaginary playmates. Learning to get along with more people. Plays cooperatively with others. Able to wash and dress self. Prints own name and draws pictures. Tolerates separation from primary caregiver. Curious about sex differences. Rituals play an important role (bedtime) (Fig. 3-6).

Meeting the preschool client's needs Use positive suggestions; avoid the use of "Don't." Be consistent and clear when describing acceptable behavior. Provide a safe environment and supervision to prevent injury. Answer questions truthfully. Follow the ritual for nap time and bedtime. Maintain the rules of conduct already set in the home.

Stage 4: School (Decreasing Dependence on Family—Learning from School and Peers)

Age: Six to 12

Characteristics Period of slow but steady physical growth. Around age 12, a rapid growth spurt indicates the transition to adolescence. Active and physically strong. At risk for injuries due to participation in sports activities and attitude of fearlessness. Enjoys being out of doors and playing with friends. Moves out from family members to seek other relationships. The "gang" becomes important. Developing basic skills—reading, writing, mathematics. Likes to solve problems; likes challenges. Developing sense of conscience, morals, and values (Fig. 3-7).

Meeting the school-age client's needs Maintain the rules of behavior already established in the home. Continue to provide a safe home environment with supervision. Reinforce rules set for bedtime; adequate rest and sleep are very important. Provide adequate nutrition. Encourage safety-conscious behavior. Reinforce responsible behavior in performing assigned chores. Honor the right to privacy. Provide choices for child to make in the routine of care. Encourage communication of feelings and emotions. Be honest when answering questions.

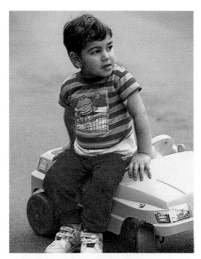

3-5 Fear of separation from primary caregiver is eventually overcome.

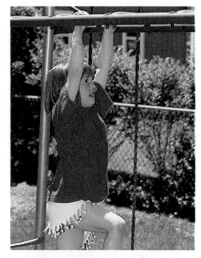

3-6 The preschooler is full of energy and eager to learn

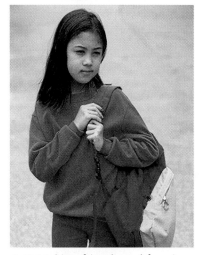

3-7 Making friends and forming new relationships is important to the school-age child.

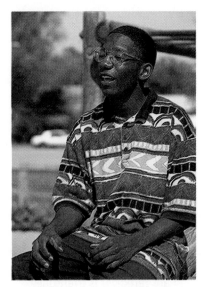

3-8 Adolescents go through many changes on their way to adulthood.

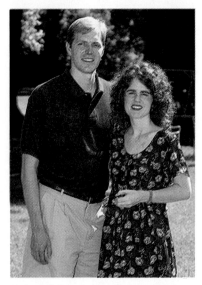

3-9 Adults must take responsibility for themselves.

Stage 5: Adolescence (The Years of Conflicts and Adjustments—Establishing Independence)

Age: 12 to 18

Characteristics The second major period of rapid physical growth. Emotional and social changes occur. Sexual characteristics develop—may be embarrassed about them. Intense loyalty to peer group, which provides a sense of belonging. Mood swings and extremes in behavior. Interacting with the opposite sex. Conflicts—wanting to be independent yet the need for dependence on the family. Achieving emotional independence from parents. Preparing for adult life—career and family (Fig. 3-8).

Meeting the adolescent client's needs Maintain the rules already set in the home. Respect the right to privacy. Continue to reinforce safety-conscious behavior. Provide opportunities for client to make choice in care routine. Answer questions honestly. Reinforce limits already established for rest and sleep. Remain calm if unacceptable behavior occurs. Be firm in reinforcing rules of acceptable behavior. Encourage communication of feelings and emotions.

Stage 6: Adulthood (Establishing and Maintaining a Meaningful Life)

Age: 18 to 65

Characteristics Physical development is complete. Accepts self and body image. Establishes an intimate bond with another through marriage or close friend of the same or opposite sex. Works in a career that is satisfying and provides financial independence. Becomes involved in community activities. Enjoys an active social life with friends. Establishes and maintains a home. Decides whether to have a child (children). If so, carries out parenting role. Accepts and adjusts to physical and emotional changes occurring in middle life. Copes with stresses of living in a positive way. May care for parents and/or grandchildren (Fig. 3-9).

Meeting the adult client's needs Assist client to maintain independence in activities of daily living as long as possible. Provide opportunities for client to make choices in the routine of care. Encourage active involvement in family life and household routine as long as possible. Encourage communication of feelings and emotions.

Stage 7: Older Adulthood (Adjusting to Change and Maintaining Independence)

Age 65 to 100 plus

Characteristics A period of many changes: physical, emotional, and social. Adjusting to and accepting the changes that occur. Adjusting to retirement and lifestyle changes due to reduced income. Adjusting to decreasing health and physical strength. Accepting and adjusting to the death of spouse, relatives, and friends. Accepting oneself as an aging person. Adjusting to the reality of death. Finding meaning in life (Fig. 3-10).

Meeting the older client's needs Maintain a clutter-free environment to prevent accidents. If necessary, use strategies discussed in Chapter 2 to communicate with hearing and visually impaired clients. Provide extra time to accomplish tasks. Allow client to do as much as possible, even though it takes more time. See Chapter 18 for more information about caring for older clients.

CHAPTER SUMMARY

- Everyone has basic human needs.

- Physiological needs must be met first.

- There are five levels of basic needs.

- There are many types of family patterns.

- The family is the most important structure in society.

- Organizations and agencies help families to meet needs.

- Knowledge of growth and development will be helpful to you in meeting the client's needs.

- There are five principles of growth and development.

- There are seven stages in human growth and development.

- Knowing what is normal for each stage will help you to understand how disease and illness affects your client.

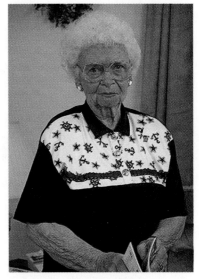

3-10 The older adult faces lots of changes and challenges.

STUDY QUESTIONS

1. List five basic needs and define each.

2. Define the word "family" using your own family as an example. Is your definition different from those in the text?

3. Explain the importance of the family in society.

4. Describe the five principles of growth and development.

5. Describe three characteristics of the following stages and how the home care aide can meet the needs of clients in these stages:
   a. toddler.
   b. adulthood.
   c. older adulthood.

4

Understanding How the Body Works

Objectives

After you read this chapter, you will be able to:

1. Describe how the body is organized.

2. List body systems and give the general functions of each.

3. Identify the important parts of each body system and their functions.

4. Discuss how body systems work together.

In order to meet your client's physiological needs, you must understand how the human body works. This knowledge is the foundation for working with sick persons and will help you to understand your client's illnesses and treatment plans.

The home care aide uses a basic understanding of **body structures** and their **functions** when giving personal care. For example, Mrs. Jimanez is recovering from a broken hip. The home care aide knows that the injury may have caused damage to other body tissues—blood vessels, muscles, nerves, and skin. The home care aide also knows that most of the body systems will be involved in recovery, since they work together to maintain health and promote recovery.

Organization of the Human Body

Cells

The cell is the basic functioning unit of the body. Cells are the smallest structures of all living things. They carry out many complicated activities. The human body is composed of trillions of cells that are so small they can only be seen through a **microscope** (Fig. 4-1).

Tissues, Membranes, and Glands

Tissues

Cells having a similar structure and function are joined together to make tissues. For example, individual muscle cells are joined together to form muscle tissue. There are four types of tissue in the human body.

1. *Muscle tissue* is able to **contract.**
2. *Nervous tissue* sends and receives messages between the body and the brain.
3. *Connective tissue* connects and supports other parts of the body.
4. *Epithelial tissue* covers the body (skin) and lines the body cavities and openings.

Membranes

Epithelial and connective tissue may also be arranged into large sheets called membranes. These structures cover body organs and line body cavities. There are three types:

1. *Mucous membrane* produces mucus and lines all openings to the outside of the body—mouth, nose, reproductive organs, etc.
2. *Serous membrane* lubricates and protects internal organs and body cavities.
3. *Cutaneous membrane* (skin) covers the entire body.

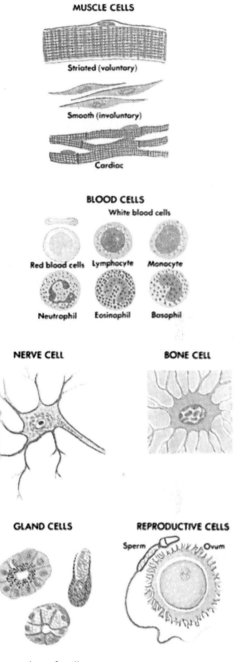

4-1 Examples of cells. *(From Thibodeau GA:* Anatomy and Physiology, *1987, Mosby.)*

body structure(s)
construction and arrangement of cells, tissues, and organs.

function(s)
action performed by any structure.

microscope
instrument for viewing objects that cannot be seen with the naked eye.

contract
to become smaller, tighter.

Glands

Glands are groups of specialized cells that manufacture and **secrete** substances into the body. **Exocrine** glands secrete substances into a duct. For example, sweat glands. **Endocrine** glands secrete **hormones** directly into the blood stream and are called ductless glands. For example, the thyroid gland secretes hormones to regulate body **metabolism.**

Organs

Organs are made up of several different types of tissue that work together to perform a specific function. They are far more complex than tissues. For example, the mouth is the first organ of the digestive system. It contains many different types of tissue, working together to begin food breakdown.

Organ Systems

An organ system is made up of many different organs working together to perform a specific function. Systems are more complex than tissues or organs. For example, the digestive system contains many organs and is responsible for nutrition and elimination.

There are many organ systems. All the systems work together and depend on one another for proper body functioning. Major organ systems are:

1. *Integumentary system* protects the body from injury.
2. *Skeletomuscular system* provides support, protection, and movement.
3. *Nervous system and senses* send and receive electrical messages and coordinate all body functions.
4. *Endocrine system* produces hormones that regulate body functions.
5. *Circulatory and lymphatic system* transports blood and tissue fluid throughout the body. Fights infection.
6. *Respiratory system* takes in **oxygen** and removes **carbon dioxide** from the body.
7. *Digestive system* responsible for nutrition and elimination of body waste.
8. *Urinary system* filters all the blood to remove dissolved waste and excess water.
9. *Reproductive system* responsible for production of offspring.

Points to Remember

- Cells are the smallest functioning unit of the body.
- Cells of similar structure and function are organized into tissues.
- Organs are made up of several types of tissues in one structure.
- Organ (body) systems are made up of many organs that perform a specific function (Fig. 4-2).

Body Cavities

The organs of the various body systems are arranged in spaces within the body. These are called body cavities. There are five major cavities (Fig. 4-3).

1. *Cranial cavity*—space inside the skull; contains the brain.
2. *Spinal cavity*—space inside the spinal column; contains the spinal cord.

---

secrete/secretion
release of a substance that serves a special function in the body.

exocrine
glands that secrete substances into a duct.

endocrine
glands that secrete hormones directly into the bloodstream.

hormones
chemicals produced by endocrine glands.

metabolism
burning of food to produce heat and energy in the body.

oxygen
gas essential for life.

carbon dioxide
gas eliminated from the lungs during exhalation.

pigment
coloring matter in the body.

Cell   Tissue

Organ

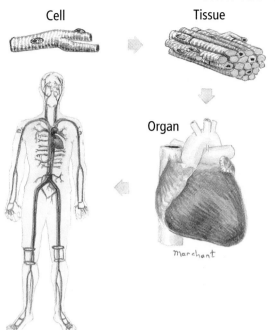

Organ System

4-2 Body organization. *(From Sorrentino, SA: Mosby's Textbook for Nursing Assistants, ed. 4, St. Louis, 1996, Mosby.)*

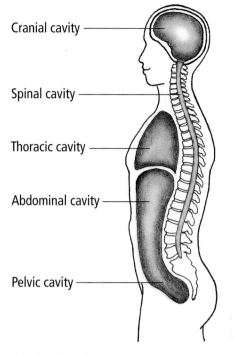

Cranial cavity

Spinal cavity

Thoracic cavity

Abdominal cavity

Pelvic cavity

4-3 Body cavities. *(From Brooks ML: Exploring Medical Language: A Student Directed Approach, ed. 3, St. Louis, 1994, Mosby–Year Book, Inc.)*

3. *Thoracic cavity*—space inside the chest; contains the heart, lungs, trachea (windpipe), and esophagus. Separated from the abdominal cavity by the diaphragm, a large, dome-shaped muscle.
4. *Abdominal cavity*—space below the thoracic cavity containing the stomach, most of the intestines, liver, gall bladder, and other organs.
5. *Pelvic cavity*—lower portion of the abdominal cavity. Surrounded by the hip bones. Contains the bladder, uterus, part of the large intestine, and rectum.

Integumentary System

Purpose: Covers the entire body and protects internal structures from damage by harmful invaders or substances; regulates body heat; relays body sensations; manufactures vitamin D for healthy bones; and holds in body fluids (Fig. 4-4).

Important Parts

Skin contains **pigment,** blood vessels, nerve endings, fatty tissue, sweat glands, oil glands, and wax glands.
Hair covers the skin to protect the skin, eyes, ears, nasal passages, and external sex organs.
Nails protect sensitive tips of fingers and toes from injury.

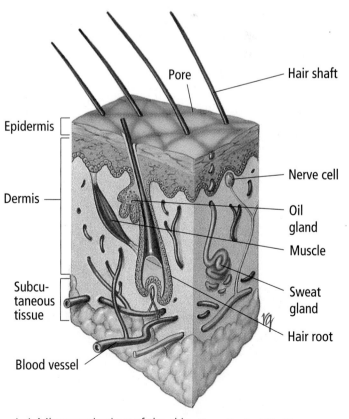

Pore

Hair shaft

Epidermis

Dermis

Nerve cell

Oil gland

Muscle

Subcutaneous tissue

Sweat gland

Hair root

Blood vessel

4-4 Microscopic view of the skin. *(From Gerdin J: Health Careers Today, ed. 2, St. Louis, 1997, Mosby.)*

Points to Remember

- The skin's color and condition can be an indication of the general health of the body.
- Fatty tissue acts as insulation to keep in body heat.
- Healthy skin is essential for a healthy body.
- Sweat glands secrete sweat to cool the body.
- The skin is the body's first line of defense against injury.
- Skin breaks down very easily in some locations when a sick person becomes unable to move easily.
- Skin is nourished from the inside with a good diet and plenty of fluids.

Do You Know?

- More money is spent on the care of skin, hair, and nails than on medical care of diseases.
- Skin is always covered with germs. Washing with soap and water is an effective method of preventing the spread of infection.
- Skin is the largest organ of the body.

Skeletomuscular System

Purpose: Acts as a framework to support the body; produces movement; maintains posture; and protects delicate internal organs (Figs. 4-5 and 4-6).

Important Parts

Long bones of arms and legs allow for movement and manufacture blood cells.

Short bones of hands, wrists, ankles, and toes allow for fine movements.

Flat bones of ribs, skull, and pelvis protect delicate organs.

Irregular bones of spinal column allow for bending and easy movement.

Joints are places where bones are joined together.

Muscles are attached to bones and cause movement to occur. Voluntary muscles are ones that we control. Involuntary muscles are ones that we cannot control, such as the heart muscle and those in internal organs.

Ligaments are tough fibrous bands that bind joints together.

Tendons are tough elastic bands that connect muscles to bones.

Cartilage is tough smooth tissue at bone ends that permits easy movement at the joints.

The Process of Movement

Movement occurs when voluntary muscles, attached to bones, contract and relax, causing a change in the joint. These muscles work in pairs. When one contracts, the other relaxes, pulling the bone and moving the joint. Ball and socket joints located in the shoulder and hip produce circular movements. Hinge joints of the elbow, knee, fingers, and toes allow movement in two directions: bending and straightening. Pivot joints such as the skull on the neck permit rotation of the head from side to side (Fig. 4-7). The brain controls movement of all muscles in the body.

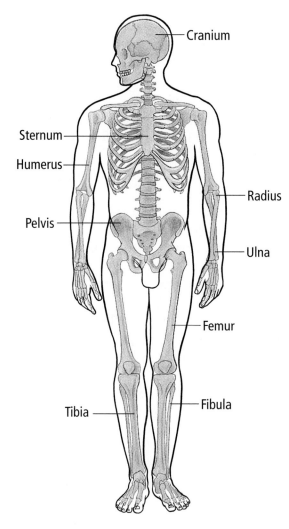

Cranium

Sternum

Humerus

Radius

Pelvis

Ulna

Femur

Tibia

Fibula

4-5 The skeletal system. *(From Thibodeau GA:* Structure and Function of the Body, *ed. 9, St. Louis, 1992, Mosby.)*

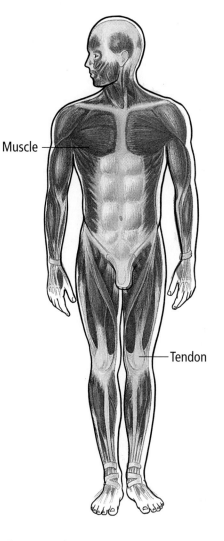

Muscle

Tendon

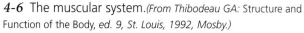

4-6 The muscular system.*(From Thibodeau GA:* Structure and Function of the Body, *ed. 9, St. Louis, 1992, Mosby.)*

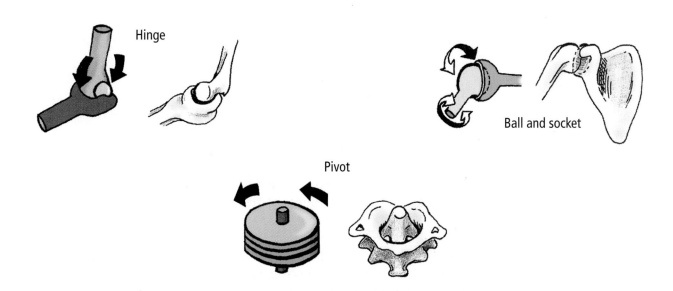

Hinge

Ball and socket

Pivot

4-7 Types of joints.

Points to Remember

- Healthy bones and muscles require foods rich in vitamins and minerals.
- Bone growth stops in early adulthood.
- Bone marrow manufactures blood cells.
- There are 206 bones and more than 600 muscles in the body.
- Large, strong muscles in arms and legs are used for lifting and moving.
- Thin layers of muscles in abdomen and back should be used for posture, not strength.
- Muscle tone refers to the readiness of a muscle to contract.
- Exercise is essential to keep muscles healthy.
- When muscles are not used, they shrink (**atrophy**) and joints become stiff.
- Lack of movement is a major cause of muscle atrophy in sick persons.
- Rings of voluntary and involuntary muscles called **sphincters** surround external body openings or openings in internal structures. For example: voluntary sphincters surround the eye and mouth; an involuntary sphincter joins the stomach and small intestine.

Do You Know?

- The smallest bones are in the inner ear and can be seen only through a microscope.
- The femur (thigh bone) is the longest and strongest bone in the body.
- Body heat is produced when voluntary muscles move.
- More facial muscles are used to frown than to smile.

Nervous System

Purpose: Controls and regulates the activities of all systems of the body to keep them functioning properly. Made up of two parts— the central nervous system and the senses (Fig. 4-8).

Central Nervous System

Important Parts

Brain contains centers that control movement, speech, sensation, learning, vision, taste, emotion, thought, alertness, balance, breathing, heart beat, and blood pressure. It sends and receives messages to and from other parts of the body.

Spinal cord is the passageway for messages going to and away from the brain.

Nerves send and receive messages for sensation and control of voluntary and involuntary muscles.

The Process of Sending and Receiving Messages

The nervous system is made up of millions of nerve cells called neurons (Fig. 4–9). Bundles of neurons are called nerves. Some nerves carry messages from the body to the spinal cord. The spinal cord then passes the message to the brain. The brain receives the message and responds.

atrophy
decrease in size or a wasting away of tissue.

sphincters
rings of voluntary and involuntary muscles that surround external and internal body openings.

It sends the message to the spinal cord. Then, other nerves carry the response back to the body. We move because nerves stimulate muscles to work.

For some activities, we can control nerve function, such as moving arms and legs. For other body activities, we cannot control nerve function, such as regulating our heart beat. A reflex is a rapid involuntary response to messages from nerve endings, such as pulling a finger away from a flame.

Points to Remember

- The nervous system is like a giant computer that regulates all body functions.
- The brain and spinal cord are protected by bones and a special cushioning fluid.
- The nervous system must have sufficient amounts of oxygen and food to function properly.
- Permanent brain damage will occur if the brain is without oxygen for more than seven (7) minutes.
- Damaged nerve tissue takes a long time to repair; sometimes it never does.

Do You Know?

- Some neurons can be almost three feet in length.
- Scientists are conducting research to better understand the functioning of the nervous system.

The Senses

The senses (sight, sound, touch, taste, and smell) are important parts of the nervous system. They receive and send information about the world around us to the brain. The brain, in turn, uses this information to help control the activities and functions of the body.

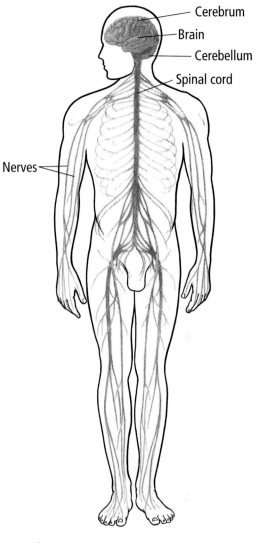

4-8 The nervous system. *(From Thibodeau GA: Structure and Function of the Body, ed. 9, St. Louis, 1992, Mosby.)*

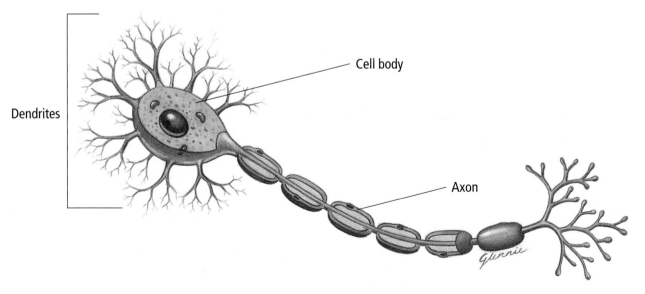

4-9 The neuron. *(From Gerdin J: Health Careers Today, ed. 2, St. Louis, 1997, Mosby.)*

Important Parts

Nerve endings in the skin receive messages of pain, heat, cold, pressure, and touch. Those in the nose and tongue receive messages of smell and taste. Nerve endings in the mouth and stomach receive messages of thirst and hunger.

Eyes and ears receive sound and light messages.

Points to Remember

- To learn about and interact with our environment, we need sense organs to receive information, nerves to transmit the information, and a functioning brain to interpret the information.
- The senses include sight, hearing, touch, taste, pain, smell, pressure, balance, temperature, position, and others.
- The brain uses information from the senses to maintain normal body functioning in an ever-changing environment.

Do You Know?

- The senses provide information to protect the body from harm caused by external forces, such as heat, cold, pressure, sun, etc.
- The senses help us to take in new information and learn new things.
- The senses help us to enjoy our world.

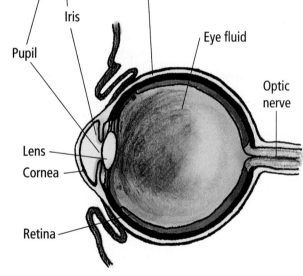

4-10 The eye.

Eyes

Purpose: Receive light rays that focus and transmit images through the nerves to the sight center of the brain (Fig. 4-10).

Important Parts

Cornea is the transparent part of the outer layer that protects the eye.

Pupil controls the amount of light entering the eye.

Lens bends the light rays to focus on the retina.

Retina contains special nerve endings for sight.

Tear glands produce tears to keep the eye moist.

Lids and lashes protect the eye from injury.

The Process of Vision

Light enters the eye through the cornea and passes through the pupil to the lens. The light rays are bent by the lens to focus on nerve endings of the retina. The nerve endings send this information to the sight center in the brain.

Points to Remember

- The eye is very delicate and protected from damage by tears, eyelids, and eyelashes.
- Eye injury and infection can lead to blindness.
- Germs can enter the eye from dirty hands, soiled wash cloths, and cosmetics.

Do You Know?

- The iris is a circular, colored muscle that automatically controls the size of the pupil to adjust the amount of light coming into the eye.
- Color is seen when light is present.

Ears

Purpose: Receive and send sound through nerves to the hearing center of the brain (Fig. 4-11).

Important Parts

Outer ear catches sound waves and sends them to the middle ear.

Ear drum, between the outer and middle ear, receives vibrations and sends them to the middle ear.

Middle ear contains three tiny bones that receive the vibrations from the ear drum and sends them to the inner ear.

Inner ear contains nerve endings for hearing and balance. Sends sound through nerves to the brain.

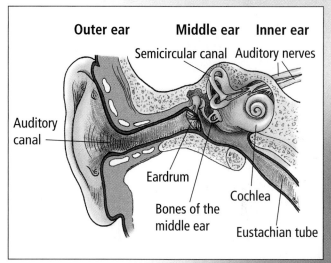

4-11 The ear.

The Process of Hearing

Sound waves enter the outer ear, causing vibrations that travel through the ear drum to the bones in the middle ear. The nerve endings in the inner ear pick up these sound waves and send them to the hearing center of the brain.

The Process of Balance

Structures in the inner ear sense the position and changes in position of the head. These messages are sent to the brain.

Points to Remember

- The auditory canal leads directly to the delicate ear drum; nothing should be placed in this area (no cotton swabs, hair pins, pencils, fingernails).
- Damage to the ear drum may cause hearing loss.

Do You Know?

- The ear receives a wide range of sounds all at once, as in music; at the same time, we understand each separate sound (drum, keyboard, voice, guitar).
- The eustachian tube connects the throat to the middle ear; it makes equal the pressure within the ear and throat; but it can also transport infections from the throat to the middle ear.
- The middle and inner ear are located in the temporal bones of the skull.

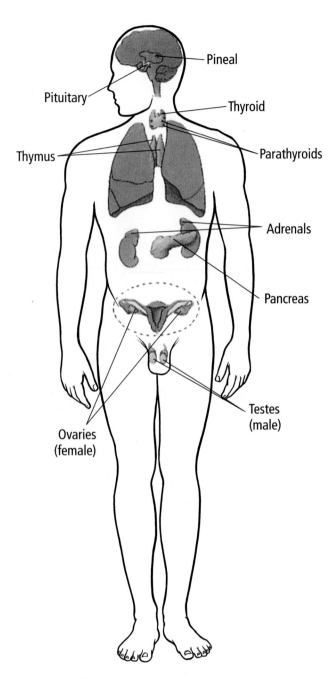

Pineal

Pituitary

Thyroid

Thymus

Parathyroids

Adrenals

Pancreas

Testes (male)

Ovaries (female)

4-12 The endocrine system. *(From Thibodeau GA:* Structure and Function of the Body, *ed. 9, St. Louis, 1992, Mosby.)*

Endocrine System

Purpose: Produces and secretes hormones from ductless glands. These hormones contain chemical messages and are responsible for human growth and development. They also control the activities of other systems, such as the reproductive system (Fig. 4-12).

Important Parts

Pituitary gland is called the "Master Gland" because it stimulates other glands to produce hormones.

Thyroid gland regulates the way food is used to provide energy.

Pancreas produces insulin in special cells of this organ. Insulin helps to break down sugar to give needed energy.

Ovaries produce female sex hormones responsible for sexual development and reproduction.

Testes produce the male sex hormone responsible for sexual development and reproduction.

Points to Remember

- Hormones are chemicals that are produced by glands.
- Hormones enter the bloodstream and regulate many important functions in our bodies.
- Hormones influence all systems of the body.
- There are 15 endocrine glands with a total weight of less than half a pound; yet, they have a powerful influence on all systems of the body.

Do You Know?

- Animal hormones can be used to replace those missing in humans.
- Hormones influence our emotions and feelings.

Circulatory System

Purpose: Delivers food and oxygen to all the cells of the body. Transports each cell's waste products to the organs responsible for removing waste (Fig. 4-13).

Important Parts

Blood, a thick red fluid, carries nutrients and oxygen to each cell of the body.

Blood vessels, called *arteries, capillaries,* and *veins,* are tubes that carry the blood to all parts of the body.

systole
contraction of heart muscle causing blood to leave the heart.

diastole
relaxation of the heart muscle causing its chambers to fill with blood.

Capillaries are tiny tubes that connect the smallest arteries with the smallest veins and supply cells with nutrients and oxygen and remove waste.

Heart, a hollow and very muscular organ, pumps blood through the blood vessels.

The Process of Circulation— the Movement of Blood

When the heart contracts, blood rich in oxygen is forced into the arteries. The arteries branch out to serve all parts of the body. The smallest arteries join with capillaries. This is where nutrients, oxygen, and other substances carried by the blood are passed to the cells of the body. The cells, in turn, pass waste products and carbon dioxide back to the capillaries. The smallest veins join larger veins to carry the blood back to the heart. Next, the blood goes to the lungs to exchange carbon dioxide with oxygen. And the process begins again (Fig. 4-14).

The heart beat—There are two parts to one beat—contracting and resting. When the muscles of the heart contract, blood is forced out of the heart (**systole**). When the heart muscle rests, blood fills the chambers of the heart (**diastole**).

The pulse—As blood is pumped from the heart, you can feel the beat in the arteries. This is called the pulse.

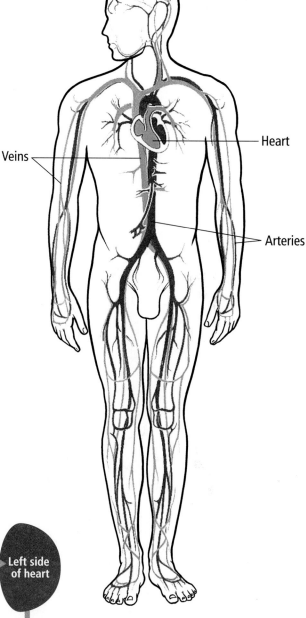

4-13 The circulatory system.
(From Thibodeau, GA: Structure and Function of the Body, *ed. 9, St. Louis, 1992, Mosby.)*

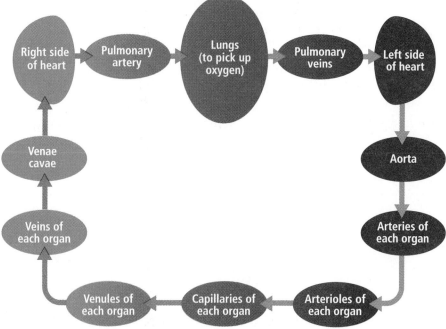

4-14 The process of circulation.

Points to Remember

- Blood distributes the oxygen we breathe, the food we eat, and other substances to the body cells. Waste products enter the blood, too, and are sent to other systems to be removed from the body.
- Blood vessels transport blood to all parts of the body.
- The action of the heart causes blood to move throughout the body in a continuous circle.
- A heart beat consists of two parts—contracting and resting.
- The circulatory system affects all the systems of the body.

Do You Know?

- The heart is an amazing organ that pumps 1,000 gallons of blood a day; it beats 100,000 times a day; it rests only between each beat.
- There are 60,000 miles of blood vessels in the human body.

Lymphatic System

Purpose: Removes excess fluids from tissues and returns them to the blood. It also filters germs and other harmful substances from the blood. This system helps to protect the body by manufacturing substances that destroy germs causing infection. The lymphatic system and the circulatory system work together to help keep the body's fluids in proper balance (Fig. 4-15).

Important Parts

Lymph, a colorless fluid, carries water and protein from the tissues to the circulatory system. *Lymph vessels,* similar in structure to veins, carry lymph to large veins that go to the heart. *Lymph nodes,* small sphere-shaped bodies, act as filters by keeping germs and other substances from spreading throughout the body. *Spleen,* the largest lymph organ of the body, manufactures white blood cells to fight infection.

Points to Remember

- Lymph vessels return excess tissue fluid to the circulatory system.
- The accumulation of lymph in the tissues is called edema.
- Lymph nodes act as the body's defense against infection; they trap infectious organisms and prevent them from traveling to other parts of the body.

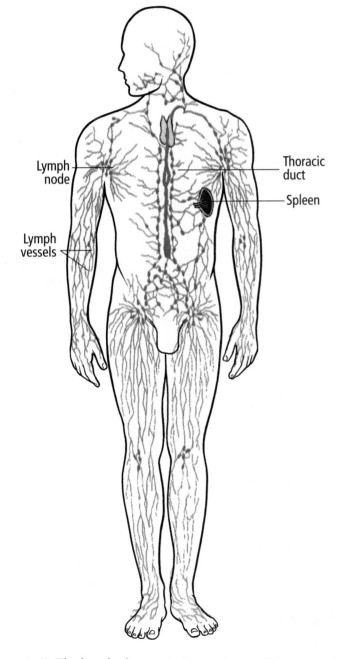

Lymph node

Lymph vessels

Thoracic duct

Spleen

4-15 The lymphatic system. *(From Thibodeau GA:* Structure and Function of the Body, *ed. 9, St. Louis, 1992, Mosby.)*

Do You Know?

- About 600 lymph nodes protect the body by filtering out harmful products.
- Tonsils and adenoids are made of lymphatic tissue and filter out germs from the air we breathe.

Respiratory System

Purpose: Carries oxygen to all the body's cells and eliminates carbon dioxide from the body. It is lined with mucous membrane. The system is divided into two parts—upper and lower respiratory tracts (Fig. 4-16).

Important Parts

- *Upper respiratory tract* contains the nose, sinus cavities, throat, eustachian tubes, larynx (voice box), epiglottis, and trachea (windpipe).
- *Lower respiratory tract* contains tubes leading to the lungs, called the right and left bronchi. The lungs (large, spongy, cone-shaped organs) contain tiny air sacs called alveoli.

Process of Respiration

There are two parts to the process of respiration—inhalation and exhalation.

Inhalation

When we breathe in (inhale), the chest expands and the diaphragm, a dome-shaped muscle, pushes down to allow more room for the lungs to expand. Air containing oxygen enters the nose, sinus cavities, and throat where it is warmed and moistened. These organs help to filter out harmful organisms and prevent them from entering other parts of the respiratory system. Next, air continues through the larynx to the trachea. The trachea transports the air to the lower respiratory tract. Tiny hairs in the trachea prevent dust and other materials from entering the lungs. Extensions of the trachea, tubes called the right and left bronchi, transport air to each lung. Branches of these tubes carry air to all parts of the lungs. At the ends of the smallest branches are the alveoli. Capillaries from the circulatory system surround the alveoli. Oxygen is exchanged for carbon dioxide between the alveoli and the capillaries.

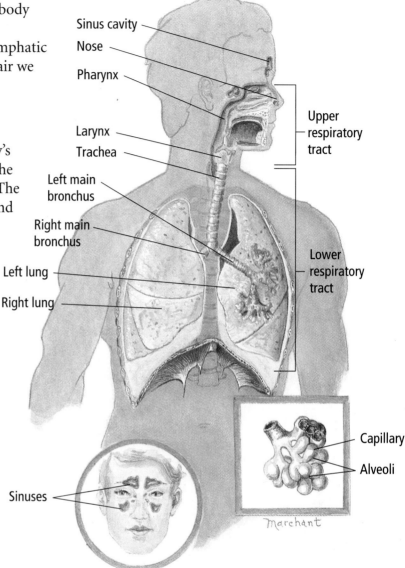

4-16 The respiratory system. *(From Sorrentino, SA: Mosby's Textbook for Nursing Assistants, ed. 4, St. Louis, 1996, Mosby.)*

digestion
complete physical and chemical breakdown of food.

feces
formed body waste discharged from the bowels.

peristalsis
rhythmic involuntary movement that occurs in hollow tubes of the body.

Exhalation

When we breathe out (exhale), the diaphragm becomes dome-shaped again and helps to force air, filled with carbon dioxide, from the lungs. Air is forced from the organs of the lower respiratory tract and through the organs of the upper respiratory tract to the outside.

Points to Remember

- The entire respiratory system is lined with delicate mucous membrane.
- Mucous membranes are the body's natural defense against germs.
- The respiratory and circulatory systems work closely together.
- The exchange of oxygen for carbon dioxide occurs in the lungs between the alveoli and capillaries.
- All cells need oxygen to survive.
- The cough reflex helps to remove material from the upper and lower respiratory tracts.
- When we swallow, the epiglottis closes to prevent food from entering the trachea.
- As air rushes over the vocal cords in the larynx during exhaling, the cords vibrate and allow speech to occur.

Do You Know?

- It takes 12 pounds of air to totally fill a person's healthy lungs.
- There are hundreds of millions of alveoli in the lungs; if they could be spread out, they would take up an area 25 times the surface of your skin.

Digestive (Gastrointestinal, G.I.) System

Purpose: Breaks down the food we eat into nutrients that can be used by the body's cells (Fig. 4-17).

Important Parts:

- *Upper digestive tract* contains the mouth, pharynx, esophagus, and stomach.
- *Small intestine* connects the stomach to the large intestine.
- *Large intestine* (colon) connects the small intestine to the end of the digestive system.
- *Other organs*, such as the liver, gallbladder, and pancreas, assist with the breakdown of food into nutrients.

4-17 The digestive system. *(From Thibodeau, GA: Structure and Function of the Body, ed. 9, St. Louis, 1992, Mosby.)*

The Process of Digestion and Absorption

Digestion starts in the mouth, where food is chewed (physical digestion) and saliva helps to moisten and break down food. The moistened food is swallowed, then goes through the esophagus to the stomach. The stomach produces chemicals called "enzymes" that continue to break down the food (chemical digestion). The action of stomach muscles causes the contents to churn. The stomach contents now enter the small intestine. Bile from the liver and gallbladder enters the small intestine. Juices from the pancreas also enter the small intestine. These chemicals break down the food to a liquid form. Capillaries in the small intestine absorb the nutrients and distribute them into the blood stream to nourish each cell in the body. The amazing process of digestion and absorption of food is completed in the small intestine.

The Process of Eliminating Solid Waste

Water and waste products of digestion enter the large intestine. As this mixture travels through the tube, much of the water is reabsorbed into the body. When waste products reach the lower part of the intestine, they become formed and are called **feces.** Feces are stored in the rectum, and water from them continues to be reabsorbed.

The process of ridding the body of feces is complex and involves the digestive, muscular, and nervous systems. The muscular walls of the large intestine contain nerves. When the rectum becomes full of feces, nerves send a message to the brain. They tell us that it is time to have a bowel movement (BM). **Peristalsis** causes the feces to move; the internal and external anal sphincters of the anus open, and feces are eliminated from the body.

Points to Remember

- The digestive system is one continuous tube.
- Mucous membrane lines the entire system (about 26 feet or 8 meters long), from mouth to anus.
- Digestion begins in the mouth and is completed in the small intestine.
- Food and fluid travel through this system by peristaltic action.
- Water is reabsorbed in the large intestine.
- Waste products are stored and eliminated by the large intestine.
- When feces remain in the large intestine and are not eliminated, they become hard and difficult to pass (constipation).

Do You Know?

- Organs of the digestive system manufacture over eight quarts of fluid in 24 hours to carry out digestive system functions.
- The liver produces bile that is stored in the gallbladder; bile helps to digest fatty foods.

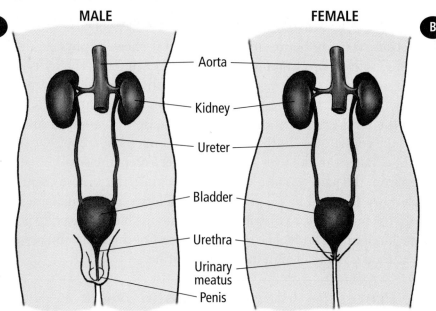

MALE   **FEMALE**

- Aorta
- Kidney
- Ureter
- Bladder
- Urethra
- Urinary meatus
- Penis

4-18 The urinary system. **A,** Male. **B,** Female.

Urinary System

Purpose: Filters out waste products from the blood and removes them from the body in the form of urine (Fig. 4-18).

Important Parts

- *Kidneys (2)* filter out liquid waste products in the blood.
- *Ureters (2)* are tubes that connect the kidneys to the bladder.
- *Bladder* receives urine from the ureters and stores it.
- *Urethra* is a tube that connects the bladder to the outside. The end of the urethra is called the urinary meatus.

The Process of Eliminating Liquid Waste (Urination)

Kidneys are constantly producing urine. Urine drips from the kidneys through the ureters to the bladder for storage. The muscular walls of the bladder contain nerves. When the muscles have stretched due to the fullness of the bladder, nerves send a message to the brain. They tell us that it is time to get rid of the urine—it is time to **urinate.** Nerves also send messages to the bladder muscles to contract. Then urine passes from the bladder through the urethra to the outside.

The entire urinary system of a normal person is free of germs. It is **sterile,** like the blood and the circulatory system. Urine, which is a product of filtered blood, is also sterile. It only becomes unsterile when it comes in contact with the outside of the body.

Points to Remember

- The urinary system maintains a balance between fluids taken in and fluids removed in the form of urine.
- Increased fluids taken in means more urine being produced; what goes in must come out! Adequate fluids are essential for health.

urinate
process of eliminating urine.

sterile
free of living germs.

- Urine is made up of water and other waste products no longer needed by the body.
- The bladder stores urine.
- Urination is a complicated process that involves the urinary system, the muscular system, and the nervous system.

Do You Know?

- Every 20 minutes, the kidneys filter all of the body's blood (5 to 6 quarts).
- The body is composed of 40% solids and 60% fluids (Fig. 4-19).
- Fluids are located inside and outside the cell and in the blood.

Reproductive System

Male

Purpose: Continues the human race by manufacturing the male sex hormone (testosterone) and sperm (the male reproductive cell). When sperm is united with the female reproductive cell, human reproduction takes place. This system is closely related to the urinary system because urine and sperm are carried by the same tube (Fig. 4-20).

Important Parts

Internal

Testes (2) produce sperm and the male sex hormone, testosterone.
Spermatic cord is a tube that connects the testes to the urethra and transports sperm.
Prostate gland surrounds the urethra below the bladder and secretes fluid to help sperm to travel.

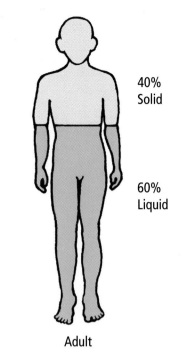

40% Solid

60% Liquid

Adult

4-19 Body composition.

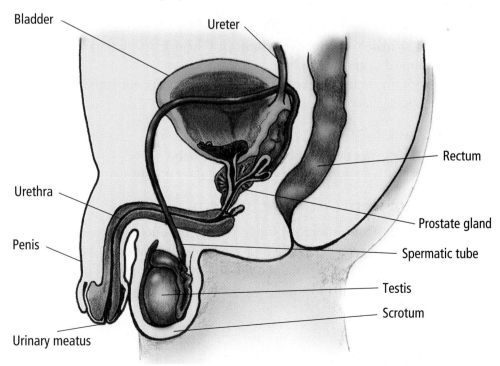

4-20 The male reproductive system.

4-21 The female reproductive system, internal structures. *(From Gerdin J:* Health Careers Today, *ed. 2, St. Louis, 1997, Mosby.)*

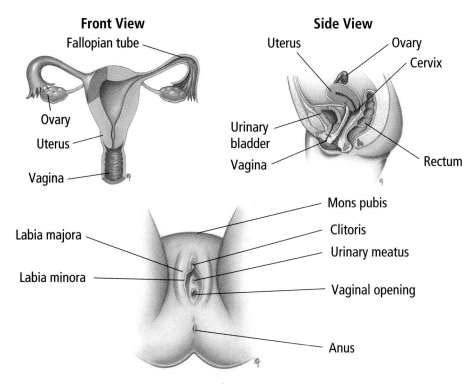

Front View
Fallopian tube
Ovary
Uterus
Vagina

Side View
Uterus
Ovary
Cervix
Urinary bladder
Vagina
Rectum

Mons pubis
Clitoris
Urinary meatus
Labia majora
Labia minora
Vaginal opening
Anus

4-22 The female reproductive system, external structures.
(From Gerdin J: Health Careers Today, *ed. 2, St. Louis, 1997, Mosby.)*

External

Penis is the male sex organ that ejects **semen.** Urine is also eliminated through the penis.

Scrotum is a sac suspended behind and on either side of the penis that contains the testes.

Points to Remember

- The male reproductive system and the urinary system are closely linked to each other.
- Sperm cannot be produced in the heat of the body; they require a cooler place—the scrotum.

Do You Know?

- Male genes determine the sex of the baby.
- Men manufacture sperm well into older adulthood.

Female Reproductive System

Purpose: Continues the human race by producing female sex hormones and ovum, the female reproductive cell. When the ovum is united with the sperm, human reproduction takes place (Figs. 4-21 and 4-22).

Important Parts

Internal

Ovaries (2) produce female sex hormones and release eggs, or ova, from puberty to menopause.

semen
fluid containing sperm.

menarche
first menstrual period.

menopause
permanent end of menstruation.

embryo
stage of human development during the first two months of pregnancy.

fetus
stage of human development from the third month of pregnancy to birth.

Fallopian tubes (2) transport ova from the ovaries to the uterus. Union of sperm and ovum takes place here.

Uterus provides nourishment and protection for growth of fetus during pregnancy. If pregnancy does not occur, the lining is shed during menstruation.

Vagina is the birth canal and organ of sexual intercourse. Products of menstruation are removed through this canal.

External

Genitalia contains the labia (large and small lips) that protect the inner organs of the system.

Perineum is the area between the vagina and anus that provides support for the organs in the pelvis. It stretches during childbirth.

Breasts (2) produce milk following childbirth to nourish infant.

The Process of Menstruation

The beginning of the menstrual cycle, or **menarche,** is the most obvious sign of physical maturity in the female. With the onset of puberty, around age 12, the body begins to produce and release hormones that allow pregnancy to occur. Each month, hormones prepare the uterus for pregnancy by developing a thick lining of blood tissue. If pregnancy does not occur, the lining breaks up and is shed through the vagina. This process, known as menstruation, occurs about every 28 days for 30 to 40 years. Around age 45 to 52, the production of hormones that cause menstruation will slowly decrease and eventually stop. This is called **menopause.**

Pregnancy

Each month, an ovary releases a mature egg (ovum) into one of the fallopian tubes. If this ovum is fertilized by a sperm, pregnancy occurs (conception). The fertilized ovum, now called an **embryo,** begins to grow as it travels through the fallopian tube on its way to the uterus. As mentioned earlier, hormones have prepared the uterus for pregnancy by lining it with a thick layer of tissue. Once the embryo reaches the uterus, it attaches itself to the lining to grow and be nourished. The body continues to produce hormones throughout the pregnancy that make sure that the growing embryo (later called a **fetus**) receives proper nourishment and has a safe place to grow. Hormones also play a role in starting labor, during childbirth, and in the adjustment to the non-pregnant state.

Points to Remember

A delicate balance of hormones controls
- menstruation
- conception
- growth of the fetus
- childbirth
- the period following childbirth
- menopause

Do You Know?

- A baby girl is born with 60,000 to 80,000 ova in her ovaries.
- The uterus, a very muscular organ, can expand from the size of a small pear to a size that holds a 7 (or more) pound baby.

CHAPTER SUMMARY

- The body is organized from the smallest structure, the cell, to groups of organs called systems.
- All body systems are connected and depend on each other to function properly.
- Internal organs are contained within five body cavities.
- Each body system has unique functions.
- The body systems and their functions are:
  1. *Integumentary system*—protects the body from injury.
  2. *Skeletomuscular system*—provides support, protection, and movement.
  3. *Nervous system and senses*—send and receive electrical messages and coordinate all body functions.
  4. *Endocrine system*—produces hormones that regulate body functions.
  5. *Circulatory and lymphatic system*—transports blood and tissue fluid throughout the body. Fights infection.
  6. *Respiratory system*—takes in oxygen and removes carbon dioxide from the body.
  7. *Digestive system*—responsible for nutrition and elimination of body waste.
  8. *Urinary system*—filters all the blood to remove dissolved waste and excess water.
  9. *Reproductive system*—responsible for production of offspring.

STUDY QUESTIONS

1. Define and give one example of each of the following:
   a. Tissue
   b. Gland
   c. Membrane
   d. Organ
   e. System
   f. Cavity
2. List the body systems, their function(s), and four important parts of each system.
3. Explain the following and tell what systems are involved:
   a. Production of urine
   b. Movement
   c. Absorption of nutrients
   d. Breathing

Working With the Ill and Disabled

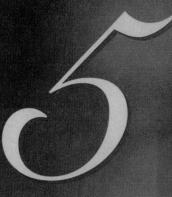

Objectives

After you read this chapter, you will be able to:

1. Define the terms health, acute illness, chronic illness, and disability.

2. Identify three effects of illness on the family.

3. Identify five effects of illness on the client.

4. Recognize your feelings about illness and disability.

5. Discuss ways the home care aide can help client and family cope with the effects of illness.

6. Explain the importance of formal and informal support systems to the client and family.

You may have heard a conversation like the one below.

Alice: "Ever since Helen first became sick a few months ago, she's been so worried about what will happen to her. She wonders how long the illness will last and how she will be able to care for herself."

Sarah: "Yes, and her daughter and son-in-law are concerned about the change in Helen. She used to be so outgoing and pleasant. Since her illness, she's become very irritable and doesn't even want to see her friends or relatives. That's really difficult for the family to understand."

This conversation is just one example of many ways people and their families react to illness. As a home care aide, you will work with a variety of clients with a range of illnesses and disabilities. Some may be short term; others may be life threatening or permanent. Some, such as a mother and her newborn child, will be healthy but need the special care a home care aide provides (Fig. 5-1). Each client and family member will react differently to illness. It is important for you to understand your client's reaction to illness because it will help you give the quality care your client needs. It will also help you to deal with the concerns the family may have over the illness.

Health and Illness

To understand what illness and disability mean, it is important to define the opposite—health.

Health means a state of physical, mental, and social well-being. It is not just the absence of disease. For example: Many people with arthritis take medicine each day and follow a special program of rest and activity. We say they are healthy because they are able to go about the routine of daily life without any problems.

Illness means the state of being sick or a change from the state of being healthy. We use the terms *disease* and *illness* to mean the same. There are two main types of illness—acute and chronic—that are based on the length and results of the illness and the type of care needed.

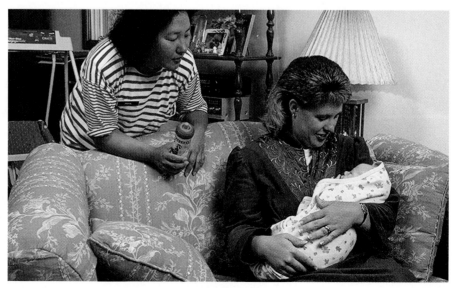

5-1 This home care aide helps mother at feeding time.

health
a state of physical, mental, and social well-being.

illness
the state of being sick.

congenital
present at birth.

genetic
inherited through the genes.

Acute Illness

- Symptoms appear suddenly and may be severe.
- The illness lasts a short time—care given at home or hospital.
- Following illness, full function usually returns.

   Examples: Common cold, sprained ankle, food poisoning.

Chronic Illness

- Symptoms do not subside, may appear gradually or may come and go.
- The illness lasts a long time, maybe a life-time—care given at home, rehabilitation center, or nursing home.
- Permanent changes in the body with decrease in ability to function.

   Examples: Diabetes, tuberculosis, Alzheimer's disease

Disability

A person who cannot perform the normal activities of daily living is said to have a disability (Fig. 5-2). This inability to function may:

- Be temporary or permanent
- Affect the ability to function physically, mentally, or both
- Be caused by illness, injury, or other factors

   Disabilities are classified as:

Physical—resulting from illness or injury to one or more body systems.

   Example: Loss of an arm or leg

Emotional—resulting from mental illness or physical condition (more information about clients with emotional disabilities is found in Chapter 20).

   Example: Depression

Developmental—resulting from illness or injury occurring before birth, during or after birth, or early childhood. Also may be **congenital** or **genetic.** Affects the ability to grow and develop at a normal rate.

   Example: Cerebral palsy

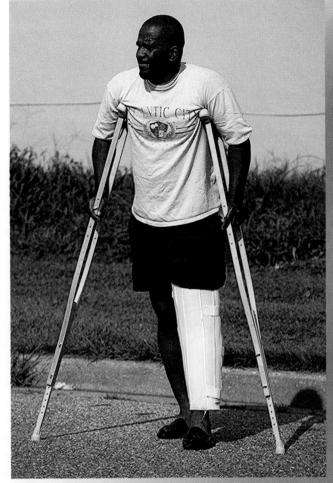

5-2 Disability may be temporary, like this person's, or permanent.

The Effects of Illness on the Family

Whether the illness is acute or chronic, or results in temporary or permanent disability, the client's family will be affected by changes that occur. Some typical effects on the family include changes in routine and income, worry and fear, disruption of plans, and changes in family members' responsibilities. Illness is never convenient. Illness does not go according to a set schedule. But it does cause changes in the lives of members of the family.

5-3 Illness may cause changes in routine.

From this...

Things to do:
1. Go to bank
2. present for Kim
3. Birthday lunch with Kim
4. pick up Joe from soccer practice

To this:

Things to do:
1. Take mom to doctor appointment
2. Rent hospital bed
3. Call home care agency for help!

Changes in Routine

One of the first responses the family may make to illness is to change the routines of everyday life. Meal times may need to be adjusted so that care can be given to the sick family member. Sometimes meals are "on your own," if all members are able to prepare for themselves. Shopping for groceries, cleaning the home, doing laundry—all these routines may be affected by illness in the family. These changes can be especially upsetting to those who have established routines in their lives. Even weekly planned recreational activities may have to be postponed, such as bowling, playing cards at the neighbors, or going to the movies (Fig. 5-3).

If the client is school aged, the routines of school are broken. Playing with friends and learning in class are not possible. If the client is an adult and employed, the routine of going to work and being with others outside the family is changed. The caregiver, who is employed, may have to change the work schedule, take a leave of absence, or even quit his or her job. When routines are disrupted, most family members experience difficulties in adjusting to these changes.

Changes in Income

When illness occurs, there is usually a loss of income and an increase in extra expenses. If the client has been the only one employed in the family, loss of income may be a serious problem. In some cases, the savings of a lifetime can be spent in a short period of time.

Worry and Fear

When one person in the family is ill, other family members are often quite worried. Sometimes their worries and fears make it difficult to concentrate on their jobs or their school work. They may also find it hard to talk about their worries, fears, and feelings. Some typical concerns include:

The unknown: How long will the illness last?
What about the future?
Will there be enough money?
Will I be able to care for this family member?

Loss:	Will there be permanent loss of function?
	Loss of income?
	Loss of companionship?
	Loss due to death?
Pain and suffering:	Seeing loved one in pain
	Feelings of helplessness
Resentment:	Too much extra work
	Additional burdens and not enough help
	Other family members not helping
	"Why me?"
Stress:	Changes in family routines
	Additional responsibilities
	Learning to care for the family member
	Not enough time in the day
	Conflicts with other family members

Disruption of Plans

Illness can also change priorities and future plans. Perhaps the family had planned a vacation away from home or an anniversary party where friends and relatives from out of town were expected. These plans may now have to be postponed or even cancelled. The effects of illness are felt by all those involved with the client and family.

Role Changes

The word *role* means the duties and responsibilities assumed by a person. When the role of the client, prior to the illness, was that of "breadwinner," another family member may need to find employment to pay the bills. If the mother or father is ill, perhaps the oldest child will become the substitute parent. Or, grandparents may take on the additional responsibilities. Mother, father, spouse, partner, significant other, child, grandparent, or friend may assume substitute roles for the ill and disabled client.

Changes in roles can result in periods of adjustment for all family members, and relationships can become strained. Each family will cope with illness and disability in its own special way. In some instances, the family bonds become stronger as each member assumes a special role and adjusts to changes in the home. In other situations, adjustments are made with difficulty or not made at all. The bonds become weak and even break under the weight of family illness and disability.

Adapting to the Need for a Home Care Aide

In most instances, the family will welcome you into the home to care for the client. The family recognizes the special skills you have and will cooperate with you in every way. Sometimes, however, a family member might react to your visits differently. The person may not trust your ability to perform the care needed. For example, a family member says: "No one can give a bed bath as well as I do." Your confident manner in performing the tasks correctly goes a long way in helping to build a sense of trust. Actions do speak louder than words.

As you progress in your career, your supervisor will help you to respond appropriately to situations where family members are having some difficulty accepting your role as caregiver. Family stress, anxiety, and worry can interfere with a good working relationship among client, family, and home care aide.

Reactions of the Client to Illness

Because each person is an individual, his/her emotions and reactions to illness will vary (Fig. 5-4). The way each responds depends on many things, including:

- age
- personality and attitude
- prior physical condition
- nature and length of condition/illness
- family support
- culture

You can play an important role in helping your client to deal with those feelings. Here are some of the common reactions to illness and/or disability:

Denial

Denial is a refusal to admit the truth. Sometimes clients use denial as a means of maintaining their emotional health because they cannot cope with what is happening to them. This helps reduce the discomfort that is felt by disturbing facts. For example, it is common for people to deny the fact that chest pain might come from a heart attack. "It's just indigestion. I'll just take some medicine and it will go away." These statements are typical of denial. The individual does not want to face the fact that he or she may have a life-threatening illness. "No, not me. The doctor must have made a mistake. It can't possibly be me." Sometimes this denial may cause a person to delay seeking needed medical treatment.

Your Role Be caring and supportive. Do not force clients to "realize" they are truly sick. Allow them to come to terms with their illness in their own way. Have a positive attitude and follow the client's plan of care to the best of your ability. If you feel that your client's denial interferes with the treatment plan, or is causing other problems, discuss this with your supervisor.

Depression

Illness can cause a person to feel **depressed,** sad, uninterested in his/her surroundings and life. One can be so tired of being sick that there is no energy left for anything else. This feeling is understandable when the client is overwhelmed by all the problems associated with illness. This type of depression is temporary and should subside as recovery progresses. However, there is always the risk that the depression may increase and the client may require psychiatric care. You must be alert for any indication that your client may be considering suicide. (See Chapter 20.)

- **Denial**
- **Withdrawal**
- **Anger**
- **Self-image**
- **Fear of over-dependence**
- **Dependence**
- **Spiritual distress**
- **Role changes**

5-4 Client reactions to illness.

---

denial
a refusal to admit the truth.

depression, depressed
a feeling of intense sadness.

Your Role Have a positive attitude when caring for the client who feels depressed. Allow the person to express his/her feelings of sadness and loss because of the illness. Remind the client of any improvements that you have observed: for example, increasing strength, appetite, or activity. Smile and be pleasant; do not become depressed yourself. On the other hand, do not minimize what the client is feeling.

Anger

Anger is a common feeling associated with illness. Clients are angry because they are sick, and they may take that feeling out on their friends and families and sometimes the home care aide.

Anger can be demonstrated as impatience. The client is irritated with the caregiver or the doctor and is impatient about all the things that he/she has to "put up with."

Clients also express frustration because they are angry about their limitations, the slowness of their progress, and their inability to control the situation.

Your Role Be calm and patient. Try not to become angry yourself. Remember, anger is a barrier to communication. You know you are doing your very best—even if nothing seems to please the client. Keep in mind that the client is angry about being sick or disabled—not with you. Discuss the situation with your supervisor to gain a better understanding of your client's individual needs and problems.

Dependence/overdependence

Sometime during an illness, most persons will be dependent on others. When you have a cold, it's nice to have someone take care of you, tuck you into bed, and fluff your pillows. However, this brief period of dependency is enjoyable only because you know you will be better and back to normal in a few days. Some chronic illnesses cause the person to become progressively weaker and increasingly dependent upon other persons for care. Clients who value their independence will become very angry and frustrated when they are dependent.

Your Role You can help clients to maintain their independence by offering choices and opportunities to try to do things on their own. Perhaps the only thing they can do is wash their face—and only if you prepare the wash cloth. Still, it is important for the client to do so, no matter how long it takes. Be careful not to become frustrated and impatient when clients' self-care takes "too long." It is very difficult to watch a client struggle in an attempt to perform self-care when you know that you could do it better and faster. Remember that you are promoting independence—a goal of care for all clients.

Some sick persons become overly dependent, helpless, and demanding. Even if they are able to become independent, they do not choose to do so. They find excuses to avoid participation in their care. It seems to you that they enjoy their dependence and all the attention that goes with it. Be careful that you do not grow to resent this individual. Do not become angry and nasty. Do not judge your client's behavior as good or bad. Follow the care plan and discuss your observations with your supervisor.

Encourage clients to be as independent as possible for as long as possible. Praise them for trying and cheer their progress.

Anxiety

Although illness itself does not cause **anxiety,** fears and worries often accompany illness. In addition to worries about money and family relationships, there are often unspoken worries. For example:

- What if there is something else wrong?
- What kind of treatment is needed?
- Will my appearance change?
- Am I going to die?

Anxiety can be so severe that it can interfere with treatment. As with denial, anxiety and fear over "what the disease could be" may cause a person to delay seeking care. Or treatment may be refused altogether. Sometimes people become so anxious about their conditions that they build a wall of silence rather than discuss their worst fears.

Your Role The home care aide can help the anxious client by carefully explaining as much as possible. For example, if the client is afraid of falling, explain in detail how you will assist him/her to get out of bed and into a chair. There should be no surprises. Be calm and confident. Carry out personal care properly.

Also, prepare the client for any problems that may develop. For example, explain that many times clients feel faint and dizzy when they get out of bed. Explain what you will do to prevent this from happening and also what you will do if the client experiences those symptoms. Knowing what to expect helps to put the client at ease.

Withdrawal

When an illness is prolonged, painful, or disfiguring, the client may avoid contact with others. Family members and visitors are turned away because the client is too sick to tolerate other persons. Other causes of withdrawal may be the side effects of treatment, depression, or anxiety. Sometimes withdrawal is forced upon clients when they are ignored or abandoned by family and friends.

Your Role Your approach to the client will vary depending on the underlying cause of the withdrawal. Discuss the client's behavior with your supervisor. Schedule periods for rest and quiet. Perform your duties calmly and efficiently. Assist the client to readjust to socialization when possible. Phone calls, letters, and cards from family and friends can prevent some of the loneliness that accompanies withdrawal. "Be there" for your client. Be attentive to spoken and unspoken needs. Observe carefully for any changes in condition and report these to your supervisor. Make certain that basic physical needs for food, fluids, exercise, rest, and elimination are being met. If depression and withdrawal are both present, be alert for risk of suicide. (See Chapter 20.)

anxiety
a state of intense worry and/or fear.

grief
physical and emotional responses associated with extreme sorrow or loss.

mourn
the process of grieving caused by great personal loss.

assistive devices
equipment used by disabled persons to help them perform activities of daily living.

Role Change

No matter what the roles of the client before the illness, there is now a change. Clients may become angry and frustrated when they cannot perform their usual roles. Family members are busy trying to keep the household running, taking the client for treatment, or dealing with medical personnel and bills. They don't always have the time or energy for the client.

Your Role The home care aide can encourage the client to participate in family discussions and activities. Arrange a schedule of care and rest periods that includes a special time for family activities. Clients need to be part of everyday family activities and decisions as much as possible.

Self-image

The way we see ourselves, our self-image, plays a very important role in how we react to the world around us. We all have an image in our mind of the perfect self, and we want the world to see us that way. When injury or illness causes a change in body image, the client may feel unattractive and worthless—even repulsive. Changes to body image can come in many forms: for example,

- loss of a limb by accident or through surgery
- loss of hair from cancer treatment
- scars from burns, cuts, or surgery
- speech problems caused by stroke

Not only do clients see themselves negatively, but they also believe that other persons do, too. Unfortunately, in some cases the client is correct.

Your Role Continue to meet the client's basic human needs—physical, psychological, and for self-esteem. Accept the client exactly as he/she is, and, if you cannot do this, perhaps another aide would be able to do so. Discuss this with your supervisor.

Be especially aware of your nonverbal communications, such as facial expressions. Any sign of disgust or revulsion on the part of the aide will cause the client to sense your rejection and feel unaccepted by you. Be matter of fact about carrying out procedures that are distasteful to you. Allow the client to use denial by refusing to participate in care. Some clients will refuse to look at their surgical incision. Most will do so, eventually—when they are ready. When denial interferes with care and progress toward the goals in the care plan, it must be reported to your supervisor.

Help clients to express their feelings about the body changes. Many clients will experience **grief** and will **mourn** what they have lost. Be a good listener. Grief causes many feelings, and it helps to talk with an understanding person.

Encourage clients to perform as much self-care as possible. This will promote independence and offer them some control. If **assistive devices** are needed, encourage their use. Help clients to dress in clothes that will minimize body changes and maximize appearance. Hair loss is easily covered by a wig or turban. Both men and women feel better when their hair and face are groomed. Assist clients to use **prostheses,** such as artificial limbs or mastectomy replacements.

Treat clients normally and encourage the family to do the same. Offer praise for their efforts in self-care and rehabilitation. Your respect and courtesy will help the client to feel worthwhile.

There are many support groups (discussed later in this chapter and throughout the text) for persons coping with changes in body image. Many people have been helped by these groups. Your supervisor can give the client and family information about specific support groups in your community.

Spiritual Distress

Within the life of every person there is a belief system that relates to birth; life; suffering; pain; one's place in the world, universe, and eternity; and death. For many people, this includes an awareness and acceptance of a creator, supreme being, supernatural force(s), or spirit(s). When illness occurs, these beliefs may be challenged and questioned. This can cause great distress and discomfort. Clients may be angry with God (or whatever name they use) and avoid their religious practices. Others may seek religious consolation through prayer and meditation. Families and clients question the meaning of suffering, life, death, and what is to come. The choice of treatment or non-treatment may cause ethical and moral questions.

Your Role How can the home care aide help? First, realize that belief systems are very personal. What has worked for you in a crisis situation might not be helpful for your client. Respect each person's right to his/her own beliefs—no matter how foreign they may seem to you. A spiritual advisor may be able to assist your client. A family member should be the one to call the appropriate advisor. If they do not know of any resource, your agency will be able to help them. Sometimes a spiritual advisor's visit is considered a sure sign of impending death. Spiritual consolation is for the living, and many view it as an important component of healing. Provide time and privacy for prayer, meditation, spiritual reading, and visits from spiritual advisors. Try to schedule personal care and activities of daily living so that clients will have the physical energy to meet their spiritual needs.

Physical Distress

Each illness or injury has its own signs, symptoms, and effects on the physical condition of the client. The amount of physical distress a client experiences depends on the type and severity of the illness or injury. The person's prior physical condition will also play a part in how much distress a person feels and how quickly they recover. For example, a young man in excellent shape may suffer less physical distress from a broken hip than an older man who already had severe arthritis.

Your Role Carefully observe your client's physical condition and symptoms. Any changes should be reported. Each individual's care plan will tell you what to watch for. Be sure to record on the client's chart what you have discussed with your supervisor. If you have any questions

prostheses
devices used by disabled persons to replace a missing body part.

about what you are to look for or are unsure of your responsibilities, ask your supervisor, so there will be no confusion.

Support Systems

Support systems are those organizations that provide assistance in times of crisis and stress and help the client and/or family to make it through the tough times. These may be informal or formal.

Informal Support Systems

Family members, neighbors, church groups, support groups, and senior citizens' clubs are examples of informal support systems. They respond when the need arises, and there is no charge for the service. For example, when Mrs. Jackson's sister became sick, the Sunday School class from her church sent meals to the home. This was a big help to Mrs. Jackson. It gave her more time to spend with her sister. Then there is Mr. Kane who has a serious heart and lung disease. He uses oxygen and only leaves his apartment to go to the doctor. His many friends do his marketing, laundry, and housecleaning. Because of his informal support system, Mr. Kane is able to be independent and remain in his own home.

Support Groups In a support group, people in similar situations come together to discuss their problems with each other. Group meetings are conducted by a leader, usually a health professional or other qualified individual. There are groups for clients and/or caregivers. Sharing similar concerns helps the client to cope with the day-to-day problems of living with illness. The client must travel to the support group meeting. Caregivers can talk with each other and a leader about the concerns of caring for a loved one on a day-to-day basis. Their frustrations, fears, and anxieties are discussed. Examples of support groups are: Alcoholics Anonymous, Children of Aging Parents, stroke clubs.

Formal Support Systems

Formal support systems are organized, structured, and charge a fee for service (Fig. 5-5). Your agency is an example of a formal support system. Other examples are: Meals On Wheels, cleaning services, shopping services, etc.

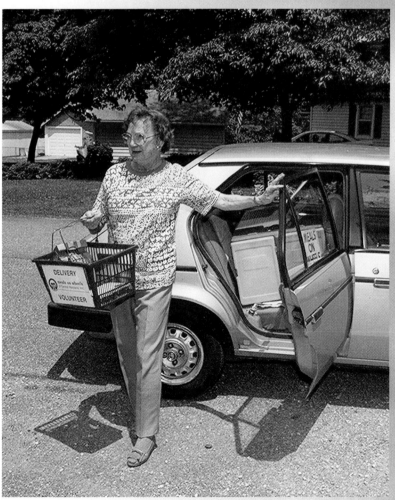

5-5 Formal support systems help a family to cope with unexpected illness or injury.

CHAPTER SUMMARY

- Health is a state of physical, mental, and social well-being, not just the absence of disease.

- Illness is described as acute or chronic.

- Disability is a lack of function and can be classified as physical, emotional, or developmental.

- Changes in roles, routines, loss of income, and disruption of plans can occur as a result of illness in the family.

- Clients experience many effects of illness, including denial, depression, anger, dependence, anxiety, withdrawal, role change, change in self-image, and spiritual and physical distress.

- You have an important role in assisting the client and family to cope with the effects of illness and disability.

- Informal and formal support systems can help the client and family to cope with the effects of illness and disability.

STUDY QUESTIONS

1. Define the terms *health, acute illness, chronic illness,* and *disability.*

2. Identify three effects of illness on the family.

3. List five reactions a client may have to illness. Discuss your role in each.

4. Identify two formal support systems available to clients in your community. Describe the services and costs.

5. Identify two informal support groups in your community. What do they offer, and how frequently do they meet?

Maintaining a Safe Environment

Objectives

After you read this chapter, you will be able to:

1. Identify 10 common hazards in the home.

2. Discuss 10 safety measures to prevent accidents in the home.

3. Identify clients at risk for accidents and injury in the home.

4. List steps to be taken in case of fire.

5. Identify personal safety precautions for the home care aide.

6. Describe procedures to be followed in a household or weather-related emergency.

Local newspaper stories tell of accidents in the home that could have been prevented. You probably have seen headlines similar to the following:

- EIGHT ROW HOMES DESTROYED BY FIRE—CARELESS SMOKING CAUSES 50 TO BE HOMELESS
- WOMAN ELECTROCUTED WHILE USING CURLING IRON IN BATHROOM
- 2-YEAR-OLD SCALDED WHILE PLAYING WITH HOT WATER FAUCETS

Most of us think that such accidents could never happen to our families. But they can happen! An accident is an unplanned and unforeseen event or circumstance. For example, a child runs and falls. Some accidents are caused by an act of nature, such as damage done by a hurricane, tornado, or earthquake. Unfortunately, many accidents are caused by carelessness, including:

- doing something we should not do—such as using a chair as a stepladder
- not doing something we should do—such as not wearing a seat belt in the car

In many cases, it is impossible to know that an accident is about to occur. Sometimes it just seems to be fate—being at the wrong place at the wrong time. However, many accidents that occur in the home can be prevented. Preventing accidents requires the development of a **habit** of safety consciousness on the job and in one's personal life. Throughout the book, principles of safety are given for each activity you perform as a home care aide. Maintaining a safe environment is very important for your client, the family, and yourself!

Becoming Safety Conscious

With this chapter, your journey begins in reinforcing and fine tuning your safety conscious behavior. But being "safety aware" never ends. It must be a lifetime habit. It means that you:

A—are **A**WARE of potentially unsafe conditions and always practice your skills safely

C—**C**ORRECT the condition or notify the appropriate person

T—**T**AKE precautions to avoid future problems

To be AWARE of potentially unsafe conditions means that we know what safety hazards are commonly found in the home. The following are typical hazards found in the home environment:

- Inadequate or dim lighting, especially near steps and stairs
- Clutter on the floor, steps, or stairs—toys, newspapers, etc.
- Frayed rugs or throw rugs that are not tacked down
- Defective electrical appliances, frayed electrical cords (Box 6-1)
- Several appliances plugged into one electrical outlet (Fig. 6-1)
- Electrical and telephone cords in the path of traffic areas
- Wobbly stairs, handrails, and furniture
- Highly waxed floors
- Portable home heaters close to curtains, drapes, newspapers, bedding, or clothing (Box 6-2)

habit
a repeated pattern of involuntary behavior or thought.

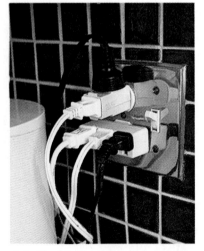

6-1 Electrical outlets should not be overloaded like this.

Box 6-1

Equipment Safety

- Check all equipment before use by yourself or client:
    - *surfaces*—free of cracks, rough or sharp edges, chips
    - *electrical cords*—intact, not frayed
    - *electrical plugs*—intact, not damaged
    - *bolts, screws*—tightened properly, not loose
- Use appliances and equipment that are in proper working condition.
- Do not use damaged or defective equipment; if you get a shock while using an appliance or equipment, notify your supervisor.
- Do not allow your client to use damaged or defective equipment.
- When in doubt about operating equipment or proper procedure for use, notify your supervisor for advice or direction.
- If unusual noise or odor is present when operating appliance or equipment, turn off immediately; notify your supervisor for further directions.
- Do not attempt to repair frayed electrical cords, appliances, or equipment.
- Do not cut off "extra" prong of the three-pronged electrical plug so that it fits into a two-pronged receptacle.

Box 6-2

Portable Home Heater Use

- Locate heater away from curtains, drapes.
- Never use heater as a drying rack or toaster or to heat food.
- Move heater only when it is not being used.
- Never place heater in doorway to obstruct passageway.
- Keep heater away from water.
- If an extension cord is needed, use only a heavy duty type.
- Freestanding electric heaters should have tip-over switches that shut off the current if the unit is knocked over.
- Use kerosene heaters only when approved by local community.
- Don't touch kerosene heater when it is operating.
- Use a protective screen in front of portable heater if children or pets are near.
- Never use gasoline or any substitute fuel for a kerosene heater.
- Store kerosene outdoors in approved container properly labeled.
- Install smoke detector in room where heater is used.
- Turn off heater when room is unoccupied or when going to sleep.

- Chairs or tables used as ladders
- Medicines, household cleaning fluids, and other chemicals within easy reach and in unmarked containers
- Incorrect tools used for household jobs
- Oily rags, old newspapers, rubbish left in piles
- Sharp objects (knives, scissors) left unprotected, within easy reach
- Spilled liquids not removed immediately

- Lit cigarette, cigar, pipe, or candles left unattended
- Electrical appliances operated near water
- Electrical wiring under rugs
- Firearms unprotected and within easy reach
- Household pets underfoot

General Rules of Safety in the Home

The following are 10 basic rules for maintaining a safe home environment:

1. Provide adequate lighting especially at steps, stairs, and uneven walking surfaces.
2. Maintain a clutter-free home (stairways, heavy traffic areas).
3. Remove frayed rugs and scatter rugs, if possible.
4. Have major gas, oil, coal, and electrical appliances (furnace, hot water heater, air conditioner) checked by a qualified person to assure proper working order.
5. Clean up spills immediately, especially liquids and grease.
6. Store gasoline and kerosene in approved containers.
7. Keep windows in working order and screens in place.
8. Maintain clean but not highly polished floors, steps, and stairs.
9. Install smoke detectors on the ceiling of each level of the home. Test every month. Replace batteries (long-life alkaline, only) every six months.
10. Set hot water heater at 120°F or lower to reduce burns due to scalding.

In addition to these 10 basic safety rules, each area in the home has its own special requirements to make it a safe place.

Client's Bedroom

The bedroom is a place where falls often occur. Your role as a home care aide is to care for your client in an environment that is as safe as possible. The following are some helpful hints to make the bedroom as "fall proof" and safe as possible:

- Remove clutter from floor and bedside.
- Arrange furniture to allow for free movement around the room.
- Provide a source of light (lamp) at or near the bedside.
- Provide a night light.
- Keep side rails on bed, if necessary.
- Position hospital bed (if used) at the lowest possible height when care is not being given.
- Remove obstacles in traffic pattern of room.

If your client is a smoker, an extra smoke detector should be installed in the bedroom and any other area in which he/she spends time. When smoking, the client should always be supervised because careless smoking is the first leading cause of fire deaths in the United States.

flammable
burns easily.

combustible
capable of catching fire and burning.

Bathroom

This area of the home can be the site of serious accidents because of the presence of electrical outlets, water, and slippery surfaces. Does the bathroom have

- hot and cold water faucets correctly marked?
- grab bars for the toilet, bathtub, and shower?
- night light in place and operating?
- non-skid mat in shower and tub?
- non-skid mat on floor, if necessary?
- soap in dish and not in tub?
- electrical appliances (fan, shaver, hair dryer, curling iron) used away from water?
- toilet secure to the floor?
- toilet seat securely attached to the toilet?

Kitchen

Many preventable accidents happen in the kitchen, especially burns and cuts. Make sure that:

- major kitchen appliances (stove, refrigerator, microwave oven) are in working order.
- fire extinguisher is in working order and located near the stove.
- small electrical appliances (toaster, coffee maker, etc.) are unplugged when not in use.
- detergents, cleaning liquids, bleach, etc., are stored separately (away from food) in clearly marked containers and out of reach of children and confused clients.
- items most frequently used are stored within easy reach.
- pan handles are turned inward and out of child's reach when cooking.
- pot holders are used, not towels or corner of apron.
- loose, long sleeves are rolled back or fastened with pins or elastic bands when cooking.
- knives and other objects are sharpened and stored properly.
- stove or microwave oven is never left unattended while cooking.
- **flammable** or **combustible** items (aerosol cans, gasoline, kerosene) are stored away from stove or other sources of heat or sparks
- aerosol sprays are never used near open flames
- microwave oven is not used when person with pacemaker is in the room

Other Areas of the Home

The following are some additional guidelines for maintaining a safe environment in other areas of the home:

Living room   Keep air space between the TV/VCR and wall.

Garage   Store pesticides and fertilizers in well-marked containers out of child's reach.

Recycle old newspapers and magazines frequently.

Basement	Remove oily rags. Provide good light source. Keep steps and handrails in good repair.
Outside	Remove snow and ice from steps and walkways as soon as possible. Use kitty litter or commercially prepared substances to melt ice. Keep steps and handrails in good repair.

Special Safety Considerations

In addition to the common hazards and safety measures previously discussed, there are special considerations for older adults, children, and confused clients. The use of oxygen in the home increases the risk of fire. Smoking is an additional hazard.

Older Adults

The normal changes that are part of the aging process (Chapter 18) make older adults candidates for accidents. Because their bones are brittle, a minor fall may cause a serious **fracture.** Slowed reaction time also puts them at risk for injury.

Falls are quite common and occur most frequently in the home. Many falls happen when the older adult trips over something. Little things—like unmended shoes, untied laces, floppy slippers, and loose drooping clothing—can cause a person to trip. Anything left on the floor—magazines, toys, electric cords, shoes, and clothing—can lead to a fall. The home care aide helps to prevent injury by being alert to potential hazards. This includes removing clutter and alerting clients and families to potentially hazardous conditions.

Children

As children grow and develop, they begin to explore the world and to try out and learn new things. Children do not have a sense of caution or awareness of danger. They take many risks during their growing years. Accidents are the leading cause of death for children and adolescents. Hints for child safety are listed in Box 6-3.

Confused Clients

Confused clients may not know their names, addresses, or phone numbers. There is a great risk that they will leave the home and wander in the neighborhood, at any time of day or night and in any type of clothing. Some protective measures are:

- Have recent, clear photos of person available.
- Have person wear an ID bracelet.
- Know where client is at all times.
- Closely supervise the client in potentially dangerous situations—smoking, shaving, cooking, bathing.
- Attach bells to ring when outside doors are opened.
- Lock doors to basements, attics, and all stairways.
- Label doors to other rooms using word and picture signs.
- Put sharp objects, weapons, chemicals, and other harmful materials in a safe place.

fracture
broken bone.

toxic
poisonous.

Box 6-3

Hints For Child Safety

- Use care to prevent burns, drownings, bumps, cuts, and falls.
- Keep dangerous items out of child's reach; use products in child resistant containers.
- Lock dangerous items in a secure place, out of child's sight and reach.
- Do not store dangerous items in cabinet under the sink.
- Keep all thin plastic wrapping material (dry cleaner, produce, grocery, or trash bags) away from children.
- Never use thin plastic material to cover mattresses or pillows; the film can cling to a child's face and cause suffocation.

- Protect against electrical shocks; cover unused outlets with safety covers.
- Disconnect all electrical appliances when not in use.
- Keep children away from open windows to prevent falls; screens will not keep a child from falling out; they are designed to keep insects out, not to keep children inside.
- Do not place furniture near windows; children may climb up to a window sill or seat.

Oxygen

Oxygen is necessary for life. We need oxygen to burn our food and convert it into energy. There must be oxygen to build a fire, and fuel burns faster in the presence of higher concentrations of oxygen. Therefore, the use of oxygen (O_2) in the home poses great risk for fire. Follow the procedures for oxygen therapy (Chapter 17) and all the safety guidelines discussed. Remember, there should NEVER be an open flame or spark-producing object near oxygen. No matches, lighters, cigarettes, pipes, electric razors, or pilot lights should be anywhere near the oxygen delivery system (Fig. 6-2). Post "No Smoking" signs on the outsides of all doors into the home. Inside the home, place signs near the source of oxygen. Know how to turn off the oxygen and what to do in the event of fire.

Smoking

Careless smoking is a major cause of home fires. An individual who falls asleep while smoking may not awaken to a smoke filled room—or be unable to leave the room without help. More people die from smoke inhalation than from burns. Flames caused by burning household furnishings are **toxic** and interfere with respiration. Smoke detectors are a necessity in every home—and especially where there is a smoker.

Smoking is risky behavior for the smoker and other family members, too. Some special safety rules include:

- Do not smoke in bed.
- Use ample ash trays to prevent butts and ashes from falling on floor.

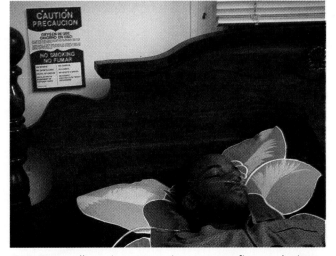

6-2 Never allow cigarettes, pipes, or any fire producing items in the same room with an oxygen delivery system!

- Do not dispose of butts and ashes in garbage; place in a large covered metal container and put outside for the embers to cool.
- Keep matches, lighters, and cigarettes out of reach of children and confused persons.
- Make sure all smoke detectors are working; test on a regular basis (every six months); replace batteries when needed.

Household Emergency Measures and Procedures

Experts agree that people who prepare for **emergencies** cope better during the **crisis** and recover more quickly. The best way to reduce risk is to think ahead. The home care aide can assist the client and family to prepare for possible emergencies.

Fire

Some causes of fire include

- smoking and matches
- misuse of electricity
- defects in heating system
- materials that ignite easily
- improper trash disposal
- improper cooking techniques
- improper ventilation
- improper use of aerosol cans (hair spray, cleaning fluids, paints, etc.)

It takes three things to start a fire (Fig. 6-3):

1. **Fuel**—any material that will burn.
2. **Source of heat**—matches, flame, spark.
3. **Supply of oxygen**—present in the air.

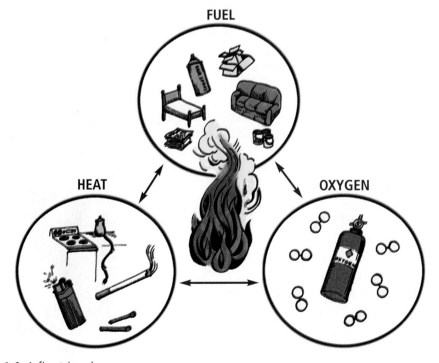

6-3 A fire triangle.

emergency (emergencies)
a serious situation that comes on suddenly and threatens life or well-being.

crisis
a critical time.

Fire can be prevented by removing any one of these three ingredients. Very tiny fires become big ones almost immediately.

Stove fires become kitchen fires, and kitchen fires become whole house fires (Box 6-4). An open, moving fire triples in size in one minute. Prevention is the key to fire safety. Most house fires occur between 8 p.m. and 8 a.m. Therefore, a working smoke detector <u>must</u> be on the ceiling of every level of the home.

The first time you enter a client's home, look for an alternate exit. Identify two escape routes from each room, just in case a fire starts. In a high rise or apartment complex, find the fire alarm box so you will be aware of its location if needed.

The number one rule in any fire is GET OUT AND GET YOUR CLIENT OUT WITHOUT ANY DELAY. Call the fire department from a nearby phone (Box 6-5). If you are in an apartment building, leave the unit and scream "FIRE" in the hallways. If there is a fire alarm system, use it. Never go back into the home for any reason. Follow the do's and don'ts listed below:

Fire Escape Do's and Don'ts

DO

- Get out with your client as fast as you can.
- Notify the fire department immediately.
- Feel door to see if it is hot. If cool, open carefully; slam door if heat and smoke rush in.
- Use alternate exit route when necessary.
- Keep doors closed to prevent smoke from entering the room.

DON'T

- Use elevators—smoke rises; elevator shafts act as chimneys.
- Waste time trying to put out a fire.
- Run if your clothing is on fire; stop, drop down, and roll to smother the flames.
- Go back into a burning structure.

Smoke is dangerous. If you encounter smoke, use an alternate escape route. If you must exit through smoke, drop and crawl on your hands and knees to the nearest exit. Take your client with you in the same way, if possible. Cover nose and mouth with a damp cloth to ease breathing, but don't waste a lot of time with this detail. Remember the number one DO rule and GET OUT.

If you are unable to get out of the building, try to call the fire department and tell them where you are—building, floor, and apartment number. If the fire is outside of the apartment, close the door of the unit and block the bottom of the door with wet towels or blankets to keep the smoke out. Move your client away from the fire to a room with a

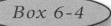

Box 6-4

Extinguishing a Small Enclosed Fire

Grease or food fire
cover pan with a lid; turn off burner

Microwave oven fire
keep door closed; push STOP switch

Oven fire
close oven door; turn off stove

Box 6-5

Reporting a Fire

REMAIN CALM
Call the fire department
(or dial 9-1-1 if in local service area)
Give the dispatcher:

1. Your name.
2. Your location (including building number, floor and apartment number, and nearest cross street).
3. Location of the fire.
4. Phone number you are calling from.

window. Close the door to that room, blocking the bottom as before. Cover your nose and mouth with a damp cloth—and your client's, too. Hang a sheet, towel, or tablecloth in the window to alert the fire fighters of your location. Don't panic. Help will come.

One of the biggest problems in fire safety is the attitude that "it can't happen to me." But that's simply not true. Each year millions of home fires in the United States cause thousands of deaths and injuries. Being alert and prepared can save lives and prevent injury.

Gas Leak

Natural gas and propane used for cooking and heating has no odor. The odor is added as a safety measure to detect leaking gas. When you smell gas in the home,

- Ventilate the area—open windows and doors.
- Check to see if the pilot lights in stove, oven, furnace, or hot water heater are on.
- Do not use anything that will produce a spark (turning on electric switches or thermostat, using matches) and cause an explosion.
- Call the gas company.

If the odor is strong,

- Leave the house.
- Call the gas company from a nearby phone.

If the odor is outdoors, call the gas company. Emergency crews are on call at all times of day and night.

Loss of Electricity

A power loss in the home may be caused by an overload to the electrical system. In this case, a fuse may need to be replaced or the circuit breaker switched on. First, turn off all appliances (except the refrigerator), and check the electrical service panel or fuse box (Fig. 6-4). Follow the instructions in Box 6-6 to restore power. This may be the responsibility of the home care aide, if no one else is available.

If the power does not come back on, call the electric company. The failure may involve several homes, the neighborhood, or a wider area. Notify your agency and follow instructions given. The extent and length of the power outage will determine the action to be taken.

Plumbing Problems

Plumbing problems are a possibility in any home with running water. A little advance knowledge may help you to deal with a gushing pipe when necessary. Knowing where the water valves are located will save time if an emergency occurs. You should know the location of the main valve that controls the flow of water into the home. Also, find the controls to sinks, tubs, and toilets.

If a leak occurs, turn off the flow of water to the fixture. Once the leak has been stopped, the appropriate person (family member, building superintendent, custodian, etc.) must be notified so repairs can be made. Notify your agency regarding the problem.

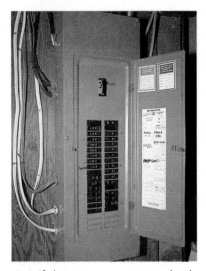

6-4 If the power goes out, check the electrical service panel to see if the circuit breaker needs to be switched on.

Box 6-6

Fuses

Fuses are protective devices that cut off the power if there is an overload or a short in the electrical system.

Replacing a blown fuse is <u>not</u> usually the responsibility of the home care aide, but there may be a time when you will have to do it.

CAUTION: DO NOT TOUCH THE MAIN ELECTRICAL PANEL IN THE HOME WHEN WATER IS PRESENT. CALL YOUR AGENCY FOR INSTRUCTIONS.

Replacing a Fuse

1. Locate main electrical service panel, usually in basement or utility room. Turn off main switch or pull out before you start.

2. Look at fuses in the panel. Check the window of each fuse plug to see if the metal strip is broken or cloudy. A broken strip indicates an overload—too many appliances in use at one time. Disconnect them. A clouded plug indicates a short circuit. The electricity is flowing from its normal path to objects that cannot handle the great amount of heat produced and may melt or catch fire (e.g., frayed electrical cord).

3. With one hand, unscrew blown fuse and replace with a new one with the same rating.

4. Restore the power.

Circuit Breakers

Circuit breakers are heat-sensing switches that shut off the electrical power if the smallest imbalance occurs.

CAUTION: DO NOT TOUCH THE MAIN ELECTRICAL PANEL IN THE HOME WHEN WATER IS PRESENT. CALL YOUR AGENCY FOR INSTRUCTIONS.

Correcting a Tripped Circuit Breaker

1. Turn off all extra appliances and big electricity users.

2. Locate main electrical service panel, usually in basement or utility room. Turn off main switch before you start.

3. Look at breaker switch. They have three positions: "On," "Off," and tripped (middle position).

4. Switch the tripped breaker to the "Off" position and then flip it to "On" again.

5. Restore the power.

Natural and Weather-Related Emergencies

Every area of the country experiences natural and weather-related emergencies. The TV news reports deep snows in the Northeast, hurricanes along the Southeast coast, floods in the Plains states, earthquakes in the West, tornadoes in the southern states. No part of the country is untouched by nature's elements. You and your client can be severely affected by these natural disasters.

Think ahead, prepare for the possibility of disasters, and know what to do if a disaster occurs.

- Prepare a disaster supply kit (Box 6-7) appropriate to your climate, seasons of the year, and past disasters.
- Have drills to prepare for possible emergencies—fire, tornado, earthquake.
- Keep in touch with your agency; they can relay information to your family and the client's family.

Box 6-7

Disaster Supply Kit

Keep the following in closet nearest to door used during evacuation:

- First aid kit
- Essential medications—protect from children
- Canned food and opener
- Bottled water
- Utensils for eating and drinking
- Extra clothing
- Rain wear, boots
- Blankets
- Battery-operated radio (extra batteries)
- Important phone numbers
- Safety matches (water proof container)
- Extra car keys

- Follow directions given by police and rescue workers—have agency notified if you are evacuated.
- Take care of your client's personal needs as best you can.
- Protect yourself and client from injury.
- Keep a two-week supply of prescription medications on hand during a "disaster time"—snow, hurricane, tornado season—and always in an earthquake zone.
- Stay tuned to TV or radio emergency broadcast system for updated news and emergency instructions.
- Water may be purified by boiling for 20 minutes.

Earthquake

- Learn how to turn off main source of water, electricity, and gas.
- Look around each room and decide where you can protect yourself from falling items.
- Position client's bed away from anything that could fall on it during an earthquake (windows, mirrors, shelves, and light fixtures).
- If a quake occurs, get under a heavy table or desk.

Hurricane/Flood

- During wind and driving rain, move away from windows.
- Close blinds, drapes, curtains.
- Stay in an interior protected room.
- Place fresh water in jugs, bottles, or buckets.
- Put possessions on a higher level.
- Prepare to evacuate when water rises rapidly.
- Call for help.
- Do not use telephone during periods of thunder and lightning.
- Have flashlights, matches, or oil lamps ready for use.
- Move cars to higher and drier location if possible.
- Remain in contact with agency, if possible.

Snow/Winter Storm

- Have sufficient amounts of food and medicine on hand.
- Have extra blanket on hand.
- Prepare car for winter travel, if necessary.
- Stay inside, keep warm, keep client warm.
- Be prepared for electrical power failure (discussed earlier).
- Remain in contact with agency.

Tornado

- Decide ahead of time the place where you will go when there is a tornado warning.
- Listen for warnings on TV and radio.
- Stay away from windows.
- Lowest level is safest; stay inside; go to basement or interior windowless room or closet.

In all of the above emergency situations, you will need a list of phone numbers readily available (Box 6-8). Keep the list next to the telephone or on the refrigerator door. If there is no telephone in the home where you are working, locate the closest one available. Keep list of phone numbers with you at all times. Complete the list during your first visit to the client.

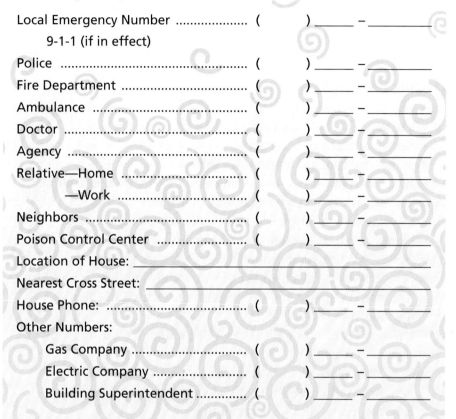

Box 6-8

Emergency Phone Numbers

Local Emergency Number .... (   ) _____ – _____
       9-1-1 (if in effect)

Police .... (   ) _____ – _____

Fire Department .... (   ) _____ – _____

Ambulance .... (   ) _____ – _____

Doctor .... (   ) _____ – _____

Agency .... (   ) _____ – _____

Relative—Home .... (   ) _____ – _____

         —Work .... (   ) _____ – _____

Neighbors .... (   ) _____ – _____

Poison Control Center .... (   ) _____ – _____

Location of House: _____

Nearest Cross Street: _____

House Phone: .... (   ) _____ – _____

Other Numbers:

   Gas Company .... (   ) _____ – _____

   Electric Company .... (   ) _____ – _____

   Building Superintendent .... (   ) _____ – _____

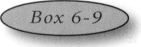

Box 6-9

Personal Safety of the Home Care Aide

Home care aides work everywhere—in the city, suburbs, country, farms, desert. You will probably travel alone to unfamiliar areas, and you must be alert to protect your own safety. Practice fire safety in your own home twice a year. Conduct EDITH (Exit Drill In The Home) with your family (Box 6-9).

List of Safety Do's and Don'ts

In Client's Home

Do

- Follow all rules of home safety.
- Keep doors locked at all times.
- Check carefully before letting a stranger into the home; always ask for identification from anyone who comes to the door.
- Shout "I'll get it," even if you are alone.
- Hang up if you receive threatening phone calls.
- Notify agency and police about threatening calls; they will tell you what to do and what records to keep.
- Call your supervisor when you arrive and leave the client's home according to your agency's policies.

EDITH Practice

Exit drills in the home

1. Everyone in bedrooms; doors closed.

2. One person sounds the alarm.

3. Each person tests the door to see if it is hot.

4. Pretend it is hot; use an alternate exit to escape.

5. Everyone meets at a designated spot. One person goes to a prearranged nearby phone to notify the fire department.

Don't
- Let strangers in to use the phone, but offer to make a call for them if there is an emergency.
- Let strangers into a security entrance of an apartment building.
- Give information over the telephone to wrong numbers.
- Let strangers (wrong number callers) know that you are alone or that your client is sick or disabled.
- Stay, if you feel unsafe in the client's home; get out.

Driving

Do
- Use your seat belt at all times.
- Keep your car in good repair.
- Make sure your spare tire is useable.
- Have enough gas in your car in case of a lengthy traffic jam or a detour; always keep your gas tank half full.
- Have money to buy gas or make a phone call if necessary.
- Plan your route; use well traveled streets; avoid unsafe areas; "safety" of the neighborhood may change according to time of day.
- Let supervisor and a member of your family know your travel route.
- Know where police and fire stations are located in client's neighborhood.
- Drive to nearest police, fire, or well-lighted gas station if you are being followed.
- Keep doors locked and windows closed while driving.
- Park in a well-lighted area and always lock car doors.
- Have key ready to unlock car door.
- Look around inside car and back seat before entering.

Don't
- Keep purse or valuables on front passenger seat.
- Pick up hitchhikers.
- Stop to help another driver; go to nearest phone and call police.
- Get out of your car until you have checked your surroundings and feel that it is safe.
- Ask strangers for directions; go to police, fire, or gas station for assistance.
- Ever let a stranger into your car.

Car Trouble

Do
- Put on emergency flashers.
- Stay in car; keep doors locked and windows rolled up.
- Place "Call Police" sign in window.
- Ask person who stops to notify police.
- Ask person in unmarked police car and in street clothes for proper identification or request a marked police vehicle.

Don't
- Leave car and walk alone on highway or unfamiliar area.
- Go in a stranger's car.

Public Transportation

Do

- Use busy, well-lighted bus, train, and subway stops.
- Wait where there are other people; stay near the group.
- Sit near the bus driver.

Don't

- Wait alone at a bus stop; try to go to a busier area.
- Get off if you feel unsafe; speak to the bus driver about your safety concerns.
- Talk to strangers; avoid eye contact.

Walking

Do

- Know where to find pay phones; always have coins to make a phone call.
- Plan your route to use well-lighted streets.
- Plan the shortest, safest route possible.
- Walk in the street at night, facing oncoming traffic.
- Carry some money in your pocket.
- Carry a whistle or personal alarm.
- Keep house and car keys in your hand.
- Walk confidently like you know where you are going.
- Check with your police department to see if they offer programs on "street safety."
- Be aware of what is going on around you.

Don't

- Walk in alleys, deserted areas, near buildings or bushes.
- Walk with strangers.
- Walk alone at night, if possible.
- Hitchhike or accept rides from strangers.
- Carry all your money in your purse or wallet.
- Carry a purse.

Arriving Home

Do

- Keep headlights on and car doors locked until you have checked parking area or garage.
- Have house or apartment key in hand.
- Leave a light on before you leave home (indoor and outdoor).
- Ask the driver to wait until you are safely inside before leaving; use a prearranged signal to indicate that it is safe to leave.

Don't

- Go inside if something seems to be wrong; instead, go to a safe place and call the police.
- Delay entering your home, especially at night.

CHAPTER SUMMARY

- A safe home environment is maintained by:
  Being aware of potentially unsafe conditions.
  Correcting unsafe conditions or notifying the appropriate person.
  Taking precautions to avoid future problems.
- The home care aide must be alert to safety risks for client, family, and self.
- Home care aides need to know the general rules for maintaining a safe home.
- Older adults, children, and confused clients require special attention to prevent injury.
- Smoking is the number one cause of home fires.
- The use of oxygen in the home poses great risk for fire.
- Planning in advance for possible household emergencies helps you to handle them more effectively.
- The number one rule in any home fire is *"Get out and get your client out without delay."*
- Prepare ahead for natural and weather-related emergencies.
- Keep a list of emergency phone numbers handy.

STUDY QUESTIONS

1. List 10 common hazards found in the home and describe how you would correct them.

2. Identify two types of clients at risk for accident/injury in the home. Describe three measures to take in preventing accidents for each type of client.

3. List steps to be taken in case of a fire.

4. What are five important safety precautions to take when traveling to and from a client's home?

5. What is the most common weather-related emergency in your area? What procedures would you take to protect yourself and your client?

Maintaining a Healthy Environment

Objectives

After you read this chapter, you will be able to:

1. Discuss the importance of a clean and well-maintained home environment to the client's health and safety.

2. Explain the role of the home care aide in maintaining a clean, healthy home environment and the usual tasks performed.

3. Select and use appropriate supplies for cleaning and maintaining the client's environment.

4. Perform basic tasks of cleaning and housekeeping of the client's immediate environment.

5. Know when to seek assistance from others—agency, client's family.

6. Teach others in the home to assist with the care of the client's environment.

Y
ou may be asking yourself, "Why does a home care aide have to maintain a clean, healthy environment? Why doesn't the aide just care for the client who is sick?" These are good questions. Consider the following client situations:

- When Brigit Kennedy, age 82, fell in the bathroom, she broke both her hip and her wrist. She had a surgical repair of her broken hip and has been discharged from the hospital to her home where she is using a wheelchair. Brigit cannot bathe, clean, cook, or do her laundry without assistance. She lives alone in a senior citizen apartment complex and has a clothes washer and a dryer. The home care aide helps Brigit with bathing, grooming, laundry, and basic housekeeping.

- Louis Roupp, age 64, lives alone in a fourth floor walk-up apartment. Because of his heart disease, he is unable to leave his home and uses oxygen most of the time. He has no strength or energy for home maintenance, cleaning, laundry, or shopping. The home care aide helps Louis with personal care and grooming. Once a week, the aide shops for food. Mr. Roupp has one meal a day from the Meals On Wheels program. He also has assistance from a cleaning service.

- Mary Helen Sawyer, age 25, has severe arthritis. The home care aide comes to Mary Helen's home daily to prepare breakfast and to help her bathe, dress, and get ready for work. The kitchen and bathroom need to be straightened and cleaned before Ms. Sawyer leaves for work in the car pool. The aide also makes Ms. Sawyer's bed and straightens the bedroom. Ms. Sawyer has a cleaning service that does all of the heavy cleaning. Her sister does the laundry on weekends.

- Father Kowalski, age 50, was in an automobile accident several months ago. He has a back injury that has caused his legs to be paralyzed. The home care aide gets Father out of bed with a mechanical lift and assists him with personal care. The housekeeper takes care of all meals and cleaning. The aide makes the bed and washes the bed linen as needed.

A Clean Environment is Important

Brigit, Louis, Mary Helen, and Father Kowalski cannot assume full responsibility for themselves or their surroundings. They have neither the strength or the ability to perform their own personal care or their own housekeeping duties. When a person is sick or disabled, care of the home is often not done or disrupted. The family may be so busy caring for the sick member that home maintenance is not a priority. Yet, a clean environment is an important part of health care. Clutter, disorder, dirt, and odors are health and safety hazards. They increase the risk for infection, disease, and accidents that can interfere with the client's recovery.

The home care aide is responsible for maintaining a clean, safe, and healthy environment. This is accomplished in many ways:

1. Performing housekeeping duties, as listed in the care plan, while the client is sick or disabled.

2. Helping the client to assume increasing responsibility for maintaining a clean, healthy environment whenever possible.

3. Teaching disorganized families to develop and carry out plans for maintaining a safe home environment.

4. Helping with home management during a crisis situation (death and/or hospitalization of a primary caregiver, suspected child abuse, sick children, etc.) until a long-term plan can be developed.

Responsibilities of the Home Care Aide

Housekeeping responsibilities include care of the client's immediate environment—usually the bedroom and the bathroom. The care plan may call for general cleaning throughout the house. If you use the kitchen, you will be expected to clean up after yourself. Specific duties will be listed on the care plan developed by your supervisor, the client, and the family. These may include dusting, vacuuming, laundry, cleaning the kitchen, and washing the dishes. If there is any question or confusion about your duties or the timing of each job, CONTACT YOUR SUPERVISOR. Do not argue with your client about your housekeeping responsibilities.

Caring for your client's environment is NOT the same as cleaning your own home. The client may want things done his/her way. Some clients may be frustrated because they must depend on you. Others may be embarrassed by all the mess in their home.

A note of caution: not all homes are like your own home. Some will be better equipped, and, as in the case of Father Kowalski, there may be full-time household help. Other times, you may be working in an environment where the resources are limited. In urban areas, a single-room-occupancy (SRO) unit may have a shared bathroom, no kitchen, and no running water in the room. In rural areas, the toilet may be outdoors, and the water may come from a hand-operated pump. Be prepared to improvise, substitute, and "make do" when necessary (Box 7-1).

Box 7-1

In the Client's Home

- Be sensitive to attitudes of client and family regarding maintaining a clean, neat home.
- "Make do" with housecleaning products available.
- Do not ask client to purchase products that you personally prefer.
- Always know products you are using—READ THE LABEL.
- If unsure about the operation of an appliance, ask the family for instructions, read the "use and care" booklet from the manufacturer, or contact your supervisor.
- Do not operate equipment you are not familiar with.
- If changes are needed in placement of furniture and storage of cleaning equipment and supplies, discuss them with the client and family; give reasons why changes would help in housekeeping tasks.
- Encourage family members to help maintain a healthy home; when needed, teach skills necessary.
- Teach family, by example, how to maintain a healthy home.
- Learn how to improvise when cleaning materials or equipment are not available.
- Do not judge client or family whose home is not up to your own personal standards of "good housekeeping."
- Do not make comments about "poor" housekeeping.
- Wear heavy duty protective gloves for cleaning or using household cleaning liquids.
- Wash your hands immediately after performing household tasks.

OLSTEN Health Care — HOME HEALTH AIDE INSTRUCTIONS

Client		Date	Case Manager

INSTRUCTIONS: Complete all tasks which are either checked or noted in special instructions. Report all changes noted to the case manager.

PERSONAL CARE		TOT. ✓	ASSISTED ✓	SELF CARE ✓
Bath	Tub			
	Shower			
	Bed			
Oral Hygiene	Routine			
	Denture Care			
Hair Care	Comb			
	Shampoo			
Grooming	Shave			
	Nails			
Eating	Feed			
	Set-up			
Dressing				
Skin Care				

VITAL SIGNS ❑ WEIGHT ❑ TEMP. ❑ PULSE ❑ RESP. ❑ BP

FREQUENCY

MEASURE INTAKE ❑ ORAL ❑ TUBE ❑ CATH CARE

OUTPUT ❑ CHECK BM ❑ MEASURE URINE ❑ MEASURE FOLEY OUTPUT

SAFETY PRECAUTIONS

ACTIVITIES		✓
Bedrest	Complete	
	Up to Bathroom	
Up as Tolerated		
Transfer Bed/Chair		
ROM		
❑ Active ❑ Passive		
Bedrest:		
Turn every hrs.		
Ambulation (amount)		
Device/Assist		

HOUSEKEEPING		✓	HOUSEKEEPING CONT'D		✓	HOUSEKEEPING CONT'D		✓	MEALS		TOT. ✓	ASSISTED ✓	SELF CARE ✓
Kitchen	Floor (clean/vacuum)		Bedrooms(s)	Floor (clean/vacuum)		Living/ Dining	Floor (clean/vacuum)		Prepare	Breakfast			
	Dishes			Dust			Dust			Lunch			
	Refrigerator			Change Linen			Wash			Dinner			
	Stove		Bathroom(s)	Floor (clean/vacuum)		Laundry	Iron		Plan				
	Garbage			Clean Fixtures					Purchase				

SPECIAL INSTRUCTIONS

SPECIAL DIET

MEDICATIONS	SELF ✓	ASST. ✓	EFFECTS TO REPORT TO CASE MANAGER

DATES REVIEWED:

REVIEWED:

7-1 The care plan. *(Courtesy Olsten Kimberly QualityCare, Melville, NY.)*

Types of Tasks to be Performed

The care plan (Fig. 7-1) lists your responsibilities for maintaining the client's environment. Both your agency and client agreed upon these services during the first visit from the case manager. Types of tasks to be performed vary according to each client's individual needs and can include any of the tasks listed below:

- *Client's bedroom*—clean immediate environment. Empty and clean the commode (Fig. 7-2). Make bed and change and launder linens as necessary. Care for client's personal laundry: hand wash in sink, or machine wash in client's home, in laundry room, or in laundromat. Dry laundry and return to proper place. Empty waste basket.
- *Client's bathroom*—may be private or shared with other family members. It may be down the hall and shared by unrelated residents of the building. Clean toilet and raised toilet seat attachment daily (Fig. 7-3). Tub and shower are cleaned after each use. In some situations, it may be necessary to clean them before your client uses them. Change and launder bath linens as necessary. Replace toilet tissue, soap, and facial tissue as needed. Empty waste basket.
- *Client's kitchen (or family kitchen)*—light cleaning of counter surfaces, dishes used by client, and utensils and appliances used by aide to prepare client's meals. Clean refrigerator, if there is no one else to do so. Clean sink and drain. Sweep floor and remove and discard trash.
- *Other areas*—vacuum carpets, dust furniture, empty ashtrays, water plants, discard trash.

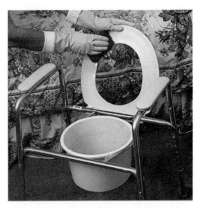

7-2 Cleaning the commode may be one of the homecare aide's duties.

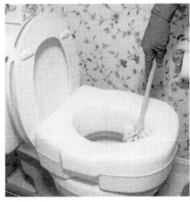

7-3 Cleaning the splash guard of a raised toilet seat.

Developing a Work Plan

Developing a work plan is important because your time in the client's home is limited. Your first priority is care of the client, so you are not able to spend a lot of time on housekeeping duties. Box 7-2 gives tips for organizing your cleaning time. An hour should be enough time to complete routine tasks. Big cleaning jobs are not your responsibility. Your agency will help the client contact a cleaning service for help in this area. Your work plan lists the jobs to be done, the schedule, and who will do each task. Typical responsibilities include the following:

Every Day Tasks:

- Washing dishes
- Cleaning kitchen counters and sink
- Sweeping floor in kitchen
- Removing trash
- Making bed
- Straightening rooms and removing clutter
- Cleaning toilet, commode, and bathroom sink

Box 7-2

Rules of Organization

- Have a cleaning plan—be flexible.
- Do each job correctly from top to bottom (except on walls), clean to dirty.
- Work around the room along the walls; come in door, turn to the right, and begin cleaning; continue until you are back at the door again.
- Try to make work easier by taking fewer steps and using a larger broom or big sponge.
- Don't try to do everything in one day.
- Do the jobs that must be done daily, plus only one of the weekly jobs.
- Post schedule of jobs and who will do each one (don't forget children).

Weekly:

- Dusting and vacuuming bedroom or client area
- Cleaning refrigerator
- Changing and laundering bed linens
- Watering plants

Follow your work plan as closely as possible, but remember to be flexible. Your client's personal physical needs come first, and sometimes you will need to adjust your plan of work. If your client has soiled the bed linens, you must change them, even if that is not on your schedule for that day. Your client may need a bath, clean clothing, and his/her personal laundry done. A work plan is just that, a plan, and plans can always be changed when necessary.

Organize your work. Straighten up as you go along. Managers in a famous fast-food restaurant chain teach their employees this easy, time and work saving rule—CUAYG, that is:

CLEAN UP AS YOU GO

Don't take extra steps; don't make extra work for yourself. Work smarter, not harder.

Once you begin a task, finish what you are doing. Begin with the worst room first. Both the kitchen and bathroom require careful cleaning. Plan to clean the kitchen daily. Toilets and sinks should be **disinfected** daily. Follow the schedule listed above, if your agency does not provide one for you. Work around the room until you are finished.

Always work from the cleanest to the dirtiest area. For example, in the bathroom, begin with the mirror and finish with the floor. If the weather is pleasant, open windows and ventilate the room as you work. Do not expose your client to a draft or chill the home unnecessarily in cold weather.

Maintaining an Uncluttered Environment

One of the easiest ways to make a home look cleaner is to eliminate clutter. However, what may look like clutter to you may be treasure to your client. Don't throw away anything without discussing it with your client and receiving permission to discard the item.

Some general rules for straightening up and reducing clutter are:

- Carry a basket or bag to collect clutter and to redistribute items to their proper location.
- Remove scraps of paper, newspapers, and old magazines; recycle.
- Remove dead leaves from plants; discard old flowers.
- Empty ash trays and waste baskets.
- Put items in their proper place—books, shoes, clothing, toys, boots, tools, etc.
- Clean counter tops; put things away.
- Check dates on containers; discard and replace outdated items.
- Check under the bed, sofa, and chairs for clutter in hiding.

Clutter is a safety hazard and is a major cause of accidental falls in the home. A magazine on the floor is as slippery as ice—so, protect your

disinfect
to destroy germs.

disinfectant
a chemical that can be applied to objects to destroy germs.

client by keeping the environment as free of clutter as possible. If you can't discard it, try to arrange the clutter as neatly as possible and move it out of the way.

Cleaning Equipment and Supplies

Television and magazine advertisements lead us to believe that we need a special cleaner for each and every housekeeping job. Not true! There are some basic cleaning supplies and tools needed. There are also some "nice to have but not always necessary" things, too.

Necessary:

- *Dust cloths*—for dusting dry surfaces; wash in soapy water after use; air dry as they may retain flammable materials from the polishing chemicals.
- *Broom*—for sweeping hard surfaced floors; shake into large, moistened bag after each use; hang to store.
- *Sponge mop*—for wet cleaning hard-surfaced floors; wash and rinse after use; stand upside down to dry; replace sponge when needed.
- *Scrub brush*—for rough surfaces; wash and rinse after use; dry with bristles down.
- *Bucket* (or two)—for cleaning and rinsing solutions; rinse and dry after use.
- *Sponges*—for washable surfaces; wash in soapy water and air dry.
- *Toilet brush*—for cleaning toilet bowl; rinse in cold water and store.
- *Dust pan and brush*—for gathering small amounts of dust from dry hard surfaces; wipe pan with damp cloth and shake brush into large, moistened bag after use.
- *Rubber gloves*—heavy duty to protect hands from irritation; hang to air dry.
- *Vacuum cleaner*—for cleaning carpets, upholstery. Follow manufacturer's instructions; empty frequently; replace filter/bags as needed; check to see that cord and plug are in good repair before each use.
- *Dish washing supplies*—cloths, brushes, detergent, scouring pads.
- *Cleaning agents:*
  - All purpose cleaners for floors, walls, counters, and other hard surfaces
  - Detergents for laundry and dish washing
  - Cleansers for scrubbing
  - Specialty cleaners for toilets, ovens, windows, tiles, etc.
  - Baking soda used to clean refrigerator, bathroom tiles, counter stains, and many other items
  - White vinegar used to clean toilets, commodes, tile, windows, mirrors, and many other items
  - **Disinfectants** are chemicals used to destroy germs; some cleaning agents are also disinfectants; bleach is a disinfectant used in certain situations (see Chapter 9).

The above items may be considered as necessary, but many homes may not have all of these supplies. When in doubt, ask your supervisor.

"Nice to have" supplies, but not necessary:

- Floor dust mop for hard floors
- Floor polisher
- Carpet sweeper
- Automatic dishwasher, clothes washer and dryer

Product Safety—A Household Concern

Incorrect use of cleaning agents can cause serious damage to the user, the surface to be cleaned, and the environment. Certain chemicals in cleaning products are thought to be **ecologically** dangerous.

The home safety hints that follow give information that will help you to avoid endangering yourself, home surfaces, or the environment.

Home Safety Hints

- Know the surface you want cleaned. Know what it's made of. Is there an outer coating or finish over another material? Ask the client if there are special cleaners to be used or any cleaners to be avoided.
- Know the cleaner. Are you using the right cleaner for the surface? The right amount of cleaner? Are you giving it the right amount of time to do the job?
- Read the label. Do you know how to use the product safely? Do you understand all the directions? Are there any potentially dangerous ingredients?
- Pay special attention to food surfaces. Do not use home cleaning products to wash dishes. Keep food away from all cleaning sprays and liquids.
- Never mix cleaning agents. For example, avoid mixing cleaners containing bleach (such as most scouring powders) and ammonia, since they react to cause poisonous fumes.
- Allow adequate ventilation when using cleaning agents. When cleaning closets or shower units, leave doors open for excess vapors to escape. Take the same precaution when using strong ammonia solutions.
- Keep aerosols away from heat. Aerosol cans are packed under pressure. Excess heat may cause them to explode. Never store at temperatures higher than 120° Fahrenheit. Keep all aerosols away from hot pipes, radiators, stoves, and ovens. Never burn aerosol cans. Do not store cans in a car's glove compartment or trunk in the hot sun. Avoid spraying aerosols near an open flame.
- Separate food, personal care, and home care aerosols. This prevents taking the wrong can by mistake.
- Keep spray cleaners away from face and eyes. Certain products contain chemicals that could irritate the lungs if inhaled. The eyes may also be injured.
- Keep all cleaning agents out of the hands of children and away from animals. Many are poisonous if taken internally. Keep containers closed. Store out of children's reach. Whenever possible, buy products with safety caps.

ecologically
relating to the environment.

microorganisms
a living plant or animal that can only be seen by a microscope.

- Purchase cleaning agents from a reliable source. These products will include information for proper use and safety. Reputable companies manufacture products that meet tough standards for durability and safety.

Cleaning the Bathroom

Unless the client has his/her own bathroom, most bathrooms are used by other family members. Sometimes a bathroom is shared by other residents of an apartment house. It is not your responsibility to clean the bathroom after use by family members or residents. It **is** your job to make sure the bathroom is clean after you or your client use it.

Keeping the bathroom clean is very important. **Microorganisms** grow and multiply rapidly in this area because there is moisture and warmth. Any materials used to clean the bathroom, such as brushes or sponges, should only be used in this area.

See the "How to" box below for daily tasks needed to keep the bathroom clean and free of harmful microorganisms.

How To Clean the Bathroom		
Task	*Materials Needed*	*Be Sure To:*
All surfaces	• Detergent and water • Disinfectant • White vinegar and water solution • Pail, soft rag, or sponge • Gloves	• Wipe toilet tank, sink, window sills, bathroom tiles, or washable wallpaper
Mirror	• Glass cleaner or white vinegar and water solution • Paper towel or newspaper	• Clean so that mirror is not streaked
Toilet bowl and seat	• Disinfectant and water • Toilet brush or sponge and pail • Gloves	• Wear gloves • Clean thoroughly: under rim of toilet bowl, under and behind toilet seat, outside toilet bowl • If used, clean plastic splash guard of raised toilet seat using brush or sponge
Tub or shower stall	• Detergent and water • Pail, soft rag, or sponge	• Clean tub or shower stall after each use by client
POINTS TO REMEMBER:	• Wear gloves when cleaning the bathroom. • Work from the cleanest area (mirrors) to the dirtiest (floor). • Clean bathroom using a disinfectant. • Keep area well ventilated and as dry as possible to prevent mildew from forming. • Do not mix ammonia with other cleaning agents.	

Cleaning the Client's Living Area

If your client has limited mobility, he or she will probably spend a lot of time in one part of the home. This area should be clean and orderly. Items frequently used by the client must be within easy reach for the client's comfort. In many cases, it is the bedroom that will be used. But sometimes it is another area, such as the living room couch or chair. In addition to the general housekeeping tasks mentioned earlier, the following should be performed each day:

- Remove clutter—old newspapers, toys, magazines
- Place reading materials and reading glasses convenient to client and off the floor
- Wash drinking cup and water pitcher; refill with fresh water and place within easy reach
- Tidy bedside table
- Empty wastebasket
- Replace items on bedside table according to client's wishes

How To Clean the Client's Living Area

Task	Materials Needed	Be Sure To:
Change bed linens	• Sheets • Pillow cases • Bedspread (optional) • Protective sheets or pads (optional) • Blankets	• Change at least once a week or more often if necessary • Change immediately when soiled, damp, or wet
Damp dust surfaces *Dust furniture*	• Damp cloth	• Dust all surfaces once weekly or more often if client has allergies
Damp mop floor *Vacuum rug*	• Damp mop • Vacuum cleaner	• Damp mop and/or vacuum rug at least once per week or more often, if necessary
Clean commode	• Disinfectant and water • Toilet brush or sponge • Pail • Gloves	• Wear gloves • Remove pail and dispose waste in toilet • Clean commode with brush and pail • Clean all surfaces of commode with disinfectant
Check supply of toilet tissue and replace as needed	• Toilet tissue	• Place toilet tissue within easy reach of client and commode
POINTS TO REMEMBER:	• Remove clutter each day to maintain a clean, safe home. • Vacuum or brush corners of chairs to remove crumbs or other pieces of food where client eats; sweep floor or vacuum rug as needed. • After cleaning, replace all personal items within easy reach of client. • Wear gloves when cleaning commode.	

- Make bed (see Chapter 12) and straighten bedding as needed
- Damp dust surfaces as needed

See the "How to" box on the facing page for other tasks to be performed in order to maintain a clean, healthy environment in the living area.

Maintaining a Clean, Orderly Kitchen

Cleaning the Kitchen

As a home care aide, you may have the responsibility to prepare and serve a meal to your client. Cleaning the kitchen after making a meal is also your job. The phrase *work smarter, not harder* is especially true. Develop a routine, and it will save you time and energy. Plan before you act. Sometimes the client's care plan calls for light cleaning in the kitchen. Typical tasks include: washing dishes; cleaning sink, counter tops, and table; and discarding spoiled food from the refrigerator.

Disposing of Household Waste

It is estimated that each person disposes of more than $1^1/_2$ pounds of paper per day. Used cans, glass bottles, wrappers from candy and gum, plastic containers, and food scraps add to the list of household waste. If these items are not recycled or disposed of each day, the environment becomes cluttered and unhealthy in a very short time.

Most communities participate in recycling programs for newspapers, cartons, glass, plastic, and aluminum cans. There are special rules and regulations that apply to recyclable items. It is important that you know what kinds of items are to be recycled and how frequently they are picked up. Obtain this information from your client, a family member, or local municipal government office.

How To Clean the Kitchen

Task	Materials Needed	Be Sure To:
Washing dishes	• Detergent or soap • Hot water	• Scrape dish to remove food • Wash in hot, soapy water • Rinse in hot water • Air dry • Wash glassware first, utensils, then cups, saucers, plates, pots, and pans
Using automatic dishwasher	• Dishwasher detergent—type and amount according to directions only	• Have family member demonstrate loading and starting, if unsure • Scrape large food particles before loading • Empty glasses and cups • Load glasses and cups, dishes • Place eating and drinking surfaces toward spray of water (usually downward) • Do not overload

Continued.

How To Clean the Kitchen—cont'd.

Task	Materials Needed	Be Sure To:
Cleaning refrigerator	• Soapy water • Baking soda solution: (3 tablespoons to 1 quart warm water) • Sponge or rags	• Dispose of food over 3 days old or food that shows signs of spoiling (odor, color change) • Remove food—one shelf at a time • Remove and wash shelves and trays with warm soapy water • Wipe inside walls with baking soda solution • Replace shelves and trays • Replace food • Place an open box or small perforated container of baking soda on shelf to absorb food odors and leave refrigerator odor free (optional)
Cleaning kitchen counters	• Hot soapy water and detergent or baking soda solution • Cloth or sponge	• Wipe counter tops after each meal • Use baking soda on a damp cloth to remove counter top stains • Wipe down food preparation surfaces with hot soapy water • Rinse and dry thoroughly
Cleaning kitchen sink (stainless steel or porcelain sink)	• Hot sudsy water	• Clean daily after meal preparation
POINTS TO REMEMBER:	• Some items should not be washed in an automatic dishwasher. They include: electrical appliances, delicate glassware, fine china, sharp knives, some types of pots and pans, and wooden bowls. These items will need to be hand washed. • Use medium heat to keep food from boiling over or splattering. • Do not open refrigerator door more often than you need; warm air causes the motor to work harder to keep the desired temperature. • Use warm, sudsy water and a cloth or sponge to wipe up cooking spills or splattered grease immediately from stove, oven, broiler, or microwave oven.	

Garbage, including food and fluids, needs to be discarded promptly to avoid odors and growth of organisms. Place garbage in a closed container lined with a plastic bag. Remove the plastic liner daily, tie, and place in a larger, closed container and store outdoors. In an apartment complex, use the garbage chute.

Some clients will have a garbage disposal unit connected to the kitchen sink. This equipment grinds up food and empties it into the sewage system. By using the garbage disposal unit, food is removed quickly and efficiently. While many food items can be removed by this method, some garbage (bones, fruit pits) will still need to be placed in containers and stored until it can be disposed. See the "How to" box on pages 95–96 for tasks to be performed to keep the kitchen clean and free of harmful microorganisms.

Laundry

If your client lives alone and is unable to wash linens, towels, and personal clothing, the care plan may call for the home care aide to perform these tasks. Clean clothing not only helps the client to feel more comfortable but also can be a morale booster. Discuss with the client or a family member preferences concerning use of detergents, softeners, or other laundry products.

How To Do the Laundry

Task	*Materials Needed*	*Be Sure To:*

Sort items to be washed	• Laundry basket	• Read the care label on clothing
		• Place items in piles according to care needed:
		  1. sturdy white
		  2. dark
		  3. colored
		  4. heavily soiled
		  5. delicate (hand or dry clean)
		• Inspect items to be washed for spots, stains, or repairs needed
		• Set aside and pre-treat spots; repair as needed
		• Empty pockets
		• Turn dark socks inside out
		• Button buttons
		• Zip zippers
		• Tie sashes and belts
		• Hook hooks
		• Treat linens soiled with body fluids (see Box 7-3)

Select correct detergent	• Detergent • Fabric softener (if used) • Bleach, if needed for stains and odors • Borax, if needed for stains and odors	• Consult client/family regarding preference • Read the directions on the package
Select correct water temperature	Use: • Hot water (130–150° F) for heavily soiled clothes, diapers, whites, and light colored cottons • Warm water (100–110° F) for moderately or lightly soiled wash and wear and permanent press fabrics • Cold water (80–100° F) for bright colors, fragile fabrics, and lightly soiled items	• Select cold water for rinse cycle • Select the proper setting for wash, rinse, and spin cycles • Read the instructions usually found on underside of the washer lid • Receive instructions from client/family regarding use of washing machine • If still unsure, contact your supervisor for directions

Continued.

How To Do the Laundry—cont'd.

Task	Materials Needed	Be Sure To:
Load the machine *Wash and dry load*		• Put water in machine, then add detergent • Mix small and large items in the load for better washing action • Do not overload; this damages items and is not efficient • Machine dry clothes • Separate lightweight and heavy items to dry more evenly • Remove permanent press items as soon as dryer stops to reduce wrinkling • Remove clothes, fold, and store in appropriate place
POINTS TO REMEMBER:	• Always wear gloves when handling linens stained with body fluids • Read the care label before selecting laundering method • Treat stains appropriately (Box 7-3) • Some items attract lint; others give off lint; separate them to avoid more work later in removing lint. • Wash heavily soiled items in a separate load. • More detergent does not always assure a clean load of laundry; read the directions on the detergent package. • Never mix chlorine bleach with ammonia because it creates a deadly gas. • Do not overload washing machine or dryer; laundry needs enough water around the items to remove soil and enough air to dry items properly. • Use cold water for washing when appropriate and especially for rinse cycle; it saves energy and prevents permanent press fabrics from wrinkling. • Discuss with your client or client's family how home laundry is usually washed; some homes may not have a washing machine; remember, your supervisor will advise you about your responsibilities if this situation occurs.	

Keeping laundry clean removes a source of potentially harmful organisms. When the client is recovering from an infection, frequent laundering of any item coming in contact with the client is necessary to prevent the spread of infection to others. Wear gloves when handling linens contaminated with body fluids. Place them in leak-proof containers. Treat and wash them as quickly as possible. Box 7-3 gives instructions for treating linens stained with body fluids.

See the "How to" box above for laundering instructions.

Controlling Household Pests

Household pests can be a source of infection, illness, and sometimes death. They can carry disease or cause illness to humans in a variety of

contamination
introduction of harmful organisms.

Box 7-3

Cleaning Linens Soiled with Body Fluids

SAFETY AND BIOHAZARD CHECK:
ALWAYS WEAR GLOVES WHEN HANDLING LINENS SOILED WITH BODY FLUIDS. STAIN REMOVAL MAY INVOLVE USE OF DANGEROUS CHEMICALS. FOLLOW LABEL INSTRUCTIONS CAREFULLY.

Ammonia is poisonous. Do not inhale fumes. Ammonia will cause burns or irritation if it comes in contact with skin or eyes. Clorine bleach is poisonous and will cause burns or irritation if it comes in contact with eyes or skin.

General rules: These directions apply to white or colorfast linens. Before treating stains, flush fabric with cold water to remove body fluids or solids on linens. Work quickly, before the stain becomes set in the fabric.

Removing Urine Stains

1. Soak in a solution of 1 quart of warm water, $\frac{1}{2}$ teaspoon liquid (hand) dishwashing detergent, and 1 Tablespoon of ammonia for 30 minutes.

2. Rinse with cool water.

3. Soak in a solution of 1 quart of warm water and 1 Tablespoon of vinegar for 1 hour.

4. Rinse with water.

5. Wash in machine using detergent and chlorine bleach according to product directions. Dry as usual.

Removing Fecal Stains

1. Soak in a solution of 1 quart warm water, $\frac{1}{2}$ teaspoon liquid (hand) dishwashing detergent, and 1 Tablespoon ammonia for 30 minutes.

2. Rinse with cold water.

3. Wash in machine using chlorine bleach and detergent according to product directions. Dry as usual.

Removing Blood Stains

1. Soak in a solution of 1 quart warm water, $\frac{1}{2}$ teaspoon liquid (hand) dishwashing detergent, and 1 Tablespoon ammonia for 15 minutes.

2. If fabric is strong enough, gently rub stain. Continue as long as stain responds to treatment.

3. Soak another 15 minutes in the solution used in step 1.

4. Soak in a solution of 1 quart warm water and 1 Tablespoon enzyme product for 30 minutes.

5. Wash in machine using chlorine bleach and detergent. Dry as usual.

ways, including bites and **contamination** of foods. Pests, such as flies, mosquitoes, ants, roaches, mice, and rats, enter the home in a variety of ways. After entering, they look for food and a place to grow and multiply.

There are two main rules for controlling pests—exclusion and sanitation.

Exclusion means keeping pests from entering the home. Keep screens repaired and in place to prevent flies and mosquitoes from entering. Seal up cracks and holes in walls or outside doors to keep out ants, mice, or roaches. If you see cracks, holes, or screens needing repair, notify your supervisor. Repairs will need to be made by someone skilled in the proper procedure.

Sanitation means performing proper techniques discussed in this chapter to remove sources of food and shelter needed for pests to grow and multiply. The following are some tips to maintain a home free of household pests:

- Refrigerate leftover cooked food immediately.
- Store all food properly—either in refrigerator or in containers with tight lids.

- Wipe up crumbs and spills immediately.
- Remove garbage promptly and place in the container with tight lid.
- Keep kitchen counters clean.
- Clean under refrigerator and stove.
- Vacuum between cushions of chair or couch where client may drop crumbs from food or snacks.
- Dust and vacuum corners, behind and under furniture to keep pests from nesting.
- Throw out vase water and wilted flowers to prevent insects from growing and breeding in stagnant water.
- Check grains, flour, and seeds for signs of insects before storing in closed containers.
- Wash fruits and vegetables before eating.
- Remove sources of moisture.

Notify your supervisor if the home shows signs of pests. Do not use any chemicals to try to control household pests.

Teaching Others

Sometimes, the home care aide will be asked to teach certain household tasks to the client or a family member. Perhaps the client has always performed all of the household duties, and, now, because of illness or disability, others must learn how to help. The home care aide can teach others to perform these tasks (Box 7-4).

When clients become disabled, they often must learn new ways to perform familiar tasks. The occupational therapist will teach the client new skills. Cleaning supplies and equipment may be adapted for your client's specific needs.

Families may need to learn to be organized and work together in home management. There are many things children can do to help out around the home (Fig. 7-4). When teaching clients or families, use the following guidelines:

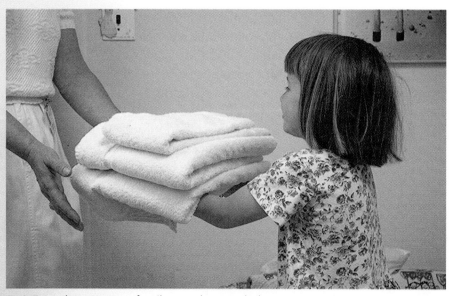

7-4 Even the youngest family member can help.

Box 7-4

Suggestions of Household Tasks

For Young Children (ages 5 and above)
- Make own bed
- Put clothing back in closet or drawer
- Put toys away
- Set the table
- Clean the table
- Pick up clutter
- Help with dishes
- Fold laundry
- Empty small wastebaskets

For older children and adolescents (including above)
- Make beds
- Help younger children make beds
- Separate recyclables and carry out trash
- Vacuum and dust
- Do laundry and dishes
- Clean bathrooms
- Clean woodwork and windows
- Clean and sweep kitchen floor
- Carry in wood and lay the fire
- Straighten closets
- Mend clothes
- Make small repairs

For all:
- Straighten and put things away
- Put away own clothes
- Hang up own things
- Clean tub or shower after use
- Restock supplies (toilet paper, paper towels, facial tissue, soap)
- Clean up after yourself

- Individualize the teaching for each family member.
- Get the person's full attention.
- Be sure the person wants to learn.
- Don't talk too fast.
- Don't teach too much at one time.
- Show and explain how to do each task—one step at a time; then have person perform the task; repeat teaching if necessary.
- Be patient; it takes time to learn to do new things.
- Give praise for attempts and success.
- Teach by example, but encourage persons to keep trying; don't do for them every time they become frustrated or fail.

CHAPTER SUMMARY

- A clean home environment contributes to the client's health and safety.

- The home care aide is responsible for maintaining a clean, safe, health environment by:
  - performing household duties.
  - helping the client to perform household tasks.
  - teaching disorganized families to care for their environment.

- Household responsibilities are listed in the care plan and may include: cleaning the client's area, bathroom, and kitchen.

- A work plan helps the home care aide to use time wisely and efficiently.

- Cleaning equipment and supplies require proper handling and storage to prevent accidents and injury.

STUDY QUESTIONS

1. Why is a clean home environment important for clients' health and safety?

2. List three ways the home care aide maintains a clean, healthy home environment. Describe three usual tasks.

3. Make a list of supplies and equipment needed to clean:
   a. the client's area or bedroom
   b. client's bathroom

4. What action would you take if:
   a. you are asked to do spring housecleaning?
   b. the washing machine is broken?
   c. you do not know how to operate the dishwasher?

5. List five guidelines to remember when teaching others to perform household tasks.

Meeting the Client's Nutritional Needs

Objectives

After you read this chapter, you will be able to:

1. Discuss the importance of nutrition in maintaining health and preventing illness.

2. List three factors influencing individual and family food habits.

3. List five foods that belong in each of the following categories: proteins, carbohydrates, and fats.

4. Discuss the role of vitamins and minerals in the diet and major food sources of these substances.

5. Describe the importance of water and dietary fiber.

6. Plan meals for the day that meet the requirements of the Food Guide Pyramid.

7. Describe food shopping for clients including: preparing list, selecting and purchasing products.

8. Discuss food preparation, including food safety.

9. Recognize the need to follow agency policy regarding client's money, expense receipts, travel, and transporting clients.

10. Feed clients who cannot feed themselves.

11. Describe the techniques for assisting clients who have difficulty eating.

12. Identify six therapeutic diets and list foods to be included or avoided.

Your body needs enough food and water in order to grow, develop, and function properly. Of course, the amount of food each person needs depends on things like age, sex, size, health, and activity level. For example, a healthy, physically active teenager needs to eat more food than an older adult who doesn't get much exercise. **Nutrition** is the process in which food is taken in and used by the body.

Function of Food

Food contains the nutrients (vitamins, minerals, dietary fiber, and water) a body needs to function 24 hours a day, every day. The human body uses the nutrients found in food for

1. *Heat and energy production.* Brendan is a soccer player. He needs lots of energy to run up and down the field to chase and move the ball. He gets very hot and sweaty during soccer games.
2. *Growth and development.* Lisa is six months pregnant. She needs food for her own body to use and for her growing fetus, too.
3. *Health and well-being.* Everyone needs the proper amount and type of nutrients. When essential nutrients are missing from the diet, **malnutrition,** weight loss, and **deficiency** disease may result. Leo has diabetes. In order to maintain a healthy body, he follows the diet ordered by his doctor.
4. *Healing and repair of body tissue.* Our bodies mend and repair injured and diseased tissue. Martha broke her leg in a fall. The doctor says it will take six to eight weeks for it to heal.

Measuring Food Energy

Food energy is measured by means of a unit called a calorie. Our daily diet should include sufficient amounts of calories from quality foods. If the food intake is less than the energy used, weight loss will occur. If the food intake is more than the energy used, weight gain will occur.

Social, Cultural, and Religious Aspects of Food

For most people, food and eating means much more than nutrition. Eating with others (family and/or friends) is a social activity, whether it be a burger and shake from the fast-food drive-in or a formal candle-light dinner. Eating with others is more enjoyable. Many social events revolve around food—picnics, fiestas, banquets, etc. Eating out can be fun, convenient, and entertaining.

Certain types of foods convey a sense of well-being. Many foods from one's childhood (sometimes called "nursery foods") provide comfort during illness and periods of stress. Everyone has heard of the curative powers of chicken soup. Most people have some special foods that just make them feel good. These will vary with the person's ethnic background, and some of these "comfort" foods may not be available to immigrants in a new environment. Most of us grew up eating the kinds of food our families have eaten for generations.

Food customs are also closely linked to religious holidays or cultural celebrations. For example, roast lamb at Easter, matzos on Passover, and Mazeo for Kwanzaa are foods that have special meaning for observers of these holidays.

nutrition
the process by which food is taken in and used by the body.

malnutrition
any disorder of nutrition.

deficiency
a lack of one or more essential nutrients in the diet.

Food Preferences

Some foods may be appetizing to you, and yet the same foods will be disgusting to someone else. A big, juicy steak may make your mouth water, but this food would offer no appeal to a vegetarian. Certain foods are not eaten for many reasons, including religious and cultural beliefs, personal taste, likes and dislikes, dietary restrictions, illness, and allergies. Generally, mealtime has many different meanings. It is a time to eat, but, in some cultures, it is the gathering of a community together to eat, relax, and communicate. For others, mealtime means "grab something to eat, gobble it down, and run out the door." For some, it means eating alone—a hot meal delivered by a volunteer from Meals On Wheels, a bowl of cereal, cold rice, etc. Many people who live alone just don't bother to prepare food; mealtime is often a frozen dinner heated in the microwave.

Some religions have rules about the kinds and amounts of food to be eaten, including food used for certain religious events and celebrations. Dietary laws indicate the regulations to follow, such as fasting, care of cooking and eating utensils, and other rules regarding food preparation. Table 8-1 outlines dietary requirements according to religious belief.

Table 8-1

Religion and Dietary Practices

Religion	Dietary Restriction
Baptist	Some groups may avoid coffee, tea, and alcohol.
Christian Scientist	Alcohol, tea, coffee not allowed.
Church of the Latter Day Saints (Mormon)	Alcohol and hot drinks, such as tea and coffee, not allowed. Meat is not forbidden, but members are encouraged to eat meat infrequently.
Greek Orthodox	Wednesday, Friday, and Lent are days of fasting. Meat and dairy products avoided during days of fast.
Islamic (Muslim/Moslem)	Alcohol, pork, and pork products are forbidden.
Judaism (Jewish faith)	Foods must be kosher (prepared according to Jewish law); meat of kosher animals, kosher fowl, and kosher fish can be eaten. Pork and shellfish cannot be eaten. Milk, milk products, and eggs from kosher animals are acceptable; milk and milk products cannot be eaten with or immediately after eating meat; milk and milk products can be eaten six hours after eating meat; milk and milk products can be a part of the same meal with meat if they are served separately and before the meat. Kosher food cannot be prepared in utensils used to prepare nonkosher food. Breads, cakes, cookies, noodles, and alcoholic beverages are not consumed during Passover.
Roman Catholic	Fasting for one hour prior to receiving Holy Communion; no meat on Ash Wednesday, Good Friday, and Fridays during Lent.
Seventh Day Adventist (Adventist)	Avoid coffee, tea, alcohol; beverages with caffeine (colas) not allowed. Some groups forbid pork and pork products, others forbid meat.

Components of Food

Food may be classified according to its basic composition.

1. Carbohydrates are composed of the chemicals carbon, hydrogen, and oxygen.
2. Proteins are composed of compounds called amino acids, which contain carbon, hydrogen, oxygen, and nitrogen. Twenty amino acids have been discovered, 11 of which are manufactured by the body. The remaining 9, called essential amino acids, must come from the food we eat.
3. Fats are composed of fatty acids that contain carbon, hydrogen, and oxygen.

Boxes 8-1, 8-2, and 8-3 give information regarding the characteristics of carbohydrates, proteins, and fats.

Vitamins

Vitamins are substances that are needed to maintain our health. Most of them cannot be produced by our bodies. Instead, they are provided by the foods that we eat. While carbohydrates, proteins, and fats contain calories, vitamins do not.

Groups of Vitamins There are two groups of vitamins—vitamins that are dissolved in fats, and vitamins that are dissolved in water.

Fat-soluble vitamins Vitamins A, D, E, and K are dissolved in fatty foods and travel with these fats to reach the cells of the body. Fat-soluble vitamins are also stored in fatty tissues and in the liver. They are not easily eliminated from the body. Unused amounts of these vitamins can build up and cause harmful effects.

Box 8-1

Carbohydrates

Function—Provides the body's major source of energy

- Supplies fiber that contributes to good digestion and elimination
- Enables the body to use proteins and fats effectively
- Supplies other nutrients, such as vitamins and vegetable proteins

Description—Fruits, vegetables, and grains

- Sugars—simple and complex sugars
- Starches—the plant's food supply stored in roots, stems, and seeds
- Fiber—part of plants that act as bulk to help the digestive system function effectively

Examples of foods

Sugars	Starches	Fiber
Table sugar	Bread	Bran
Honey	Pasta	Nuts
Fruit	Rice	Seeds
Fruit juices	Grits	Popcorn
Dried fruits	Potatoes	Raw fruits with skins

Digestion—Begins in the mouth

- Carbohydrates are broken down more rapidly than proteins or fats; therefore, carbohydrates are a quicker source of energy

Amount Needed—Daily intake should be about 55% of food consumed

Energy Produced—Yields four calories per gram

From: Birchenall, JM, and Streight, ME: Health occupations, exploration and career planning, *St Louis, 1989, Mosby.*

Box 8-2

Proteins

Function—Builds and repairs body tissue

- Maintains healthy muscle
- Helps to defend the body against disease
- Promotes growth

Description—High-quality protein contains all nine essential amino acids

- Lower-quality protein does not contain all nine essential amino acids
- Therefore, these foods must be eaten with high-quality proteins to increase their effectiveness

Examples of foods

High Quality		Lower Quality	
Milk	Yogurt	Cereals	Taco shells
Meat	Cheese	Bread	Spaghetti
Fish	Eggs	Vegetables	Matzos
Poultry	Legumes		
	(dried beans and peas)		

Digestion—Begins in the stomach and is completed in the small intestine; while it is not a quick source of energy, protein intake is essential for energy production

Amount Needed—Daily intake should be about 15% of food consumed

Energy Produced—Yields four calories per gram

From: Birchenall, JM, and Streight, ME: Health occupations, exploration and career planning, St Louis, 1989, Mosby.

Box 8-3

Fats

Function—Provides a highly concentrated source of energy, more than twice the amount of carbohydrate or protein

- Carries fat-soluble vitamins—A, D, E, and K
- Essential for healthy skin and nervous system
- Holds vital organs in place and acts as a protection from injury
- Provides flavor to food and sense of satisfaction of fullness

Description—Fatty acids are either produced by the body or must come from foods (essential fatty acids)

- Essential fatty acids are in two categories— saturated and unsaturated.
- Saturated fats contain all the hydrogen possible and are solid at room temperature (Note: Cholesterol is a chemical in the blood, digestive juices, and tissue; it is found in saturated fats)
- Unsaturated fats contain less hydrogen and become liquid at room temperature

Examples of foods

Saturated Fat	Unsaturated Fat
Butter	Fish
Lard	Vegetable oil
Chocolate	Nuts
Lunch meat	Peanut butter

Digestion—Begins in the small intestine; fats are broken down slowly by action of bile and other enzymes in the small intestine; a high-fat diet will cause the stomach to empty more slowly

Amount Needed—Daily intake should be no more than 30% of food consumed

Energy Produced—Yields nine calories per gram

From: Birchenall, JM, and Streight, ME: Health occupations, exploration and career planning, St Louis, 1989, Mosby.

As the home care aide, you will be responsible for selecting nutritious foods and preparing meals for your client. Table 8-2 lists the major functions and food sources of vitamins A, D, E, and K. By using the information in this table, you will be able to select and prepare foods that supply natural forms of these important vitamins.

Water-soluble vitamins Vitamins B and C are dissolved by water in the cells of our bodies. Water-soluble vitamins cannot be stored. Excess amounts of these vitamins are eliminated from the body through urine and feces. When foods high in the B vitamins and vitamin C are cooked, some of the vitamins are lost through cooking water and heat.

Because these vitamins are not stored in our bodies, it is important to provide your client with foods rich in the B and C vitamins each day. Table 8-3 describes the functions of each vitamin and lists good food sources.

Taking Vitamins The best way to "take" vitamins is through a varied, well-balanced diet rich in natural sources of fat-soluble and water-soluble vitamins. Sometimes, because of poor appetite or other problems caused by illness, your client may not be receiving the desired amount of vitamins in food. When this happens, the physician may prescribe vitamin supplements to the diet.

Taking large doses of vitamins without medical supervision can produce harmful results and may interfere with the effectiveness of other medications being taken. So, the natural way of taking vitamins, through the food we eat, is the best way.

Minerals

Minerals are chemicals that come from water and the ground. Minerals become a part of the plant foods we eat because plants are nourished by soil, commercially prepared fertilizers, and water. Animal products are also good sources of minerals, since animals eat plants and consume water, too. Both plants and animal sources help us satisfy our needs for minerals.

Table 8-2

Fat-Soluble Vitamins

Vitamin	Major Functions	Food Source
Vitamin A	• Promotes growth • Prevents dry skin • Promotes good vision • Helps body resist infection	milk, liver, yellow and green leafy vegetables (carrots, sweet potatoes, spinach, greens), broccoli, and fruits (apricots and cantaloupe)
Vitamin D	• Keeps bones strong and healthy • Helps body absorb and use calcium and phosphorus	milk with vitamin D, fish oils, tuna fish, and salmon
Vitamin E	• Protects cells from harmful substances • Helps prevent cell destruction	vegetable oils, green leafy vegetables, and asparagus
Vitamin K	• Clots blood	green leafy vegetables, peas, green beans, and liver

Minerals are required in the daily diet for strong bones and teeth, nerve and muscle function, water balance, and other essential body functions. The best way to get adequate amounts of minerals is by eating a balanced diet of protein, carbohydrates, and fats. Taking mineral supplements without medical supervision is dangerous because of possible harmful reactions.

Table 8-4 lists the key minerals and their food sources.

Table 8-3

Water-Soluble Vitamins

Vitamin	Purpose	Food Source
Thiamin	• Promotes healthy nerves • Helps body use carbohydrates, proteins, and fats	pork products, whole grains and enriched grains, breads and cereals, organ meats
Riboflavin	• Keeps skin and mucous membranes healthy • Helps body use carbohydrates, proteins, and fats	milk and milk products, enriched breads and cereals, meats, and eggs
Niacin	• Keeps skin and gastrointestinal tract healthy • Helps body use carbohydrates, proteins, and fats	enriched breads and cereals, tuna and other fish, beef, chicken, and turkey
B-12	• Keeps nervous system healthy • Helps body use proteins	organ meats, oysters, clams, eggs, beef, pork
Vitamin C	• Helps to heal wounds • Promotes healthy teeth, gums, bones, and skin	citrus fruits, broccoli, strawberries

Table 8-4

Minerals

Mineral	Purpose	Food Source
Calcium	• Helps to strengthen bone and teeth • Helps in blood clotting • Helps muscles to function	milk, cheese, canned fish, yogurt, and tofu
Phosphorus	• Helps to strengthen bone and teeth	milk, cheese, eggs, and meat
Iron	• Carries oxygen in the blood	red meat, egg yolks, spinach, broccoli, seafood
Iodine	• Helps thyroid gland function	iodized salt, seafood, and shellfish
Sodium	• Transmits nerve impulses • Maintains body fluid balance	table salt and processed foods
Potassium	• Promotes healthy function of nerves and heart	bananas, orange juice, other fruits and vegetables and milk

dehydrated/dehydration
excessive water loss from body tissues resulting from not enough fluid intake.

Water

The human body is composed of about 60% water. Water is essential to life because it helps carry proteins, carbohydrates, fats, vitamins, and minerals to each cell. It also helps carry waste products to various organs to be excreted from the body. Water helps keep the body at a constant temperature.

The Body's Need for Water Adults can survive without eating food about eight weeks because they use the nutrients that have been stored in the body. But the body cannot store water. Therefore, we can survive only a few days without drinking water.

Fluid Balance A normal adult must consume four to six cups (1000–1500 milliliters) of water a day to maintain health. Besides drinking water, liquids such as milk, coffee, tea, juice, and soup also provide water. Other foods, including fruits and vegetables, supply additional water. The body also produces water when digestive juices are made to help break down food. The total amount of water taken into the body each day is almost 8 to 12 cups (2500 milliliters) from all sources. Because water cannot be stored, it is eliminated from the body in the form of urine, feces, perspiration, and in the air we exhale (Fig. 8-1 and Table 8-5).

The phrase *What goes in, must come out* is very true about water. For proper balance, the water we take in (intake) must be removed

Table 8-5

Examples of Intake and Output

Intake

- Liquids
    water
    coffee, tea, soda
    juices
    milk
    clear soup
- Fruits, vegetables
    grapefruit
    orange
    watermelon
    cucumbers
    tomatoes
- Digestive juices

Output

- Urine
- Feces
- Perspiration
- Respiration

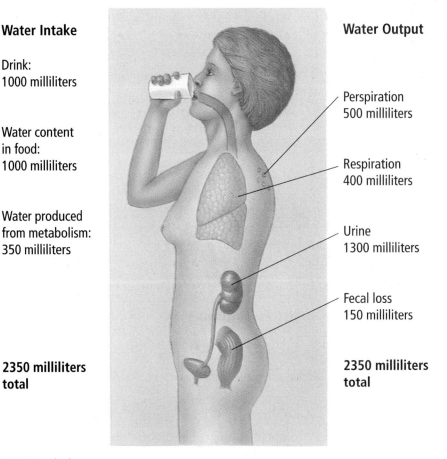

Water Intake

Drink:
1000 milliliters

Water content
in food:
1000 milliliters

Water produced
from metabolism:
350 milliliters

**2350 milliliters
total**

Water Output

Perspiration
500 milliliters

Respiration
400 milliliters

Urine
1300 milliliters

Fecal loss
150 milliliters

**2350 milliliters
total**

8-1 Water balance. *(From Wardlaw G, et al: Contemporary Nutrition: Issues and Insights, ed 2, 1994, St Louis, Mosby–Year Book, Inc.)*

(output). If enough water is not taken in, the person becomes **dehydrated,** and serious problems can occur if not treated immediately. If the output is much smaller than the intake, water has accumulated in body tissues (Fig. 8-2). In Chapter 14, procedures used to measure fluid intake and output will be discussed.

Dietary Fiber

Commonly called "roughage," dietary fiber produces bulk needed for proper elimination of solid waste products from the bowel. Dietary fibers are substances found in foods, such as wheat bran, citrus fruits, oat products, beans, and vegetables. They are parts of plant structures that absorb water. By holding water, dietary fiber helps to enlarge and soften feces. Therefore, elimination of feces becomes easier. A diet high in dietary fiber and adequate amounts of water helps prevent constipation.

Excellent sources of dietary fiber include kidney and lima beans, citrus fruits, cereals with wheat and oat brans, popped popcorn, dried figs, prunes and dates, corn, and baked potatoes with skins.

The Food Guide Pyramid

The U.S. Department of Agriculture has developed a food guide to assist us in planning a variety of nutritious meals each day. The Food Guide Pyramid gives the food groups and the number of servings needed for each (Fig. 8-3). Remember, food requirements depend upon the person's age and energy needs (Table 8-6). For example, an older adult who has little activity needs less calories than a growing, active teenager.

The Guide calls for most of the energy sources to come from carbohydrates—grains, fruits, and vegetables. Fats, oils, and sweets provide the least amount of nutrients but the largest amount of calories. They appear at the tip of the Pyramid and are to be used sparingly. By following the Food Guide Pyramid, the needs for all nutrients will be met. The following list is the plan for adults over the age of 25:

- Six to 11 servings from the Bread, Cereal, Rice, and Pasta Group
- Three to five servings from the Vegetable Group
- Two to four servings from the Fruit Group
- Two to three servings from the Milk, Yogurt, and Cheese Group
- Two to three servings from the Meat, Poultry, Fish, Dry Beans, Eggs, and Nuts Group

Note: For children, teenagers, pregnant women, nursing mothers, and adults under 25, the Food Guide Pyramid recommends three servings from the Milk, Yogurt, and Cheese Group. Box 8-4 lists the amount of different foods that equal one serving.

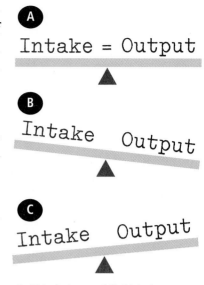

8-2 Variations of fluid balance. *A,* Fluid balance. *B,* Dehydration. *C,* Fluid accumulates in the body (retention).

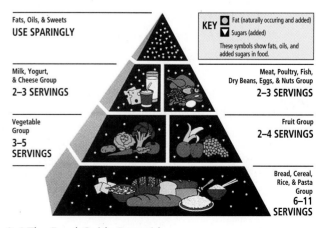

8-3 The Food Guide Pyramid.

Table 8-6

Amount of Servings Needed Daily

Calorie level*	Women and Some Older Adults about 1600	Children, Teen Girls, Active Women, Most Men about 2200	Teen Boys and Active Men about 2800
Bread group	6	9	11
Vegetable group	3	4	5
Fruit group	2	3	4
Milk group	2–3**	2–3**	2–3**
Meat group	2	2	3
	(for a total of 5 ounces)	(for a total of 6 ounces)	(for a total of 7 ounces)

These are the calorie levels if you choose low-fat, lean foods from the five major food groups and use foods from the fats and sweets group sparingly.

*** Women who are pregnant or breast-feeding, teenagers, and young adults to age 24 need three servings.*

Source: United States Department of Agriculture, 1992.

Box 8-4

What Is One Serving?

Bread, Cereal, Rice, and Pasta

- 1 slice of bread
- 3–4 crackers
- 1/2 cup cooked cereal
- 1 cup dry cereal
- 1/2 cup cooked rice or pasta

Fruit

- 1 melon wedge
- 1 medium size whole fruit
- 3/4 cup fruit juice
- 1/2 cup cooked or canned fruit
- 1/4 cup dried fruit (raisins, prunes, figs)

Vegetable

- 3/4 cup of vegetable juice
- 1 cup raw leafy vegetables
- 1/2 cup chopped or cut raw vegetables
- 1/2 cup cooked vegetables
- 1 small potato

Meat, Poultry, Fish, Dry Beans, Eggs, and Nuts

- 2 1/2–3 ounces cooked lean meat, poultry, or fish
- 1/2 cup cooked dry beans
- 1 egg
- 2 tablespoons peanut butter
- 1/2 cup nuts

Milk, Yogurt, and Cheese

- 1 cup milk
- 1 1/2 ounces natural cheese
- 2 ounces processed cheese
- 2 cups cottage cheese
- 1 cup yogurt

Fats and Sweets

- Use sparingly

Planning the Menu Using the Food Guide Pyramid

So far, you know the food sources of proteins, carbohydrates, fats, vitamins, minerals, dietary fiber, and the value of water in the diet. You know the food groups of the Pyramid. The next step is to put this information into practical use. When planning your client's menus, consider the following:

- *Food preferences*—
  know the likes and dislikes of the person
- *Meal patterns*—
  know when main meal and lighter meals and snacks are usually eaten
- *Variety*—
  select different foods within each food group every day for variety in flavors, textures, colors, and shapes
- *Moderation*—
  use fats, oils, and sweets sparingly
- *Balance*—
  choose foods from each of the groups according to the requirements of the Pyramid
- *Fluids*—
  meet the needs for adequate fluid intake: a minimum of four to six cups (1000–1500 milliliters) a day

Before planning the menu, discuss food likes and dislikes with your client. This is important to know so that you include foods that the client likes to eat. The most successful menu is one that the client enjoys eating and also provides the necessary nutrients. You can plan a good, nutritionally balanced meal; but, if the client doesn't eat it, your work has been in vain. Some clients prefer to eat the main meal in the evening. Others are used to having this meal at noon. Perhaps some prefer a lighter breakfast with snacks in mid-morning and mid-afternoon. Plan according to these preferences, too (Fig. 8-4).

Choosing foods from all the groups provides that balance of nutrients so necessary for good nutrition. Varying the foods within each group allows for different tastes, textures, and colors. Variety helps to make each meal more interesting, attractive, and less boring to the client.

Many of your clients will have well-established food habits. For example, Mr. Humphrey has eaten the same food for breakfast for the past 25 years—two cups of coffee and a doughnut. This food habit will be very difficult to change—perhaps impossible. Your challenge is to add foods for the remaining meals, including snacks, to make up for the lack of a well-balanced breakfast.

Planning the menu to include adequate amounts of fluid is essential for good health. Some clients prefer to drink fluids with the meal. But others will tell you that they

☑ Food Preferences
☑ Meal Patterns
☑ Variety
☑ Moderation
☑ Balance
☑ Fluids

8-4 Planning the menu involves many factors.

become too full and can't finish their food if fluids are served during the meal. Be sure to provide water, milk, fruit juices, and other fluids during the day to meet the daily fluid requirement of four to six cups.

Table 8-7 gives a meal plan for a day using the Food Guide Pyramid for an adult with no dietary limitations.

Shopping for Food

The home care aide may do the food shopping, if the client cannot and there is no one else to assume this responsibility. Assisting the client to shop may be part of the care plan. You may go to the market alone or you might be taking the client to the market. Whatever the case, be sure that you understand and follow the policy of your agency regarding handling clients' money and transporting clients in cars. This is very important because you and the agency could be held legally responsible if there are any losses, injuries, or accidents involving you and the client. Be sure that you follow rules and regulations of the agency.

Table 8-7

Meal Plan for a Day Using Food Guide Pyramid

Breakfast	Serving	Group
Orange juice	3/4 cup	1 Fruit
Dry cereal—plain	3/4 cup	1 Bread, cereal
Milk—1%	1/2 cup	1/2 Milk, yogurt
Raisin toast	1 slice	1 Bread, cereal
Margarine	1 teaspoon	1 Fats, oils
Coffee	1 cup	
Mid-morning		
Water	1 cup	

Lunch

Turkey sandwich		
whole wheat bread	2 slices	2 Bread, cereal
sliced turkey breast	2 ounces	1 Meat
mayonnaise	1 teaspoon	1 Fats, oil
Carrot sticks	1/2 cup	1 Vegetable
Apple—medium size	1	1 Fruit
Water	1 cup	

Afternoon Snack

Crackers—whole grain	3–4 small	1 Bread
Cheese	1 1/2 ounces	1 Milk, cheese
Milk	1/2 cup	1/2 Milk

Dinner	Serving	Group
Broiled flounder	3 ounces	1 Meat
Broccoli, cooked	1/2 cup	1 Vegetable
Rice	1/2 cup	1 Bread
Tomato and lettuce salad		
lettuce, shredded	1 cup	1 Vegetable
tomato	1/2 cup	1 Vegetable
oil and vinegar dressing		1 Fats, oil
Sliced peaches	1/2 cup	1 Fruit
Tea		1 cup

Evening Snack

Pudding	1 cup	1 Milk

Totals for the Day		Recommended Totals
Bread Group	6	6–11 servings
Fruit Group	3	2–4 servings
Vegetables Group	3	3–5 servings
Meat Group	2	2–3 servings
Milk Group	3	2–3 servings
Fats Group	4 teaspoons	sparingly
Fluids	5 3/4	4–6 cups (1000 to 1500 milliliters)

Think of food shopping as a challenge. Your goal will be to get the most for your client's money by:

- purchasing the best quality, most healthful foods
- staying within the food budget

Prepare Shopping List

Preparation for shopping begins with menu planning and preparing a shopping list. Each time you use up an item, write it on a list. This way there is a continuing record of what is needed. Keep the list in the same place, and encourage your client to use it when possible. On marketing day, rewrite the list to include:

- items needed and replaced frequently, such as milk, soap, toilet tissue, etc.
- sale items listed in newspaper advertisements and supermarket circulars
- items needed because of dietary needs or restrictions, such as sugar substitute, low-sodium or low-fat foods

Try to write the list according to the layout of the store, so you won't waste time and energy running all over the market. The time allotted for shopping may be limited, so do the job quickly and thoroughly. Use the list so you won't forget anything your client needs. Coupons can help to save money. Keep these with the market list.

Read Labels

Read the label to help you choose foods that can be used to make up a healthful diet. For example, too much saturated fat and cholesterol can increase the level of cholesterol in the blood (a risk for heart disease). Large amounts of sodium can increase the risk for high blood pressure. A food label (Fig. 8-5) may give several types of information, including:

- **Open dates.** This helps to determine the freshness of the food. There are three commonly used dates (Fig. 8-5):
  1. **Sell by…** This is the last recommended date of sale. Most products will keep about three days beyond the date stamped.
  2. **Best if used by…** This is the last date that the manufacturer will guarantee full freshness and quality.
  3. **Expiration date…** This is the last date the product can be safely used. The date appears after the statement, "Do not use after (date)."

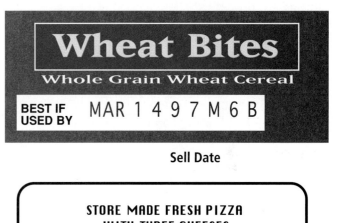

128 P1007C
EXP JUN .26
Expiration Date

Wheat Bites
Whole Grain Wheat Cereal

BEST IF USED BY   MAR 1 4 9 7 M 6 B

Sell Date

STORE MADE FRESH PIZZA WITH THREE CHEESES

HIGH GLUTEN FLOUR, YEAST, SALT, WATER,,
SUGAR, TOMATOES, PEPPER, GARLIC
SEASONINGS,
MOZZARELLA PROVOLONE PARMESAN
HEATING INSTS PRE HEAT OVEN 400DEGREES
PLACE ON PAN OR FOIL

HEAT FOR FIFTEEN MINUTES

SLICE & ENJOY

[USE IMMEDIATELY OR FREEZE]

NET WEIGHT 1 PD 4 OZ

| PACKED ON May 28, 97 | | SELL BY Jun 01, 97 |
| NET WT/CT | UNIT PRICE | TOTAL PRICE $2.50 |

KEEP REFRIGERATED

Freshness Date

8-5 Food labels.

Wheat Crackers

INGREDIENTS: ENRICHED WHEAT FLOUR CONTAINING NIACIN, REDUCED IRON, THIAMINE MONONITRATE (VITAMIN B1) AND RIBOFLAVIN (VITAMIN B2), VEGETABLE SHORTENING (PARTIALLY HYDROGENATED SOYBEAN AND COTTONSEED OILS), GRAHAM FLOUR, SUGAR, TOASTED WHOLE WHEAT, SESAME SEEDS, SALT, CORN SYRUP, LEAVENING (SODIUM BICARBONATE, SODIUM ACID PYROPHOSPHATE, MONOCALCIUM PHOSPHATE), DEHYDRATED ONIONS, MALT, WHEY, ARTIFICIAL COLOR.

Bitesize Wheat Cereal

Ingredients: Whole wheat, sugar, sorbitol, gelatin, Vitamins and Minerals: iron, niacinamide, zinc oxide, pyridoxine hydrachloride,(vitamin B6), riboflavin (vitamin B2), thiamin hydrochloride (vitamin B1) folic acid and vitamin B12. To maintain quality, BHT has been added to the packaging.

Pink Grapefruit Juice Cocktail

Ingredients: Pink Grapefruit Juice from Concentrate, Filtered Water, High Fructose Corn Syrup, Pectin, Citric Acid, Natural Grapefruit Flavor, Vitamin C (Ascorbic Acid), Canthaxanthin (Color).

8-6 Contents labels.

Serving size —

Calories from serving —

Nutrients In each serving:

Fat

Carbohy-drates

Proteins

Vitamins

Minerals

Nutrition Facts	
Serving Size 1 packet (35g)	
Servings Per Container 10	
Amount Per Serving	
Calories 130 Calories from Fat 15	
	% Daily Value*
Total Fat 1.5g	2%
Saturated Fat 0.5g	3%
Polyunsaturated Fat 0.5g	
Monounsaturated Fat 0.5g	
Cholesterol 0mg	0%
Sodium 105mg	4%
Total Carbohydrate 26g	9%
Dietary Fiber 3g	11%
Soluble Fiber 1g	
Sugars 11g	
Protein 4g	
Vitamin A	15%
Vitamin C	0%
Calcium	15%
Iron	30%
Thiamin	20%
Riboflavin	10%
Niacin	15%
Vitamin B6	20%
Folate	20%

* Percent Daily Values are based on a 2,000 calorie diet. Your daily values may be higher or lower depending on your calorie needs:

	Calories:	2,000	2,500
Total Fat	Less than	65g	80g
Sat Fat	Less than	20g	25g
Cholesterol	Less than	300mg	300mg
Sodium	Less than	2,400mg	2,400mg
Total Carbohydrate		300g	375g
Dietary Fiber		25g	30g

More nutrients may be listed on some labels

— Calories from fat

Percent of daily value listed for vitamins and minerals to meet daily requirements

g = grams (about 28g = 1 ounce)
mg = milligram (1000mg = 1 gram)

8-7 A Nutrition Facts label.

- *Contents.* This label is found on processed foods and lists the ingredients in the product (Fig. 8-6). The contents are listed in descending order. That is, the first ingredient listed is present in the largest amount. For example, an orange juice container label only lists one ingredient—orange juice—while the label for orange drink lists water, high fructose syrup, citric acid, and orange juice.
- *Nutrition facts.* This label contains nutrition information and is required on almost all packaged foods. This information can be used to help in planning a healthy diet. Fig. 8-7 shows a nutrition label and how to read it. Terms used on food labels are defined in Box 8-5.
- *Size of product.* This label tells the total amount of the product you are purchasing. For example, five pounds of potatoes, 500 napkins, one dozen eggs.

Compare Prices

There are several ways to compare prices. Most supermarkets display **unit prices** on the shelf above or below the products for sale. The unit price will vary. Items may be priced according to:

- *weight,* as coffee by the pound, or sugar by the kilogram
- *volume,* as milk by the quart or soda by the liter
- *count,* as tea bags by the hundred or toilet tissue by the sheet

Check prices by comparing cost, unit for unit, according to what amount has been posted on the supermarket shelf. Also, check the ingredients in the product. When buying frozen meals, compare the serving size and the contents.

Box 8-5

Food Label Terms

Terms used on the food label must meet the definitions established by the U.S. Food and Drug Administration:

- **Light or lite**—One third fewer calories or 50% less fat per serving than the regular product
- **Low fat**—Three grams of fat or less per serving
- **Fat free**—Less than one gram of fat per serving
- **Low cholesterol**—20 milligrams or less of cholesterol and two grams or less of saturated fat per serving
- **Cholesterol free**—Less than two milligrams of cholesterol and two grams or less of saturated fat per serving
- **Low calorie**—40 calories or less per serving
- **Calorie free**—Less than five calories per serving
- **Reduced or less sodium**—At least 25% less per serving than the regular product
- **Light in sodium**—Less than 50% of sodium in regular product per serving
- **Low sodium**—140 milligrams or less of sodium per serving
- **Very low sodium**—35 milligrams or less of sodium per serving
- **Sodium free**—Less than 5 milligrams of sodium per serving
- **High fiber**—Five grams of fiber or more
- **Good source**—serving contains 10% to 19% of daily value for a particular nutrient
- **High in**—Serving has 20% or more of daily value

Buying in quantity can be very economical. But this isn't always practical for clients who live alone. They may not be able to use or store large quantities of food.

Buy food in its "original" form. Usually, the more a food is processed, the greater the cost. Do most of your shopping in the "outside aisles" of the supermarket for fresh and frozen foods.

Shop for Freshness

Try to buy foods that are "in season": such as apples in the fall, berries in the spring and summer. Today, we are able to buy produce grown in other countries—foods that are "in season" in another part of the world. When these products are "on special" at the market, they are usually fresh and a good buy.

Farmers' markets and "green grocers" offer freshly picked produce right from the grower. This is an opportunity to obtain the freshest fruits and vegetables available.

unit prices
a method of pricing food.

When shopping at the supermarket, always check the dates on food before making a purchase. Also, check the appearance of the food. Does it look and smell fresh? Frozen foods should be solid, and refrigerated foods should be cold. Purchase refrigerated and frozen foods last to prevent warming and thawing.

When you shop, include some food from each of the groups found in the Food Guide Pyramid.

Returning to the Client's Home

Be certain that you have the market receipt, the correct change, and the marketing list. You will give these to your client as a record of your purchases and expenditures. Keep records in the same place, and always follow your agency's procedures regarding client's money and receipts.

Food Storage

Proper storage is essential to maintain the quality and the safety of food. Meat, poultry, and fish must be refrigerated or frozen until used. Thaw in the refrigerator or microwave, never at room temperature. Recommended storage times are different for each product. Quality cannot be maintained if foods are improperly stored. For example, if the bag inside a cereal box is not closed tightly, the product becomes limp and soggy, and the quality is poor. Try to use items before the expiration date. Some recommendations about storage are listed in Table 8-8.

Preparing Food

Your goal in preparing food is to promote the client's nutrition according to the care plan. Certainly, you want to prepare food that the client is able to eat and that will be enjoyable. Color, flavor, and variety make a meal appealing to see, smell, and taste. Use cooking methods that will preserve color and taste, as well as vitamins and minerals. Don't add unnecessary and unwanted ingredients, such as

Table 8-8

Food Storage Guidelines

Freezer—temperature 0° F	Refrigerator—temperature 34–40° F at all times	Pantry
• Use moisture-proof wrap; label and date all packages	• Wrap perishable foods to prevent mingling of tastes and odors	• Use cool, dry storage areas; avoid damp and hot locations
• Keep a list of freezer contents; any foods stored beyond appropriate time (quality and safety may be questionable) should be discarded	• Wrap raw meat loosely	• Date packages not already dated
	• Refrigerate leftovers immediately; wrap tightly to prevent drying; use within 2–3 days	• Keep foods in moisture-proof containers (except for fresh produce)
• Foods should not be stored any longer than one month beyond recommended time	• Keep eggs cold; store inside refrigerator, not on the door	• If pests are a problem, store dry goods (cereal, pasta, etc.) in glass or heavy plastic storage containers

large quantities of salt, sugar, and fats. Try to offer variety in the meals, as no one wants to eat the same thing every day. If the choice of available foods is limited, try to vary the methods of preparation. Potatoes can be baked, mashed, boiled, or fried. They can be served hot, cold, and in stews and soups. The use of the same food each day does not have to be boring. Table 8-9 offers some suggestions for choosing healthy foods.

Table 8-9

Smart Food Choices

Breads, Cereals, Rice, and Pasta Group

- Choose whole grain breads and flour
- Use cereals where sugar is listed on the label as a third ingredient or lower
- Do not add salt to cooking water for pasta and rice
- Avoid creamed sauces on pastas and large amounts of butter or margarine on bread

Fruits and Vegetables

- Eat fruits without sugar or whipped toppings
- The best choice is whole fruit; then choose fruit juice over fruit drink or soda
- Steam or microwave fresh vegetables; season with herbs, pepper, or lemon juice
- To boost fiber, leave skin on potatoes, tomatoes, apples, pears, and peaches

Milk, Yogurt, and Cheese

- Use skim or 1% milk
- Replace cream in recipes with evaporated milk
- Nonfat yogurt is a good substitute for sour cream
- Limit high-fat cheeses (cheddar, American, Swiss, and cream)
- Use small amounts of sharp cheese as flavoring
- Select nonfat cottage cheese

Meat, Poultry, Fish, Dry Beans, Eggs, and Nuts

- Serve 3-ounce portions (the size of a deck of cards)
- Use cooking methods that let the fat drain away—grilling, broiling, roasting, and baking; trim fat from meats and remove skin from poultry before cooking
- Select lean cuts of meat
- Limit breaded and fried chicken and seafood
- Use ground turkey instead of ground beef
- Limit:
  organ meats (liver)—high in cholesterol
  smoked fish—high in sodium
  eggs to 3–4 per week—high in cholesterol
  lunch meats, cold cuts, hot dogs, and sausage—high in sodium and fat

Fats, Oils, and Sweets

- Limit intake
- Always use oils by the level teaspoon
- Use nonstick cooking sprays
- Select fat-free and reduced-calorie salad dressings
- Try herb vinegars and lemon juice on salads instead of salad dressing
- Use jams and jellies (if allowed) instead of butter

Frozen and Canned Foods

- Read labels and select products with less than 400 calories, 800 milligrams sodium, and 15 grams of fat
- When serving a frozen dinner, add a green salad, fresh fruit, and skim milk for a complete meal
- Frozen yogurt and ice milk are lower in fat than premium ice creams
- Avoid canned soups that are high in fat and sodium

The agency staff dietitian will be able to help you with special dietary needs for your clients.

bacteria
microorganisms causing disease.

Food Safety

Over the past few years, the number of deaths caused by harmful **bacteria** in meat and poultry has been steadily rising. Because of this, the U.S. Department of Agriculture developed rules regarding the safe handling and cooking of meat and poultry.

Labels on uncooked meat and poultry outline four steps for safety of meat and poultry:

1. Store properly (as discussed earlier in this chapter).
2. Avoid cross contamination by keeping raw meats and poultry separate from other foods. Wash all work surfaces (including cutting boards), utensils, and hands after touching raw meat or poultry.
3. Cook thoroughly. Meat and poultry should be fully cooked. Hamburgers should not be pink on the interior.
4. Keep hot foods hot and cold foods cold until serving. Refrigerate leftovers immediately or discard.

Always wash your hands thoroughly with warm water and soap before you begin meal preparation. If you are interrupted—to give client care, answer the phone, blow your nose, whatever—wash your hands <u>AGAIN</u> before resuming your food duties (see Chapter 9—Hand Washing).

Serving the Food

Before serving the meal, help your client to use the toilet, commode, or bed pan and to wash his/her hands. Make sure the bed pan or urinal is stored properly after use. Assist with oral hygiene (Chapter 13) if appropriate.

The food should be attractively arranged on the plate. Try not to serve foods that are all one color, such as white fish, white potatoes, and white cauliflower. This is not appealing to the eye. Carrots or green beans instead of cauliflower would liven up the appearance of the dish. Try your best to make things look good. Set the table with the proper utensils. If your client uses adaptive eating utensils, such as a plate guard or built up silverware (Fig. 8-8), place these properly and within easy use. Cut the food and assist the client as required. Encourage the client to be as independent as possible.

If your client stays in bed, take the food to him/her on a tray. You can substitute a baking sheet for a tray or cut a cardboard box to make a tray (Fig. 8-9). Set the tray as you would set the table. Don't forget napkins. Use several napkins or paper towels because it is not easy to eat in bed and be neat.

Feeding the Client

If your client is unable to feed himself/herself, assist with feeding. See Procedure 8-1—Feeding the Client.

Special Situations

Many clients have problems eating because of missing teeth or illness resulting in poor appetite or trouble swallowing. Some clients are so tired that they just do not have the energy to eat. These situations pro-

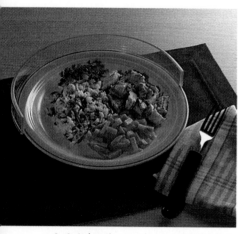

8-8 Adaptive eating utensils and plateguard. *(Courtesy S & S Worldwide, Colchester, Conn.)*

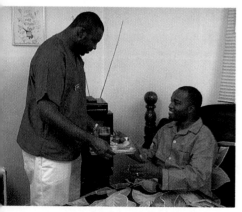

8-9 A cookie sheet can be substituted for a tray.

Procedure 8-1

Feeding the Client

Materials Needed

- Utensils: knife, fork, spoon
- Dishes, bowls, cup, glass
- Napkins (2)
- Towel or bib
- Straws
- Adaptive supplies:
    Plate guard
    Special utensils
    Universal cup holder
    Bed tray

Procedure

1. Explain what you are going to do.
2. Wash your hands.
3. Obtain materials listed above.
4. Prepare client for mealtime:
   - Offer to assist with toileting
   - Offer to assist client to wash hands
   - Position client to sit up
     - in bed
     - in a chair
   - Place table or bed tray over client's lap so he/she can see and reach the food
5. Drape napkin across client's chest and under the chin.
6. Serve food on tray, if needed.
7. Sit near the client.
8. Explain what is being served.
9. Cut food, butter bread, pour and prepare liquids as needed.
10. Ask the client what he/she would like to eat first.
11. Encourage client to do as much self-feeding as possible.
12. Feed client one bite at a time. Use a spoon and fill only half full according to ability to chew and swallow.
13. Alternate solids and liquids. Use a straw for drinking.
14. Talk pleasantly with client and encourage him/her to eat. Offer praise.
15. When client is finished, wipe client's mouth and then remove tray (if used).
16. Wash client's hands and face. Remove napkin or bib.
17. Offer oral hygiene.
18. Make sure client is safe and comfortable.
19. Note amount eaten and record in care plan according to percent of food consumed (100% =all; 50% = half).
20. Wash your hands.
21. Wash dishes and utensils used for meal.
22. Clean and straighten kitchen.

vide opportunities for the home care aide to adjust the menu or method of food preparation so that the client is more likely to eat. A client with many missing teeth will probably not be able to eat a raw apple. By adjusting the menu to substitute applesauce, one of the requirements of the food group of the Pyramid will be met.

The client who is blind may or may not require adjustments to the menu or method of food preparation. But this person will need to know where foods are placed on the plate in order to select what to eat.

Poor Appetite

Mrs. DiMattia has just returned home from the hospital following gallbladder surgery. She says that they removed her appetite at the same time they removed her gallbladder! Looking at the big plate of food makes her "sick."

anorexia
loss of appetite

The term used to describe a loss of appetite is **anorexia.** There are many reasons for this complaint. The illness itself, medical treatments such as cancer therapies, worry, anxiety, or fear can result in lack of interest in eating. Box 8-6 gives some advice for preparing and serving foods for clients with poor appetites.

Difficulty Chewing and Swallowing

The home care aide's client, Mr. Carver, is 89 years old and has no teeth. His daughter insists that he wear the full set of dentures that has just been repaired to fit properly. But when his daughter leaves the apartment, Mr. Carver takes out the dentures and refuses to wear them.

Difficulty chewing can be caused by many factors, as in the case of Mr. Carver. Poorly fitting dentures, missing teeth, or a sore mouth can make chewing very difficult. Also, chewing takes a lot of energy. Clients whose illnesses result in low energy levels may find chewing to be exhausting.

The act of swallowing is a complex process that requires coordination of the nerves and muscles of the throat. Saliva helps lubricate food so that swallowing takes place without effort. When clients do not produce enough saliva or have illnesses that affect nerves and muscles of the throat, swallowing becomes difficult. The speech therapist may teach your client techniques to help improve swallowing. Your encouragement to use these techniques is important. Box 8-7 gives information about ways to plan and prepare meals for the client who has difficulty chewing or swallowing.

Clients With Low Energy Levels

Mr. Fong has great difficulty breathing. "I have such a hard time breathing that I haven't any strength to do anything else."

For clients whose illnesses cause severe fatigue to occur, energy must be conserved so that activities of daily living, like eating, can be performed with as little effort as possible. Drinking, chewing, and swallowing require a lot of energy. Lifting a fork or cup, reaching for the salt shaker—these actions take energy to perform. Usually, the morning

Box 8-6

The Client With Poor Appetite

- Make meals attractive, colorful
- Offer small meals and snacks frequently
- Select foods and snacks high in nutrients and calories
- Prepare snacks in advance and have them readily available
- Avoid foods high in fat, which can cause a feeling of fullness
- Give high calorie liquids in place of plain water or diet soda
- Serve foods at desired temperature—may need to be cool or warm rather than cold or hot

- Give liquids 30–60 minutes before a meal rather than with a meal, which fills stomach quickly
- Provide companionship while client is eating if he/she is alone
- Do not force foods; if a food is not appealing today, try it again another day
- Serve the same foods each day if the client wants to eat them
- Record and report unusual difficulties in eating to your supervisor

hours are best for clients with low energy because energy reserves are at their highest point. Therefore, breakfast may become the best meal of the day.

Other helpful hints for the low-energy client are listed in Box 8-8.

The Blind Client

Mohammed has been blind since birth. He can feed himself, but he says, "I like to eat all my vegetables first, then the rest of the food."

Box 8-7

The Client with Difficulty Chewing and Swallowing

Chewing

- Select ground meats—beef, turkey, lamb, ham
- Include high-calorie, high-protein drinks
- Prepare foods such as eggs, fish, and cheese for sources of high protein
- Use food processor or blender to soften or puree food
- Include soups or puddings
- Cut food in small pieces
- High fiber foods (vegetables, bran cereals) must be soft
- Be patient with client; don't rush

Swallowing

- Have client sit upright, slightly forward, with chin tilted down, if condition permits
- Have client lower the chin during the swallowing process
- Select foods with similar textures for ease in chewing and swallowing—thick, soft foods are easier to swallow
- Thicken liquids to ease swallowing process
  - Add commercially available thickening agents to hot liquids
  - Add gelatin to cold liquids
- Have client remain in sitting position for 20–30 minutes following the meal
- Record and report unusual difficulties in eating to your supervisor

---

Box 8-8

The Client With Low Energy Levels

- Allow plenty of time to eat
- Encourage a rest period for about $1/2$ hour before and after eating
- Serve small meals at least six times a day
- Select foods high in nutrient value
- Select foods that do not require a lot of chewing
- Use blender to puree food
- Provide a straw to eliminate the need to lift cup or glass
- Cut food into small pieces
- Butter the bread; pour liquids
- Assist with feeding as needed
- Prepare nutritious drinks, such as milk shakes
- Use liquid dietary supplements, if ordered by the doctor
- Prepare foods in advance that can be served without delay
- Use the microwave, if available, to reduce time spent in cooking or reheating foods
- Use cups, glasses, and eating utensils that are light and easy to handle; place each within easy reach
- Record and report unusual difficulties in eating to your supervisor

Mealtime can be a pleasant experience for your blind client if you take the following steps:

- Explain where foods are on the plate; describe the plate as a clock; "the broccoli is at 3 o'clock, the baked flounder is at 6 o'clock, and the mashed potatoes are at 9 o'clock."
- Keep utensils, napkin, cup, glass, salt shaker, etc., in the same location on the table or tray.
- Avoid the urge to "help" the client unless he/she requests your assistance.

Special Diets to Meet Special Needs

Treatment of the client's illness may include changes in the diet. This is called nutritional therapy. In combination with other types of treatment—such as medications, physical therapy, and speech therapy—nutritional therapy contributes to the client's recovering process.

The type of diet ordered by the doctor depends upon the nutritional needs of the client. Perhaps there are problems with the way the food is digested or absorbed. Or the body requires increased amounts of certain nutrients so that the healing of tissues can take place. Nutritional therapy is an important part of the client's overall plan of care.

Modifying the Diet

The Food Guide Pyramid forms the foundation for modifying the diet to meet the client's needs. In fact, the diet ordered by the doctor should be as similar as possible to the client's regular diet. Changes may need to be made in the frequency of meals, the quantity of certain types of foods, and/or the texture or digestibility of the foods consumed. The dietitian meets with the client and family to discuss the client's food preferences and explain the dietary changes needed. The dietitian will also answer questions concerning food selection, preparation, and serving. When teaching the client and family about the modifications needed, the dietitian considers food preferences, existing diet, cultural and religious requirements, budget, and kitchen facilities available.

Your Role in Nutritional Therapy

Nutritional therapy is an important part of the care plan. Your responsibility is to prepare meals according to the diet plan. Because you will visit the client more frequently than other staff members, you can observe and record information about how the diet is being tolerated. Accurate record keeping of the food eaten and fluids consumed is very important. The dietitian may need to visit again to review the diet modifications. Table 8-10 provides information about therapeutic diets frequently used for clients. Remember, the food groups of the Pyramid form the foundation for each of the diets listed. The kinds of foods selected or the method of food preparation will vary according to the specific diet.

Table 8-10

Therapeutic Diets

Name	Purpose	Foods
Regular	Provide all nutrients	*Include:* All food groups of Pyramid. *Avoid:* None.
Soft	Provide foods that are easy to chew, swallow, and digest	*Include:* All food groups of Pyramid that have been strained, chopped, and/or pureed. *Avoid:* High-fiber foods, seeds.
Bland	Promote easy digestion and avoid irritation to digestive system	*Include:* All food groups of Pyramid. *Avoid:* Highly seasoned foods, pepper, coffee, alcohol, high-fiber foods, seeds.
High Calorie	Increase caloric intake	*Include:* All food groups of Pyramid. Add nourishing snacks with high nutrient and caloric value, such as milk shakes. *Avoid:* None.
Low Calorie	Decrease caloric intake	*Include:* All food groups of Pyramid. Choose high-nutrient, low-fat foods: skim milk, yogurt, fresh fruits and vegetables, lean meats. *Avoid:* Foods high in fat, sodas, fried foods, beer, gravies.
Sodium Restricted	Limit sodium intake	*Include:* All food groups of Pyramid. Choose fresh fruits and vegetables, but limit cheese, milk, bakery bread. *Avoid:* Table and cooking salts, lunch meat, bacon, canned vegetables and soups, salted butter and margarine, commercially prepared frozen dinners.
Diabetic	Regulate the amount of carbohydrates in the diet	*Include:* All food groups of Pyramid but use lists of food called "Exchange Lists" (available from the agency's dietitian). *Avoid:* Table sugar, honey, carbonated sodas, alcoholic beverages.
Low Residue	Limit the amount of residue in the colon after digestion and absorption of food occurs	*Include:* All food groups of Pyramid. Milk, refined bread, canned or cooked fruit, and vegetable juices. *Avoid:* Whole grain breads and cereals; potato skins, corn, fried foods, seeds, and nuts.
High residue	Increase the amount of residue in the colon to stimulate peristalsis	*Include:* All food groups of Pyramid. Whole grain breads and cereals, fruits, vegetables, and high-fiber foods such as popped corn. *Avoid:* None.
Low Fat	Limit the amount of fat in the diet	*Include:* All food groups of Pyramid. Skim milk, lean meat, fish and poultry, low-fat cottage cheese, fruits, and vegetables. *Avoid:* Fried foods, cooking oil, cheese, butter, margarine, ice cream, salad dressings, eggs, gravies, bacon, lunch meat, and avocados.
Low Cholesterol	Reduce the amount of cholesterol in the blood	*Include:* All food groups of Pyramid. Skim milk, lean meat, fish, poultry, fruits, and vegetables. *Avoid:* Foods and fats that come from animals, such as liver, bacon and bacon fat, egg yolks, butter, cheese, mayonnaise, sour cream, and ice cream.

No matter what type of diet your client receives, balance, variety, and moderation are keys to healthy eating. The following tips can help you to provide good nutrition for your client:

- Serve a variety of nutrient-rich foods
- Use the Food Guide Pyramid as a reference in meal planning
- Serve whole grains, fruits, and vegetables according to diet requirements
- Offer moderate portions of food
- Avoid too much sugar and sodium
- Encourage adequate fluid intake
- Avoid too much fat, saturated fat, and cholesterol

CHAPTER SUMMARY

- Good nutrition is an important part of maintaining health.
- Many factors influence food selection—likes and dislikes, culture, religion, physical condition, income.
- Foods are classified as carbohydrates, proteins, fats:
  - Carbohydrates include sugars, starches, and fiber
  - Milk, meat, eggs, and legumes are good sources of protein
  - Fats are found in butter, oils, nuts, and chocolate
- Vitamins and minerals must be consumed daily for good health.
- Water is essential for life; the normal adult must drink four to six cups of water each day.
- Fiber helps to promote proper bowel function.
- The Food Guide Pyramid is a resource for meal planning.
- The home care aide may be responsible for the client's food shopping.
- Prepare foods according to recommendations included in this chapter; proper food handling and storage are essential to maintaining the quality and safety of food.
- Follow agency policy regarding client's money, expense receipts, travel, and transportation of clients.
- Assist client to eat according to the care plan and the client's individual needs.
- Nutritional therapy is an important part of the care plan; prepare meals according to this plan.

STUDY QUESTIONS

1. How does good nutrition help to maintain health and prevent illness?

2. List three factors that influence individual and family food habits.

3. From the foods listed below, identify which are good sources of carbohydrate, protein, or fat:

orange juice	butter	milk
oatmeal	carrots	olive oil
turkey	hamburger	flounder
bacon	bread	potato chips
bagel	cream cheese	yogurt
ice cream	strawberries	tuna fish

4. Prepare a chart listing the vitamins and minerals. Include their functions and three food sources of each.

5. Explain why water and dietary fiber are needed in the diet each day.

6. Plan a weekly menu using the Food Guide Pyramid.

7. Using the weekly menu, prepare the shopping list. Discuss with your classmates.

8. Describe storage of
   a. fresh ground beef
   b. dry boxed cereal
   c. leftover turkey
   d. eggs

9. Review your agency's written policies regarding
   a. handling clients' money
   b. traveling and transporting clients

10. Describe the step-by-step procedure for feeding clients.

11. Describe what you would do for clients who have difficulty chewing and swallowing.

12. Identify foods to be included or avoided for the following therapeutic diets:
    a. Sodium restricted
    b. Diabetic
    c. High residue
    d. Bland
    e. Low cholesterol

9 Preventing Infection/Medical Asepsis

Objectives

After you read this chapter, you will be able to:

1. Discuss microorganisms, pathogens, and nonpathogens.

2. Describe the cycle of infection.

3. Identify four ways infection can be spread.

4. Discuss the terms *medical asepsis, surgical asepsis,* and *universal precautions.*

5. Demonstrate correct practice of universal precautions in a client's home.

6. Demonstrate correct hand-washing technique.

7. Apply nonsterile gloves and remove contaminated gloves.

8. Describe the importance of following CDC and OSHA regulations about blood-borne pathogens.

9. Understand methods of disinfection in the home.

10. Demonstrate correct use of mask and moisture-resistant gown or apron.

The Waters' twins came home from kindergarten coughing and sneezing. They had no appetite, complained about runny, sore noses, and felt hot and sick. Their mother took their temperatures, called the doctor, and followed instructions for treating their symptoms.

The twins were home from school for several days. Grandma Waters took care of the children while their parents went to work.

About a week later, Grandpa Waters began to cough, sneeze, and have a runny nose. "It's all your fault," he told his wife. "You brought those darned germs home, and now I feel awful."

Infection occurs when harmful organisms enter the body and grow, causing illness or disease. Microorganisms are small living plants or animals that can only be seen through a microscope. Even though we cannot see them, they are everywhere—on our skin, under the nails, on clothing, in food, in water, and in the air we breathe. Animals and insects also carry microorganisms (Fig. 9-1).

Microorganisms

Many microorganisms are **nonpathogenic,** meaning that they do not usually produce an infection. Some nonpathogens are helpful and are used in the production of certain foods, such as bread, cheese, yogurt, beer, and wine. Other nonpathogens live in and on the human body and cause no harm. Some of these are also helpful. For example, the E. coli is a bacteria that normally lives in the bowel. This organism assists with bowel function and the manufacture of vitamin K in the body. (But E. coli can cause serious infection if it invades other parts of the body, such as the urinary bladder, upper digestive tract, or surgical wounds.)

There is, however, another group of microorganisms, known as pathogens, or **pathogenic** organisms, which are harmful and capable of producing illness known as infectious disease.

Growth of Microorganisms

As living substances, microorganisms must have the following to live and grow:

- *Host*—a person, animal, or food on which to live.
- *Warmth*—microorganisms grow best at body temperature; extreme heat will destroy microorganisms and cold will slow their growth, but will not prevent it; food stored in the refrigerator too long eventually becomes "spoiled" due to the action of growing microorganisms.
- *Darkness*—microorganisms thrive in dark places, but light can destroy them.
- *Oxygen*—is necessary to living organisms and needed by **aerobic** organisms; other microorganisms thrive where there is little or no oxygen; these are called **anaerobic** organisms.

infection
occurs when harmful organisms enter the body and grow, causing illness or disease.

nonpathogenic
usually not capable of causing or producing a disease.

pathogenic
capable of causing or producing a disease.

aerobic
able to live in the presence of oxygen.

anaerobic
able to live without air or oxygen.

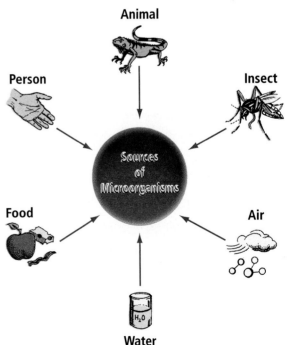

9-1 Microorganisms come from many sources.

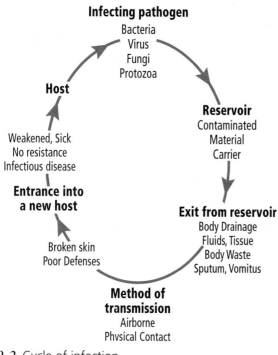

Infecting pathogen
Bacteria
Virus
Fungi
Protozoa

Host

Weakened, Sick
No resistance
Infectious disease

**Entrance into
a new host**

Broken skin
Poor Defenses

Reservoir
Contaminated
Material
Carrier

Exit from reservoir
Body Drainage
Fluids, Tissue
Body Waste
Sputum, Vomitus

**Method of
transmission**
Airborne
Physical Contact

9-2 Cycle of infection.

AIDS
abbreviation for acquired immunodeficiency syndrome.

hepatitis B
an infectious disease of the liver
spread through contact with
blood and caused by a virus.

reservoir
a place where a pathogen is
stored, can live, and grow.

carrier
a person or animal who spreads
disease to others but does not
become ill.

sputum
material coughed up from the
lungs and spit out through
the mouth.

vomitus
material expelled from the
stomach when vomiting.

transmitted
passed from one person or
place to another.

- *Moisture*—microorganisms grow in moist areas.
- *Food*—as living things, microorganisms need food to multiply; that food may be leftover green beans in the back of the refrigerator or the tissues of the human body.

Pathogenic microorganisms flourish where it is warm, dark, and moist with oxygen and a food supply. Can you think of any places in the body that act as a suitable home for pathogens? How about the mouth, throat, and nose? These and other body tissues meet all the requirements needed by pathogens to set up housekeeping and to cause an infection.

The Cycle of Infection

In order for a pathogenic microorganism to cause an infection, a definite cycle or chain of infection occurs (Fig. 9-2). This cycle includes six parts as follows:

1. The Pathogenic Organism

The most common groups of pathogenic microorganisms include:

- *Bacteria*—one-celled microscopic plants that multiply very quickly (Fig. 9-3). There are many types of bacteria. Bacteria commonly found in the client's environment are:
  - *streptococcus*—may cause wound, heart, respiratory, and other infections
  - *staphylococcus*— may cause wound and soft tissue infections

  The term *strep infection* is used when the streptococcus organism is the cause of the disease. Likewise, the term *staph infection* refers to a disease resulting from an invasion of one of the staphy lococcal organisms.
- *Viruses*—the smallest known living disease-producing organisms. They cause many illnesses, ranging from the common cold and influenza to **AIDS** and **hepatitis B.**

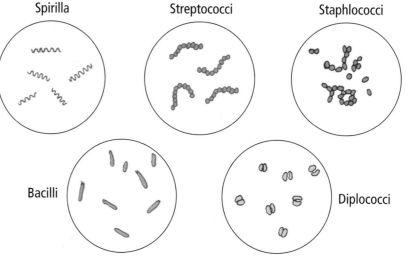

Spirilla

Streptococci

Staphlococci

Bacilli

Diplococci

9-3 Types of bacteria.

- *Fungi*—tiny plants that live on other plants or animals and can cause disease. Fungi (singular form of word is fungus) are very plentiful in the environment; they can be seen growing on old bread or oranges. We might describe that food as being moldy. Among the diseases caused by fungi are athlete's foot and vaginal yeast infections.
- *Protozoa*—one-celled microscopic organisms that usually live in water and can cause disease. Infectious diseases caused by protozoa include malaria and a type of pneumonia associated with AIDS.

2. Reservoir of Infection

The place where the pathogen is stored, lives, and grows is called a **reservoir.** Examples of reservoirs are persons with infectious diseases, soiled tissues and linens, client supplies, and equipment such as thermometers, bedpans, commodes. Another reservoir may be a **carrier,** a person or animal who does not become ill but who spreads the disease to others.

3. Exit From the Reservoir of Infection

The pathogen must escape from the original host in order to cause disease in another host. Pathogens can be found in body fluids—such as blood, urine, semen, saliva, **sputum, vomitus**—and in mucous membranes, tissues, and organs of the body. Secretions from the eyes, ears, nose, vagina, or penis may also contain pathogens. Of course, draining sores and infected wounds are excellent sources of pathogens.

4. Method of Transmission

Organisms are **transmitted** by means of many routes—through direct or indirect contact, in the air, by animals and insects, and by food and water.

Direct Contact Microorganisms are transmitted through direct contact with the person who is infected, including sexual contact. It is said that the 10 greatest carriers of disease are the fingers (Fig. 9-4). Touching body secretions and handling body fluids without protecting your hands are ways to carry pathogens from the infected person to yourself. *Examples:* Syphilis and gonorrhea.

Indirect Contact Organisms can be transmitted through contact with items used by the infected person. Using another person's washcloth, towel, razor, toothbrush, and comb can result in microorganisms being transferred from the infected person to yourself without any direct personal contact. Drinking from the client's cup or glass or handling used tissues are ways organisms travel from one person to another. *Example:* The common cold.

Air Some pathogens travel through the air in tiny droplets of water or dust. When we breathe in this air, organisms enter our respiratory systems. If we sneeze without covering the nose and mouth with a tissue, millions of organisms enter the air. Breathing in this air can cause pathogens to enter the body. *Example:* Tuberculosis.

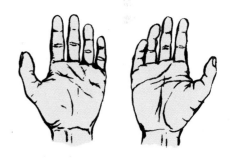

9-4 The ten greatest carriers of disease.

catheters
hollow, flexible tubes made of soft plastic or rubber that can be inserted into the body to withdraw or to insert fluids.

intravenous (IV) infusions
administration of nutrients or medications through a vein or veins.

contaminated
dirty, exposed to harmful organisms, making the object unsafe for use as intended.

medical asepsis
use of techniques and practices to prevent the spread of pathogenic organisms.

Animals and Insects Transmission of disease can occur through animals and insects. They carry organisms from place to place. Flies, mosquitoes, rats, mice, and ticks are examples of common carriers of disease. *Examples:* Malaria and Lyme Disease.

Food and Water Eating contaminated food or undercooked meat or poultry, eating unrefrigerated leftovers, or drinking unsafe water are ways in which organisms travel from source to human. Proper preparation and storage of food are discussed in Chapter 8. *Example:* Diarrhea.

5. Entrance Into a New Host

The pathogen must find a way to enter the body of the new host. Remember that the first line of defense is the skin. When skin is broken from a cut, a surgical wound, by injection, or from a bedsore, there is the opportunity for infection. Drainage tubes and **catheters** are often the route by which pathogens invade the body. **Intravenous (IV) infusions** provide a direct line through the skin and into the blood and may be used by pathogenic microorganisms as a "superhighway" for entrance into the host.

6. Host

Microorganisms are all around us, but most of us do not have an infection. That is because we have resistance to many microorganisms. But when pathogens increase in numbers and strength and body defenses cannot destroy them, an infection may occur. Some signs and symptoms of infection are listed in Box 9-1. Be alert for these symptoms in your client and report them to your supervisor immediately.

Some people are more susceptible to infection than others. Factors that place persons at risk for infection include:

- age—either the very old or the very young
- great stress
- chronic or acute illness
- inadequate nutrition
- poor living conditions
- poor personal hygiene

If the host acts as a good place for pathogens to live and multiply, the cycle of infection will be complete and ready to start all over again.

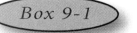

Box 9-1

Signs and Symptoms of Infection

1. Redness of tissue
2. Swelling of area
3. Pain in area
4. Warmth in area (warm to touch)
5. Fever, chills, and headache
6. Nausea, vomiting, diarrhea
7. Coughing
8. Skin rash
9. Pus or foul-smelling drainage from a wound or body opening
10. Fatigue

If your client develops any of these symptoms, notify your supervisor.

Breaking the Cycle of Infection

Protecting the client from becoming a new host is an important role for every home care aide. The cycle of infection must be broken to prevent the transmission of a pathogen from one host to another. The organism can be removed, destroyed, or blocked in its progress through the cycle. Keep clean things "clean" and dispose of **contaminated** materials promptly. Follow all practices of good housekeeping and other measures (listed in this chapter) to prevent the spread of disease.

Preventing the Spread of Disease

Practicing good personal hygiene is important in combating the spread of disease. Maintaining your own health is essential, so you don't become a host for disease-producing organisms. Using proper techniques of housekeeping, including food preparation and storage, also help to prevent the spread of disease. See Chapters 7 and 8.

Box 9-2 lists 10 common sense rules to follow in preventing the transmission of disease.

Medical Asepsis

The practice of **medical asepsis** is the use of techniques and practices to prevent the spread of pathogenic organisms from one person or place to another person or place. Medical asepsis is also known as clean technique.

Hand washing is a key component in the practice of medical asepsis. Experts on infection control often say that hand washing is one of the most effective ways of preventing the spread of infection. Establish a place in the client's home where you can keep all of your supplies for hand washing. This may be next to the kitchen sink and/or on top of the toilet tank in the bathroom. If running water is not available, you and your supervisor will need to find a way for you to carry out this technique. Bar soap should not be used. Ask your client to get liquid soap, or bring your own to be kept at your "special handwashing place." These materials are for your use only.

Box 9-2

Ten Common Sense Rules to Prevent Transmission of Disease

1. Wash your hands after using the bathroom.
2. Wash your hands before and after handling or preparing food and before and after eating.
3. Cover your nose and mouth when coughing, sneezing, and blowing.
4. Wash your hands after coughing, sneezing, or blowing nose.
5. Do not use another's soiled drinking or eating utensils.
6. Do not use another's personal items, such as toothbrush, razor, wash cloth, or towels.
7. Practice good personal hygiene, and maintain good grooming habits.
8. Wash raw fruits and vegetables before eating or serving.
9. Prepare and store food properly.
10. Use good housekeeping practices to eliminate household pests and maintain a clean environment.

Procedure 9-1

Hand Washing

Materials Needed

- Liquid soap in a pump container
- Paper towels—remove from the roll and separate four individual towels
- Warm running water
- Wastebasket
- Hand lotion, if desired

Procedure

1. Collect all materials at the sink (Fig. 9-5).

2. Remove your wristwatch or push it up onto your forearm about four to five inches. Remove rings.

3. Stand back from the sink so that your clothing does not become wet.

4. Turn on the faucet. Adjust the water to a comfortable temperature.

5. Completely wet hands and wrists under the running water. Always keep your fingers and hands below your elbows to prevent dirty water from contaminating your arms (Fig. 9-6).

6. Apply soap to your hands.

7. Lather hands well by rubbing the palms together (Fig. 9-7). Spread lather over the entire area of your hands and wrists. Get soap under your nails and between your fingers.

8. Use a rotating and rubbing motion (friction) for 30 seconds.

   a. Vigorously rub one hand against the other and around wrist. Repeat with the other hand and wrist (Fig. 9-8).

   b. Wash between fingers by interlacing them (Fig. 9-9).

   c. Rub your fingernails against the palms of your hands to clean this area.

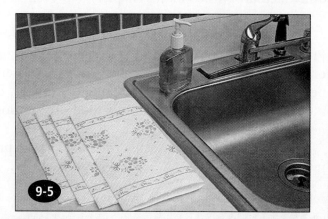

9-5

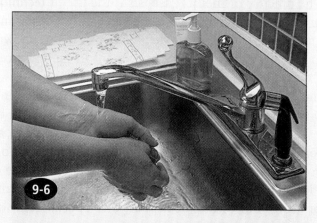

9-6

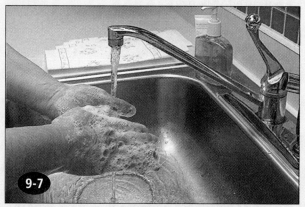

9-7

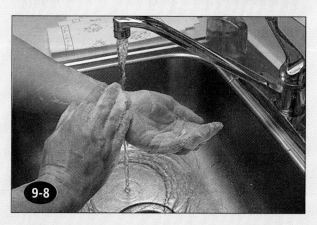

9-8

Procedure 9-1 cont'd.

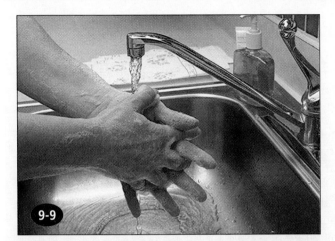

9-9

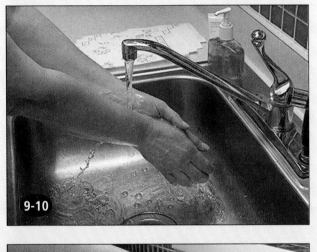

9-10

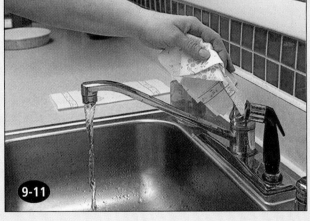

9-11

9. Wash at least two inches above your wrists.

10. Rinse well, under the running water, one hand at a time. Rinse from two inches above the wrist. Keep hands and fingers below the elbows so water flows from the finger tips directly into the sink (Fig. 9–10).

11. Dry your hands and wrists with paper towels.

12. Drop the used paper towels into the wastebasket.

13. Turn off the faucets using another dry paper towel (Fig. 9-11).

14. Discard towel.

15. Apply hand lotion, if desired.

The inside of the sink and the faucets are considered to be contaminated. Do not touch these areas when hand washing. After you have washed your hands, turn off the water using a dry paper towel. Procedure 9-1 gives the steps needed for proper hand washing. Other medical aseptic practices are listed in Table 9-1.

Table 9-1

Breaking the Cycle of Infection Through Medical Asepsis

Step in Cycle	Home Care Aide Activity
1. Pathogenic organism	Keep environment clean. Practice disinfection.
2. Reservoir of infection	Eliminate reservoir, when possible. Use gloves to handle contaminated material (e.g. tissues, sanitary napkins). Double bag and discard into covered trash container to keep animals out of trash. Empty bedpan, urinal, and commode promptly. Disinfect properly. Remove and treat soiled linens promptly. Keep client clean; bathe when necessary. Clean refrigerator; discard leftovers.
3. Exit from reservoir of infection	Block exit. Do not cough or sneeze on client or permit anyone to sneeze or cough on you. Teach client to cough into tissue and to discard in plastic bag. Do not go to work if you have an open, draining sore anywhere on your body. Notify supervisor if you have an infection. Seek advice about caring for clients when you have an infection. Wear gloves when handling body fluids. Wear other personal protective equipment (PPE) as needed. Place soiled linens in plastic bags. Wear gloves when doing laundry contaminated with body fluids.
4. Method of transmission	WASH HANDS. Clients should have their own personal care items—linens, razors, toothbrush, etc. No sharing. Do not let client care items touch floor. Discard or disinfect any items that touch the floor. Do not let soiled linen touch your uniform. Keep drainage bags and tubes off the floor. Do not shake linens when changing the bed. Do not put linen on the floor. Cover nose and mouth when sneezing. Discourage people with infections, especially colds and flu, from visiting the client. Keep window and door screens in place to prevent entrance of insects. Drink safe water only. Prepare and store food properly. Keep clean and contaminated items apart.
5. Entrance into a new host	Protect client's skin. Keep clean, dry, and prevent breakdown. Wear gloves if there is a risk of exposure to blood or other body fluids. Dispose of "sharps" properly—into a puncture-proof container (e.g., coffee can or plastic milk jug) according to agency and/or local community policy.
6. Host	Maintain and encourage healthy practices—good nutrition, sufficient rest. Avoid persons with infections.

Surgical Asepsis

With surgical asepsis, **sterile** equipment and supplies are used. The term *sterile* means free from all microorganisms, pathogens, and nonpathogens. Sterile technique is a specialized skill used during surgical procedures, injections, and other **invasive** procedures. Sterile technique is usually not the responsibility of the home care aide.

Universal Precautions

Universal precautions is a method of infection control by which all human blood and body fluids are treated as though they are infected with pathogens. In other words, every client is treated as if he/she has a potentially infectious disease. Hand washing is a vital part of the practice of universal precautions, along with the proper use of gloves. Gloves are always worn when there is risk of direct contact with body fluids or moist body surfaces. They are used to protect

- you from infectious disease
- the client from you (sometimes health care workers bring infection to clients)

Hand washing is always done BEFORE and AFTER using gloves. Other rules for hand washing are listed in Box 9-3. Explain the reasons for using gloves to both the client and family. When applying and removing gloves, follow Procedure 9-2 (See page 138).

> ### Box 9-3
>
> ## *Rules for Hand Washing*
>
> - Wash your hands
>   - when you arrive in the client's home.
>   - before and after you give "hands on" care or have personal contact with a client or his/her personal care items.
>   - during care if you are interrupted for any reason.
>   - between tasks or procedures.
>   - after using the toilet.
>   - when you cough, sneeze, or blow your nose.
>   - before and after meals.
>   - before and after handling food.
>   - if your hands become contaminated with body fluids.
>   - before you leave the client's home.
>   - before and after using gloves.
> - For a 60-second hand wash, sing the song "Yankee Doodle" twice.
> - Keep nails short, and remove jewelry from fingers.
> - Rings and long fingernails may harbor pathogenic organisms.

Protecting Against Blood-borne Diseases

Health care workers can be exposed to blood and other infectious body fluids while caring for patients and clients. If proper precautions are not taken, **blood-borne pathogens** may be transmitted from client to health care worker and lead to disease, perhaps even death. The health care worker, in turn, can spread the disease to his/her family and/or friends.

HIV and HBV

Human immunodeficiency virus (**HIV**) and Hepatitis B virus (HBV) are two pathogens carried by blood. HIV can eventually lead to AIDS and death. Hepatitis B virus attacks the liver and can lead to chronic liver disease and death. At the present time, there are no cures for these diseases.

The HIV is a more fragile virus than the HBV. Fragile means that the HIV virus is more easily destroyed when it is outside the body in blood or other body fluids. Hepatitis B virus, however, is very strong. It resists normal hygiene practices employed to destroy organisms. In fact, this virus can live for more than one week in dried saliva or blood on clothing or surfaces.

sterile
free from all living organisms.

invasive
entering the body.

universal precautions
an approach to infection control designed to prevent the spread of blood-borne diseases.

blood-borne pathogens
pathogenic microorganisms that are present in human blood and can cause disease in humans.

HIV
abbreviation for human immunodeficiency virus.

Applying Gloves and Removing Contaminated Gloves

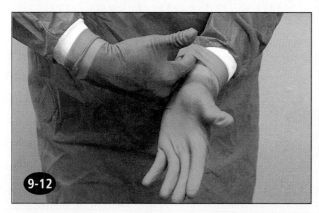

9-12

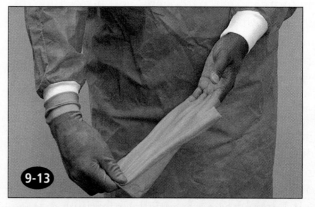

9-13

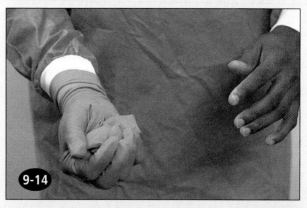

9-14

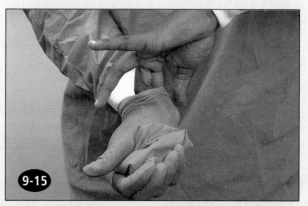

9-15

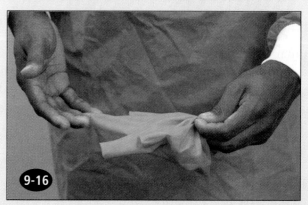

9-16

Applying Gloves

Materials Needed

- Pair of gloves (available from agency)

Procedure

1. Wash your hands.
2. Dry hands thoroughly.
3. Inspect gloves for tears or perforations.
4. Put gloves on when ready to begin client care.

Removing Contaminated Gloves

Procedure

With both hands still gloved,

1. Use right hand to grasp the glove on the left hand. Grasp the outer surface of the glove only—just below the wrist cuff (Fig. 9-12).
2. Pull the left glove downward until it is off and turned inside out (Fig. 9-13).
3. Continue holding the left glove in your right hand (Fig. 9-14).
4. Insert two fingers of your left hand inside the cuff of the right glove. Do not touch the outside of the glove with your bare hand (Fig. 9-15).
5. Pull the right glove down and inside out and completely over the left glove (Fig. 9-16).
6. Deposit both gloves into the proper container.
7. Wash your hands.

Every year, hundreds of thousands of people in the United States become infected with HBV. Many become carriers of this blood-borne disease. The number of HIV-infected persons has increased rapidly. About one million Americans have HIV, which damages the immune system and leads to AIDS.

Federal Regulations   Because of the rapid increase in the numbers of persons with HIV and HBV, the federal government has issued regulations to safeguard health care workers who come in contact with body fluids. Doctors, nurses, dentists, emergency medical workers, and home care workers are examples of health care personnel who may be at risk.

The U.S. Government's Centers for Disease Control and Prevention (CDC) and Occupational Safety and Health Administration (OSHA) require health care workers to protect themselves against exposure to blood-borne diseases.

Sometimes a health care worker accidentally comes in direct contact with the client's blood or other potentially infectious material. This is called an **exposure incident.** Blood-borne pathogens can enter the health care worker's body through several routes—the eye, mouth, other mucous membranes, tiny breaks in the skin, especially the hands or around the fingernails, or **parenteral** contact. OSHA requires that the exposure incident be reported immediately to the employer. This allows treatment to begin without delay. It also helps to prevent the spread of disease to others. During your training program, you will learn how to protect yourself from the possibility of being exposed to harmful organisms.

Health Care Employer's Responsibilities   The OSHA regulations require that health care employers:

- Provide hepatitis B immunizations for at-risk employees at no cost to the employee.
- Establish, in writing, tasks and procedures to be used when employees are working with clients.
- Establish procedures to eliminate or reduce employee exposure to blood-borne diseases.
- Provide employee training about hazards, precautions, and procedures when working with clients.
- Establish procedures for employees who have had an exposure incident to possible blood-borne pathogens.
- Require employees to use **personal protective equipment** that the agency provides.

Home Care Aide's Responsibilities   The federal OSHA regulations also affect you, the home care aide. They are designed to help to eliminate or reduce your exposure to HIV and HBV. Rules and regulations are only effective if they are carried out properly. Therefore, for your own protection, it is essential that you:

1. Treat all blood, body fluids, and waste as if they are infectious (universal precautions) (Box 9-4).
2. Use correct techniques for hand washing, handling body secretions, and disposing of wastes.

exposure incident
a specific eye, mouth, other mucous membrane non-intact skin or parenteral contact with blood or other potentially infectious material that results from the performance of an employee's duties.

parenteral
piercing mucous membranes or skin through needle sticks, human bites, cuts, and scrapes.

personal protective equipment (PPE)
specialized clothing or equipment worn by an employee for protection against a hazard.

3. Use appropriate personal protective equipment (Box 9-5).
4. Obtain hepatitis B vaccination.
5. Attend training sessions provided by your employer.
6. Report, immediately, to your employer any exposure incident.
7. Notify your agency when you are ill and unable to work so that you do not transmit your illness to your client and family.

Box 9-6 gives additional information about ways to protect yourself.

Box 9-4

Basic Rules for Universal Precautions

- Wear gloves when there is a chance of being in contact with client's blood, semen, vaginal secretions, or other body fluids.

- Wear gloves when the skin of your hands is broken or irritated.

- Wash hands before applying gloves and immediately after removing gloves.

- Wash hands immediately after being contaminated with blood or other body fluids.

- Clean up blood or body fluid spills immediately with bleach and water solution (1:10); remember to prepare solution daily.

- Do not handle used "sharps" such as needles.

- Ask client to place used "sharps" in puncture-resistant container or Biohazard Needle Box container provided by your agency or community. (Fig. 9-17)

- Wear personal protective equipment as required by your agency.

- Avoid splashing when disposing of contents of bedpan, urinal, or commode; if splashing occurs, clean area immediately.

- Wear gloves when disposing of soiled sanitary napkins or tampons.

- Do not eat, drink, apply cosmetics, or handle contact lenses in areas where exposure to blood or other potentially infectious materials is possible.

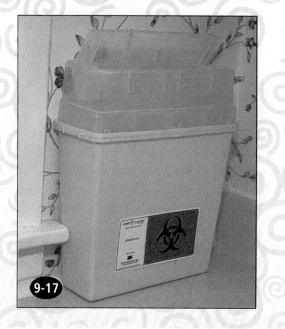

9-17

Box 9-5

Personal Protective Equipment (PPE) for Blood-borne Diseases

Gloves—Use when there is risk of direct contact with body fluids or moist body surfaces or when the skin of your hands is broken or irritated.

Plastic aprons or moisture-resistant gowns—Use when there is a risk of body fluids splashing onto clothing and/or skin.

Mask—Use when there is risk of spraying or splashing of body substances into nose and mouth.

Protective eyewear—Use when there is risk of body substances spraying into eyes.

Box 9-6

Basic Rules to Protect Yourself in the Client's Home

- Remember that your fingers are the 10 best carriers of disease.
- Wear gloves if you have cuts on your hands, chapped hands, or other breaks in the skin.
- Wear gloves when cleaning up blood and body fluids.
- Wear gloves when touching mucous membranes.
- Wear gloves when using disinfecting solutions.
- Wash your hands before and after using gloves.
- Wash your hands before and after giving personal care to client even if gloves are worn.
- Treat all blood, body fluids, and waste as if they are infectious.
- Wear protective clothing, as required (gloves, mask, etc.).
- Use proper techniques to avoid spattering of body fluids and waste.
- Dispose of body fluids and waste according to agency policy.
- Do not handle client's used needle and syringe; ask client to dispose of them in puncture-resistant container.
- Do not recap, bend, or break a needle after use.
- Wear heavy rubber gloves when removing trash.
- Wash hands even after removing rubber gloves.
- Contact your supervisor, when in doubt about proper procedures.

Additional Precautions CDC has recommended that hospitals and other institutions follow an infection control practice known as *Standard Precautions*. Standard Precautions are designed to reduce the risk of transmitting blood-borne and other pathogens from known and unknown sources of infection in hospitals. Standard precautions apply to:

- blood
- all body fluids, secretions and excretions except sweat regardless of whether or not they contain visible blood
- nonintact skin
- mucous membranes

If your agency uses Standard Precautions in home care, you will be given additional guidelines for their use.

Sterilization and Disinfection

Sterilization is the process used to destroy all living microorganisms—both nonpathogenic and pathogenic. Disinfection is the process that retards or inhibits the growth of pathogens. Sterilization and disinfection are methods used to prevent the spread of microorganisms and to reduce the spread of disease. While disinfection destroys most pathogens, it usually does not destroy all of them.

Equipment, materials, linens, towels, clothing—anything used by the client or health care worker can be sterilized or disinfected. In health care institutions, specially trained workers using complicated equipment keep all departments supplied with sterile materials. But in the client's home, this equipment is usually not available. It is very difficult to destroy all

Procedure 9-3

Disinfecting Using Wet Heat

Materials Needed

- Items to be disinfected—cleaned and dried
- Clean pot—large enough to hold items and lid
- Clean lid for pot
- Cold water
- Clock or timer
- Stove, hot plate, or other source of heat
- Pot holder

Procedure

1. Wash your hands.
2. Place items in pot so that all surfaces will be in contact with water.
3. Cover items with water. Provide some space at top of pot for steam to escape.
4. Place lid on top of pot.
5. Place covered pot on stove or other source of heat. Be sure bottom of pot is in full contact with heat source.
6. Turn pot handle(s) to the side(s).
7. Turn on heat and bring water to a boil. *Do not open lid any time during this process (steps 7 through 10).* Steam begins to escape from sides of pot.
8. Boil for 20 minutes.
9. Turn off heat.
10. Allow water and contents to cool.
11. Remove cover with potholder.
12. Remove disinfected item. Place on clean towel to air dry. Store properly.
13. Wash, dry, and return disinfecting supplies to appropriate location.
14. Wash your hands.

Procedure 9-4

Disinfecting Using Dry Heat

Materials Needed

- Items to be disinfected—cloth wrapped dressings or other items
- Flat pan of metal (pie tin) or ovenware
- Oven
- Timer or clock
- Pot holder

Procedure

1. Wash your hands.
2. Place cloth-wrapped dressings in flat pan.
3. Place flat pan in the oven.
4. Turn on oven to 350° F.
5. Bake for 1 hour. *Do not open oven while items are baking.*
6. Turn off oven and allow items to cool.
7. Remove flat pan using pot holder.
8. Unwrap cloth carefully without touching dressings.
9. Return items to appropriate location.
10. Wash your hands.

spores and viruses without using special sterilization equipment. Fortunately, many items now can be purchased for home care use in sterile packages that are disposable after use.

Disinfection in the Home

Usually, you will not be responsible for sterilizing equipment or other materials in the home. But you will be responsible for disinfecting equipment used by the client and performing housekeeping tasks to disinfect various areas in the home. See Chapter 7 for more information.

Wet and Dry Heat

The usual methods of disinfection are by wet and dry heat (boiling water and baking) and by chemicals. The method used depends on the type of item to be disinfected. For example, glassware is disinfected using wet heat, whereas dressings are disinfected using dry heat. Urinals are chemically disinfected. If in doubt about the correct method of disinfecting items in your client's home, contact your supervisor. Procedures 9-3 and 9-4 describe wet and dry disinfection.

Chemical Disinfection

The most common, least expensive chemical solution used in the home is soap or detergent and hot water. Friction caused by scrubbing surfaces with a brush or the rotating action of the automatic dishwasher or clothes washer loosens microorganisms from surfaces. Heat from the hot water solution helps to destroy pathogens.

Other solutions can be made by diluting chemicals with water. For example, OSHA standards require a bleach solution made with water to treat blood and body fluids because it destroys blood-borne pathogens. Therefore, it is important that you know the correct method of preparing this solution. See Procedure 9-5—Making Bleach Solution.

Cleaning the client's bedpan, urinal, toilet, or commode with a vinegar and water solution will disinfect these items and prevent offensive odors. See Procedure 9-6—Making Vinegar Solution.

Commercially prepared disinfectants are also available. Before using these products, remember to READ THE LABELS for instructions on proper use and precautions. Box 9-7 gives information about household disinfecting solutions and their uses. Procedure 9-7 gives steps to follow when disinfecting with household solutions.

Procedure 9-5

Making Bleach Solution

Materials Needed
- Household bleach
- Water
- Plastic container with cap
- Label
- Pen or pencil (for writing label)
- Measuring cup
- Rubber utility gloves (for cleaning)

Procedure

1. Wash your hands.
2. Put on rubber utility gloves.
3. Measure 10 cups of water, and pour into container.
4. Measure 1 cup of household bleach, and pour into container.
5. Place cap on container and shake to mix solution.
6. Prepare label, "Bleach Solution 1:10," date, and put on container (Fig. 9-18).
7. Store in closed cabinet out of reach of children and away from foods. Return materials to appropriate location.
8. Remove and rinse gloves. Hang to dry.
9. Wash your hands.

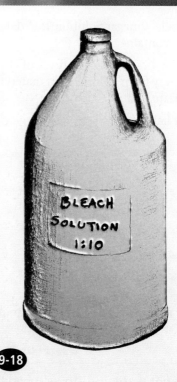

9-18

Procedure 9-6

Making Vinegar Solution

Materials Needed

- White vinegar
- Water
- Plastic container with cap
- Label
- Pen or pencil (for writing label)
- Measuring cup

Procedure

1. Wash your hands.
2. Measure 3 cups of water, and pour into container.
3. Measure 1 cup of white vinegar, and pour into container.
4. Place cap on container, and shake to mix solution.
5. Prepare label, "Vinegar Solution 1:3," date, and put on container.
6. Store in closed cabinet out of reach of children and away from food. Return materials to appropriate location.
7. Wash your hands.

Procedure 9-7

Disinfecting with Household Solutions

Materials Needed

- Items to be disinfected
- Plastic pan
- Container with solution (bleach 1:10; vinegar 1:3; or commercial solution)
- Detergent and warm water
- Paper towels
- Rubber utility gloves
- Timer

Procedure

1. Wash your hands.
2. Put on rubber utility gloves.
3. Wash items with detergent.
4. Rinse items with warm water.
5. Pour solution into plastic pan.
6. Submerge washed items in solution for 10 minutes.
7. Remove items.
8. Rinse well with hot water.
9. Lay items on paper towel to dry or hang on towel rack or shower rail to dry.
10. Clean area and return materials to appropriate location.
11. Remove and rinse gloves. Hang to dry.
12. Wash your hands.

Box 9-7

Household Disinfecting Solutions

Solution	Used For
Detergent and hot water	Towels, bed linens, clothing, dishes, drinking glasses/cups, eating utensils, pots, pans
Bleach and water	Bathroom and kitchen surfaces, blood, body fluids, feces, vomitus stained clothing, toilet
Vinegar and water	Urinal, bedpan, toilet, commode, surfaces in shower, tub, and kitchen
Commercial disinfectants	Toilet, bathtub, shower, sink, and other surfaces in bathroom; floors, sink, and other surfaces in kitchen

Isolation Precautions

There may be times when the client's illness requires other precautions to be taken, in addition to the procedures already discussed. When the client has a highly contagious disease, isolation is necessary to decrease the chance of spreading the disease to caregivers and others. Or, perhaps a member of the family has an illness that could be spread to the client whose immune system is not working well. Protecting the client from the chance of infection is another reason for using isolation procedures.

The care plan will indicate what procedures are necessary to protect you and your client. Your supervisor will give special instructions concerning these procedures, including the use and disposal of protective personal equipment such as masks and gowns.

Personal Protective Equipment

The most common equipment used in the home are gloves, masks, and moisture-resistant aprons or gowns.

Gloves are used as protection against pathogens from the client entering the home care aide. Examples of activities that require the use of gloves include: changing linens or clothing soiled with body fluids, giving personal care where there is risk of coming in contact with the client's blood, caring for the client's mouth, and performing certain housekeeping tasks, such as removing trash. Gloves are **ALWAYS** worn when there is contact or risk of contact with body fluids. If you have cuts, chapped hands, or other skin problems, notify your employer. Gloves must be worn.

Before putting on gloves, remove all jewelry and keep your nails short. Rings and long fingernails can tear gloves. Discard disposable gloves immediately after use. Use a new pair of disposable gloves each time. If gloves are required to give your client care, the agency will provide them for your use.

Masks are used to cover the nose and mouth of the wearer. When the client's illness is spread by airborne pathogens, wearing a mask acts as a barrier to prevent organisms from entering the caregiver's respiratory system. Masks and protective eyewear are used when there is a chance of splashing or spraying body fluids into the mouth, nose, or eyes. A mask should be worn no more than 20 to 30 minutes. After that time, the mask usually becomes damp or wet due to breathing. It is no longer an effective barrier and is considered to be contaminated. See Procedure 9-8—Applying a Mask and Removing a Contaminated Mask.

Moisture resistant gowns or aprons are used when there is a chance of soiling clothing with blood, other body fluids, or wastes while giving client care. Gowns used in the home are usually disposable and are discarded into the trash container in the client's room. See Procedure 9-9—Applying a Gown and Removing a Contaminated Gown and Box 9-8 for the sequence for removing contaminated personal protective equipment.

Applying a Mask and Removing a Contaminated Mask

Applying Mask

Materials Needed

- Disposable mask (from agency)

Procedure

1. Wash your hands.

2. Pick up mask by top strings (or upper elastic band).

3. Position mask over nose and mouth (Fig. 9-19) with top strings over ears. Tie strings behind head (or position elastic band over ears and high up on head).

4. Tie lower strings (or position lower elastic band low on back of head, under ears).

Removing Contaminated Mask

Procedure

1. Wash your hands.

2. Untie lower strings of mask (or pull lower elastic band up to top of head).

3. Untie upper strings and remove mask while still holding strings (or lift both elastic bands over head and remove mask) (Fig. 9-20).

4. Discard mask in proper container.

5. Wash your hands.

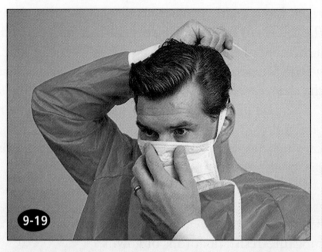

9-19

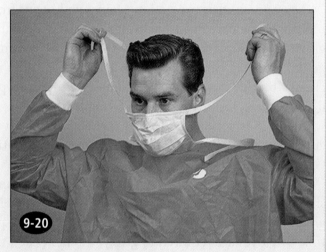

9-20

Box 9-8

Sequence for Removing Contaminated Personal Protective Equipment

1. Remove contaminated gloves and discard. Hands are the most contaminated.

2. Remove mask and discard.

3. Remove gown and discard.

4. Wash your hands.

Removing Contaminated Material

Contaminated material is removed from the client's room through a process known as double bagging. Trash or linens are placed in a plastic bag inside the room. This is known as the "dirty" bag. Another person, outside the client's room, holds open another plastic bag (the "clean" bag) ready to receive the contaminated material. See Procedure 9-10—Double Bagging.

Procedure 9-9

Applying a Gown and Removing a Contaminated Gown

Applying Gown

Materials Needed

- Disposable, moisture-resistant gown (from agency)

Procedure

1. Wash your hands.
2. Insert arms into sleeves of gown with opening in the back.
3. Tie the neck strings (or close Velcro strips).
4. Close the back opening by overlapping one side of gown over the other.
5. Tie at waist (or close Velcro strips).
6. Give client care.

Removing Contaminated Gown

Procedure

1. Untie waist strings.
2. Untie neck strings.
3. Pull gown down from the shoulder with neck ties (Fig. 9-21).
4. Leaning forward, turn the gown inside out while removing it. Do not touch the outside of the gown. This surface is contaminated (Fig. 9-22).
5. Keeping one hand inside the sleeve of the gown, use it to pull off the other sleeve. Do the same on the other side.
6. Roll up the gown into a ball. Keep contaminated area inside (Fig. 9-23).
7. Discard into proper container (Fig. 9-24).
8. Wash your hands.

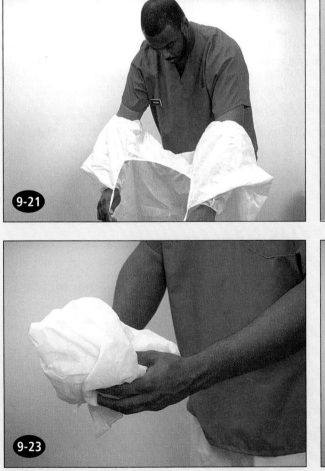
9-21

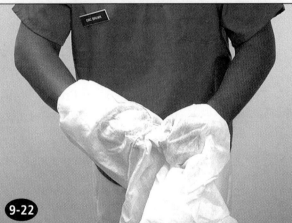
9-22

9-23

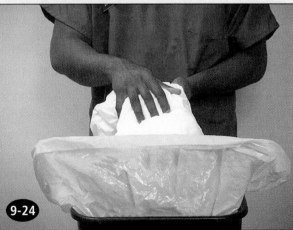
9-24

Double Bagging

Materials Needed
- Two plastic bags—one "clean," one "dirty"
- Isolation gown
- Gloves
- Helper (family member)

Procedure

1. Position helper with "clean" bag outside door of client's room. If you are alone, place clean, open bag in doorway, and go ahead with procedure.

2. Wash your hands.

3. Apply gown and gloves.

4.. Enter room. Take "dirty" bag in.

5. Place contaminated materials in "dirty" bag. Seal.

6. Ask person with "clean" bag to open it so you can insert second bag. Have helper seal "clean" bag. If alone, place "dirty" bag in "clean" bag but do not seal until hands are clean.

7. Remove gloves, gown. Discard in proper container.

8. Wash your hands.

9. Dispose of double-bagged material appropriately.

CHAPTER SUMMARY

- The home care aide has an important role to play in preventing infection.
- Pathogenic microorganisms produce disease as they travel through the cycle of infection.
- Medical asepsis and universal precautions are used in the home to prevent the spread of disease.
- Proper hand-washing techniques is one of the most effective ways of preventing infection.
- Universal precautions **MUST** be used whenever there is risk of contact with blood or body fluids.
- It is always important to follow CDC, OSHA, and your agency's regulations concerning blood-borne pathogens.

STUDY QUESTIONS

1. List four requirements for microorganisms to live and grow.
2. Describe the cycle of infection, and give two methods for blocking each part.
3. Define the following terms:
   a. medical asepsis.
   b. surgical asepsis.
   c. universal precautions.
   d. bloodborne pathogens.
4. List five rules to follow when there is risk of exposure to blood-borne pathogens.
5. Describe how to prepare a bleach solution for use in the home.

Observing, Reporting, and Recording

Objectives

After you read this chapter, you will be able to:

1. Discuss three purposes of the client care record.

2. Discuss the responsibilities of the home care aide to accurately observe, record, and report information about the client, family, and home environment.

3. Describe the three types of observation methods.

4. List five general rules for recording information on the client's care record.

5. Describe five points to remember when telephoning your supervisor to report your client's condition.

6. Identify the meanings of 10 of each of the following used in medical terminology: prefixes, suffixes, root words, and abbreviations.

7. Discuss the steps in reporting and recording an incident.

observe/observation
act of watching carefully and attentively.

care record
a permanent written record of client's progress during illness and rehabilitation; also contains information about client care.

Ms. Clarke has been visiting her client, Mr. Smirnoff for six months. Twice a week, she gives him a shower, straightens his bedroom, and makes a lunch before leaving for her next assignment. Mr. Smirnoff lives alone and uses a walker to get around his small apartment.

The care plan indicates that he has poor circulation in his legs. Yesterday, while giving the shower, Ms. Clarke noticed a reddened area the size of a quarter and hot to touch on the heel of his left foot. When she asked him about it, he said it was sore, especially when he put on his shoe. Ms. Clarke recorded her observations on the care plan and notified her supervisor, who, in turn, contacted a physician. "Because of Ms. Clarke's accurate observations and prompt reporting, I was able to start treatment immediately to avoid serious complications," said the physician.

Three of the most important responsibilities of the home care aide are observing, reporting, and recording information accurately. The home care team relies on you to be an excellent observer of the client, family, and home environment. Because more time is usually spent by you with the client than other home care team members, the home care aide becomes the vital communication link between what occurs in the home and what information is known by the agency (Fig. 10-1).

The word **observe** means to watch carefully and attentively. This is a way of gathering information about something. In Chapter 2, general principles of communications were discussed. People communicate in various ways: verbal, nonverbal, and written. Just as communication is a continuous process, observation also must be a process that is constantly being used.

During the first visit, you will be gathering new information about your client, the client's family, and the home environment. Then, with each visit, you will build on this information by observing any changes in your client, client's family, and home environment.

10-1 The home care aide—a vital link.

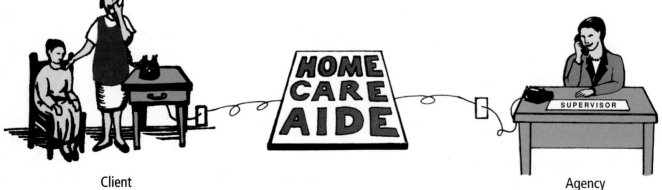

Client   Agency

Observing the Client

When you observe your client, you will be using your senses to gather information on your client's condition.

There are three types of observations—OBJECTIVE, SUBJECTIVE, and VITAL SIGNS. The OBJECTIVE method of observation means that the person is using one or more body senses to gather information.

> *Sight*—seeing the bruise on the client's arm
> *Sound*—hearing two family members argue about financial problems
> *Smell*—smelling the odor of spoiled food in the refrigerator
> *Touch*—touching the client's reddened skin

Another way of obtaining information is called the SUBJECTIVE method. This means that someone tells you information that you cannot observe. For example, your client says that he has a dull pain in the right shoulder and is dizzy. Or, a family member tells you that the client has been very depressed.

VITAL SIGNS means a group of four important indicators about the body's condition. They are temperature, pulse, respirations, and blood pressure. Vital signs are discussed in detail, including procedures, in Chapter 16.

You will use all three methods of gathering information. For clients who are infants, children, and others who are not able to tell you about their symptoms, your powers of observation are especially important. Developing your observation skills takes time and practice. As you continue in your career as a home care aide, your observation skills will sharpen and improve.

Observation Guidelines

Listed in Box 10-1 (See pages 152–153) are guidelines to help you perform a head-to-toe observation of the client .

The Client's Care Record

Every client has a **care record.** This is a permanent written record containing information about the client's progress during illness and rehabilitation. The care record serves many purposes:

- to document the work done, the quality of care, and client progress according to the care plan
- for communication between care providers
- as a basis for evaluating the plan of care and changing the plan accordingly
- to recall information at a later time, or if the client is discharged and then readmitted to agency services
- as a record for billing to obtain reimbursement for services from care providers

It is also a legal document, and its contents are confidential. In order to protect the client's privacy, most of the medical record is kept in the agency offices. (See information about confidential communications and client's Bill of Rights in Chapter 2.)

Some part of the client record will be located in the home for your use. The particular type of form will vary from agency to agency, but

Box 10-1

Guidelines for Head-to-toe Observation

I. OVERALL APPEARANCE

A. Consciousness
Alert	Confused
Does not react	Drowsy
Slow to react	Listless

B. Grooming
Clean	Dirty
Untidy	

C. Skin
Pale	Yellow
Clammy	Dry
Rough	Red
Bruises	Rashes
Open sores	Scaly patches

D. Mood
Cheerful	Withdrawn
Anxious	Sullen
Hostile	Demanding
Agitated	Irritable
Angry	Sad

II. HEAD TO TOE

A. Head and Neck

1. Hair and Scalp
Clean	Matted
Oily	Dandruff
Dirty	Dry
Sores	

2. Eyes
Bright	Red
Sensitive to light	Sees well
Dull	Glassy
Discharge	Sees poorly
Blind	

3. Ears
Discharge	Pain
Hears well	Difficulty hearing
Deaf	

4. Nose
Dry	Discharge
Bleeding	Stopped up

5. Mouth
Odor	Bluish or pale lips
Discharge	Sores
Difficulty chewing	Condition of
Difficulty swallowing	teeth/dentures
Gums—red, bleeding	

6. Speech
Normal for	Slurred
individual	Unable to speak
Difficulty talking	

7. Breath
Slow	Noisy
Coughing	Painful
Rapid	Difficulty breathing

8. Neck
Swelling	Difficulty swallowing
Pain	

B. Arms, Wrists, Hands, and Fingers
Bruises	Cuts
Rashes	Swelling
Cold	Pale or bluish fingernails

Movement
Easy	Difficult
Painful	Shaking
Twitching	
No movement—one side or both sides	

Strength
Weakness—general or one sided
Difficulty holding objects
Loss of strength

Feeling
Numbness	Tingling sensation
Pain	

C. Chest and Abdomen
Bruises	Cuts
Rashes	Swelling
Pain	

Breasts
Lumps	Discharge from nipple
Soreness	Pain
Irritation of skin under breast	

D. Pubic Area

Bruises	Cuts
Rashes	Swelling
Pain	Lumps

1. Female

Vaginal discharge

Odor	Swelling in groin area
Color	

Menstruation

Odor	Large amount
Pain	Blood clots

2. Male

Penis and Scrotum

Discharge	Odor
Swelling	Lumps
Pain	Swelling in groin

E. Legs, Ankles, Feet, and Toes

Bruises	Cuts
Rashes	Swelling
Pain	Bluish toenails
Sores	

Movement

Easy	Difficult
Painful	Shaking
Twitching	No movement

Strength

Weakness	Loss of strength

Feeling

Numbness	Tingling
Pain	

F. Upper and Lower Back and Buttocks

Bruises	Sores
Scaly patches	Dry skin
Redness	Pain
Swelling	

III. OTHER

A. Activities of Daily Living

Performs ADL without assistance
With assistance
Cannot perform

Personal Care: bathing, hair care, brushing teeth, shaving
Toileting: toilet, commode, urinal, bedpan
Eating: in bed, in room, in kitchen, other area
Moving: sitting, standing, walking

B. Appetite

Fluids	Thirsty
Foods	Drinks
Eats	Poor

C. Elimination

1. Urine

Pale or red	Dark amber
Odor	Small amount
Large amount	Painful urination
Difficulty urinating	Frequent urination
Incontinence	

2. Feces

Black, tarry	Bloody
Clay colored	Watery
Diarrhea	Odor
Difficulty moving bowels	
Painful movements	
Frequent movements	
Incontinence	

D. Equipment Needed by the Client

Wheelchair	Walker
Oxygen	Catheter
Commode	Cane
Hospital bed	

E. Pain

Dull	Aching
Stabbing	Comes and goes
Severe	
Location	

you will use an assignment sheet (sometimes called a client record or daily care plan) in the home. Most agencies require the home care aide to **chart** completed assignments on a check list form. The check list may be designed to record the care given in just one day, or it may cover a longer period of time (Fig. 10-2).

Recording on the Client's Record

Document the tasks performed by initialing or checking off the appropriate area on the check list. At the bottom of the list, or on the back of the form, there will be space for recording anything that does not fit into the usual daily routine. Always use this special area to record:

- Deviations from normal, as described in Box 10-1
- Medical emergencies, as described in Chapter 23
- Household emergencies, as described in Chapter 6
- Calls to supervisor, instructions followed, and results

Other forms that may be used in the home include:

- Identifying information record—client's name, address, phone number, responsible person to call in an emergency, etc. (Fig. 10-3)
- Intake and Output record (I and O sheet—see page 252)
- Daily weight record

These records will be reviewed by your supervisor and returned to the agency offices when they are fully completed. New forms are available from your supervisor. Follow agency policy regarding confidentiality of records found in the client's home.

Other home care providers (therapists, nurses, social workers, etc.) will bring their own records to complete. These forms, too, will become a part of the client's record kept by the agency.

Remember, the client's record is a legal document that may be used as evidence in court. Therefore, it is important that your charting is accurate. Record what you did and what you observed. Do not record what you thought, guessed, or how you felt about your work or observations. Be sure to follow the basic rules for recording listed below.

- Always record the correct date and time.
- Do not erase; draw a line through your mistake; write "error" above it; place your initials and date next to the word *error*; rewrite your entry.
- Always use ink.
- Write legibly or print entry.
- Record phone calls to your supervisor.
- Use agency-approved abbreviations and medical terminology.
- Record only the facts.
- Document client's response to care.
- Record what the client tells you; use direct quotes; don't record what you think they told you.
- Be concise.
- Use correct spelling and proper English.
- Don't leave blank lines or empty spaces that someone else could fill in; print N/A (not applicable) in the space(s) that is not used. Sign your initials or full name and title according to agency policy.

chart
to record in writing information on client's record.

document
to describe in writing observations or action taken; also called recording or charting.

WEEKLY CLIENT CARE RECORD

Client _____

Address _____

City _____ State _____ Zip _____

Phone (day) _____ (eve.) _____

Employee _____

Title _____

Soc. Sec. No. _____

Week Ending _____ / _____ / _____

Fill in the date for each day.

Write your initials in the box which corresponds to each task performed.

	DATE							
DAY		Mon.	Tue.	Wed.	Th.	Fri.	Sat.	Sun.
TIME ARRIVED								

PERSONAL CARE:

	Mon.	Tue.	Wed.	Th.	Fri.	Sat.	Sun.
Bath ❏ Bed ❏ Chair ❏ Shower ❏ Tub							
Perineal Care							
Hair ❏ Groom ❏ Shampoo							
Mouthcare ❏ Denture Care							
Shave							
Nail Care ❏ Clean ❏ File							
Foot Care							
Special Skin Care							
Dressing ❏ Assist ❏ Complete							
Toileting ❏ Bed Pan ❏ Commode							
Other instructions: _____							

CLIENT ACTIVITIES:

Transfer Activity Instructions: _____

	Mon.	Tue.	Wed.	Th.	Fri.	Sat.	Sun.
Assist with walking ❏ Cane ❏ Walker ❏ Crutches							
Assist with exercises ❏ ROM ❏ Other (specify)							
Wheelchair activities							
Other instructions: _____							

OTHER FUNCTIONS:

	Mon.	Tue.	Wed.	Th.	Fri.	Sat.	Sun.
Temp. ❏ Oral ❏ Rectal ❏ Underarm							
Pulse							
Respirations							
Blood Pressure							
Weigh Client							
Record Intake/Output (use special form)							

10-2 Check list—client care record.

Continued.

	Mon.	Tue.	Wed.	Th.	Fri.	Sat.	Sun.
OTHER FUNCTIONS:							
Prepare and serve meal/snack							
Special diet (Specify)							
Assist with feeding							
Medications reminder							
Ostomy care							
Incontinent care							
Record bowel movements							
Change in condition (office was notified)							
Other instructions: _____							
HOUSEHOLD SERVICES:							
Change/make client's bed							
Clean client's room							
Clean bathroom							
Clean kitchen; wash dishes							
Vacuum, sweep, dust							
Client laundry							
Marketing							
Errands (specify) _____							
Other instructions: _____							
DEPARTURE TIME							
TOTAL HOURS							

I certify that the hours shown represent my true total hours worked.

Signature _____ Title _____ Date _____

Return form to Home Care Agency weekly.

Notify Home Care Agency if your client's condition has changed since your last visit.

10-2—cont'd. Check list—client care record.

ABC Home Care Agency
Client Identification Record

Client Name _____

    Address _____

    _____

    Phone _____   Account No. _____

    Religion _____   Age _____

    Place of Employment _____

        Occupation _____

        Social Security No. _____

Diagnosis _____

Date of Initial Service _____

Physician Name _____

    Phone _____

Pharmacy Name _____

    Phone _____

Advance Directives   Yes _____   No _____

Emergency Contact _____   Phone _____

HEALTH INSURANCE

    Primary Insurer _____

        Phone _____

    Secondary Insurer _____

        Phone _____

R.N. Signature _____

10-3 Identifying information record.

Reporting to the Agency

The agency should be notified when you observe changes in the client's physical or mental condition. Also, report any client complaints about his/her physical condition or care. Anything that seems unusual or out of the ordinary should be reported. Before you call, have a pen and paper ready so that you can write the instructions you receive.

When you call your supervisor to report information about your client, give the following information:

1. Your name
2. Client's name, address, phone number
3. Your observations, for example:
   - What you saw—
     client is crying.
   - What you heard the client say—
     "I feel sick to my stomach. I don't want to get up, let me sleep."
   - What you felt (to the touch)—
     client's skin is hot and dry.
   - What you smelled (if anything)—
     fruity odor to breath.
4. How long client has had the problem

Stay on the telephone and write down the instructions you receive from your supervisor. Repeat the instructions to your supervisor to avoid any confusion or misunderstanding. Do not hang up the phone until your supervisor tells you to do so. Always record your calls to your supervisor, and write the instructions on the client's record. Follow instructions from your supervisor, and record the results on the care record. If you need to report your activities to your supervisor, do so promptly. In the example above, you may be instructed to take the client's temperature, pulse, and respirations. Do it immediately, and call the results into the agency immediately. Again, record and report your observations.

Written records are very important legal documents that provide evidence of care given by you, your supervisor, and your agency.

Incident Reports

Sometimes, an unexpected event (**incident**) occurs in the client's home or even in the agency offices. An incident usually involves an accident or injury. For example, you may fall and be injured; the client may fall; a visitor may fall—any one of a number of unusual events may happen. When anything of this nature occurs, notify your supervisor immediately and then fill out a form known as an Incident Report. This special form is available from your supervisor. It is important to record incidents according to your agency policy to protect the client, the agency, and yourself. Complete the Incident Report as soon after the event as possible, while everything is fresh in your mind. Fig. 10-4 shows a sample Incident Report form.

incident
an unexpected event.

Olsten
Kimberly QualityCare℠

CONFIDENTIAL—DO NOT DUPLICATE
Quality Assurance Material • Attorney/Client Communication

BRANCH #	BRANCH NAME (CITY)		PHONE ( )

BRANCH ADDRESS:	STREET	CITY	STATE	ZIP

CLIENT NAME	AGE	SEX ☐ M ☐ F

CLIENT ADDRESS:	STREET	CITY	STATE	ZIP

PRIMARY DIAGNOSIS	ICD-P CODE	MENTAL STATUS
		☐ Alert/Oriented ☐ Uncooperative
		☐ Confused ☐ Sedated
		☐ Cognitively Impaired

DATE OF INCIDENT	TIME AM PM	DATE REPORTED	REPORTED BY WHOM (INCLUDE NAME AND/OR FACILITY)

SERVICES PROVIDED
☐ RN ☐ LPN/LVN ☐ PT/OT/SLP ☐ MSW ☐ HHA/PCW ☐ HMK/Companion   SERVICE FREQUENCY   # of hrs/visits/day: # of days/visits/wk:

PRODUCT LINE
☐ Agency ☐ Private ☐ Rehab ☐ HME ☐ Pharmacy ☐ Peds ☐ IV ☐ Staffing ☐ Facility Private Duty
☐ Other (specify):

Type of Occurrence: Enter Incident Report Code: ☐ ☐ ☐ ☐ **(See reverse side of form)**

CAREGIVER/EMPLOYEE PRESENT? ☐ Yes ☐ No	CAREGIVER /EMPLOYEE NAME	TITLE

CLIENT INJURED? ☐ Yes ☐ No	SEVERITY OF INJURY? ☐ Minor ☐ Major ☐ Death ☐ Unknown	WAS TREATMENT REQUIRED ☐ Yes ☐ No	WHERE TREATED? ☐ Home ☐ ER ☐ MD Office ☐ Admitted to Hospital

WAS PHYSICIAN NOTIFIED? ☐ Yes ☐ No IF YES:	PHYSICIAN NAME	DATE NOTIFIED	TIME

PHYSICIAN'S FINDINGS RELATED TO INCIDENT

Describe the incident. (**Investigate details. Be specific [who, what, when, how, why].**) Attach Client Incident Report Supplement form if more space is needed. _____

Follow-up Actions Taken (with client, MD, case manager or others): _____

Submit white and yellow copies to Professional Services within 48 hours of incident—retain pink copy in a locked file in the branch.

Supervisor Completing Report Signature/Title:	Date:
Branch Director Reviewing Report Signature:	Date:

CLIENT INCIDENT REPORT
SIDE 1

©1995 Olsten Kimberly QualityCare
HCL 1018   2/95

10-4 Incident Report form. *(Courtesy Olsten Kimberly QualityCare, Melville, NY.)*

Medical Terminology

In order to record information correctly, you must understand the special language of medicine—medical terminology. A brief introduction to medical terminology follows.

Some medical terms are very old and originate from Latin or Greek words. For example:

Humerus, from Greek, meaning upper arm bone.
Vertebra, from Latin, meaning one of the bones of the spine.

Some medical terms come from the names of the persons who discovered or described the medical condition. For example, Alzheimer's disease was named after Alois Alzheimer, a German neurologist born in 1864.

Another type of medical term is an acronym—a name formed from the first letters of several words, such as **AIDS** from *Acquired Immuno Deficiency Syndrome.*

Word Parts

Most medical terms are made up of several word parts. There are four components that may be found in medical terms:

1. **word roots (wr)**
2. **suffixes (s)**
3. **prefixes (p)**
4. combining vowels (cv)

Word Roots One part of the medical term that is always present is the root. This is the word base to which other parts are attached. The root gives the basic meaning of the word. For example, in the word *microscope,* the root is *scope.* A *scope* is an instrument for viewing. In the term *arthritis,* the root is *arthr,* meaning *joint.*

Suffixes A suffix is attached to the end of the word root to modify the word root. Suffixes are used to describe disease conditions, diagnostic tools and techniques, and various treatments. To understand or analyze a medical term, begin with the suffix. For example, in the term *arthritis,* the suffix *itis* modifies the word root *arthr.* The suffix *itis* means inflammation. Therefore, *arthr+itis=inflammation of the joint.*

Try it yourself. Analyze the term *dermatitis. Dermat* is the word root. It means *skin,* and *itis* is the suffix, meaning *inflammation.* Therefore, *dermat+itis=inflammation of the skin.*

Prefixes Other words may have a prefix attached to the beginning of a word root that will also modify the meaning of the word root. In the example *microscope,* the word root is modified by the prefix *micro.* The prefix *micro* means very small. Therefore, *micro+scope=instrument for viewing something that is very small.* In the term *thermometer,* the prefix *thermo* means *heat,* and the word root *meter* means instrument to measure. Therefore *thermo+meter=instrument to measure heat.* Note: Not all medical terms will have prefixes.

word root
the word part that is the core of the term; contains the basic meaning of the word.

suffix
a word part attached to the end of the word root to modify its meaning.

prefix
the word part attached to the beginning of a word root to modify its meaning.

Combining Vowels Combining vowels are used to connect roots to suffixes and roots to other roots. They make the words easier to say. The vowel that is used most often is "o." For example, in order to combine the word root *arthr* and the suffix *scope,* it is necessary to add the combining vowel *o.* Therefore *arthr+o+scope=arthroscope,* an instrument for examining the joints. Without the combining vowel, it would be very difficult to pronounce the term arthroscope. In fact, word roots are usually listed in their combining form, that is, with the combining vowel attached or in parenthesis.

A few rules to remember about combining vowels are:

1. Use a combining vowel between word roots even if the root begins with a vowel.
2. Drop the combining vowel before a suffix that begins with a vowel.

Example

OSTE/ O/ ARTHR/ ITIS

OSTE/O	is the combining form of the word root that means bone. The combining vowel is used between the word roots.
ARTHR/O	is the combining form of the word root that means joint.
ITIS	is the suffix that means inflammation. Since it begins with the vowel *I,* the combining vowel is not used.

So, the term osteoarthritis means inflammation of the bones and joints.

Listed in Table 10-1 is a small sample of medical word components that, when combined, form terms commonly used in health care. A medical dictionary is a valuable resource for your use.

Abbreviations

Many medical phrases and word combinations are used repeatedly. In order to save time and space in written communication, abbreviations are used. Some abbreviations are standard, that is, in common use and understood by health workers. However, some agencies will use abbreviations that are exclusive to that employer only. Ask your supervisor if your agency has such a list.

If you do not know whether an abbreviation is acceptable, you should write the complete phrase so the record is accurate and easily understood. Listed in Table 10-2 are some abbreviations in common use.

Table 10-1

Medical Word Components

WORD ROOT (combining form)	MEANING	EXAMPLE of USE	WORD ROOT	MEANING	EXAMPLE of USE
abdomin/o	abdomen	abdominal	urethr/o	urethra	urethral
arteri/o	artery	arteriosclerosis	urin/o	urine	urinalysis
arthr/o	joint	arthritis	vascul/o	blood vessel	vascular
ather/o	yellowish, fatty plaque; fatty substance	atherosclerosis	**SUFFIX**		
			-algia	pain	neuralgia
bronch/o	bronchial tubes	bronchitis	-ectomy	surgical removal	tonsillectomy
card, cardi/o	heart	cardiac	-emesis	vomiting	hematemesis
chem/o	chemical, drug	chemotherapy	-emia	blood condition	uremia
cerebr/o	cerebrum	cerebral	-itis	inflammation	hepatitis
col/o	bowel	colostomy	-meter	measuring instrument	thermometer
cyan/o	bluish color	cyanosis	-osis	abnormal condition	cyanosis
cyst/o	urinary bladder	cystoscope			
enter/o	intestines	enteritis	-pnea	breathing	apnea
gastr/o	stomach	gastrostomy	-rrhage, -rrhagia	excessive flow	hemorrhage
glyc/o	sugar	glycosuria			
hem/o, hema, hemat/o	blood	hemocyte	-stomy, ostomy	new opening	colostomy
hepat/o	liver	hepatitis	-tomy	cutting, incision	tracheotomy
mast/o	breast	mastectomy	-uria	urine, urination	hematuria
nephr/o	kidney	nephritis	**PREFIX**		
neur/o	nerve	neuralgia	a, an	without	apnea
oste/o	bone	osteoporosis	ab-	away from	abduct
phleb/o	vein	phlebitis	ad-	toward	adduction
pneumon/o	lung, air	pneumonia	dys-	painful, difficult	dysuria
rect/o	rectum	rectal	hyper-	over, above, excessive	hyperglycemia
therm/o	heat	thermometer	hypo-	under, below normal	hypoglycemia
thromb/o	blood clot	thrombo-phlebitis			
			micro-	small	microscope
trache/o	trachea	tracheostomy	post-	after	postoperative
ur/o	urine, urinary tract, voiding	uremia	pre-	before	preoperative
			trans-	across	transurethral

Table 10-2

Abbreviations

ABBREVIATION	MEANING	ABBREVIATION	MEANING
abd	abdomen	OT	occupational therapy
ac	before meals	pc	after meals
ADL	activities of daily living	po	by mouth
ad lib	as desired	prn	as required
bid	twice a day	PROM	passive range of motion
BP	blood pressure	PT	physical therapy
c̄	with	qd	every day
Ca	cancer	qid	four times a day
cc	cubic centimeter	qod	every other day
c/o	complains of	qs	sufficient quantity, as much as necessary
h or hr	hour	ROM	range of motion
H₂O	water	s̄	without
I & O	intake and output	Tbsp	tablespoon
IV	intravenous	tid	three times a day
meds	medications	TPR	temperature, pulse, respirations
ml	milliliter	tsp	teaspoon
N/A	not applicable	w/c	wheelchair
NPO	nothing by mouth	wt	weight
O₂	oxygen		
OOB	out of bed		

CHAPTER SUMMARY

- Observing, reporting, and recording information accurately are important responsibilities of the home care aide.
- The home care aide is a vital communication link between the home and the agency.
- There are three types of observation methods: objective, subjective, and vital signs.
- Observations are recorded on the client's care record.
- All client records are legal documents. Their contents are confidential.
- Follow the general rules for recording information on the client's care record.
- Notify the agency when changes in the client's physical or mental condition or behavior are observed.

- When calling your supervisor, give precise and accurate information.
- Follow agency policy regarding telephone communications and incident reports.
- Medical terminology is the special language used by health care workers.

STUDY QUESTIONS

1. Why do agencies keep client records?

2. What is meant by:
   a. Subjective observations? Give three examples.
   b. Objective observations? Give three examples.
   c. Vital signs?

3. List 10 observations that must be recorded and reported to your supervisor.

4. List five rules to be followed when recording information on the client's care record.

5. Immediately after lunch, your client vomits everything she ate and complains of sharp pains in her abdomen. With a classmate, act out a phone call to your supervisor. Document your observations and phone call.

6. Identify the prefix, word root, and suffix and give the meaning of the following words:
   a. osteoarthritis
   b. colostomy
   c. thrombophlebitis
   d. neuralgia
   e. glycosuria
   f. mastectomy
   g. hyperglycemia
   h. hepatitis
   i. hypothermia
   j. gastrostomy

7. Write the meaning of the abbreviations in italics:
   a. *OOB tid*
   b. *NPO* from midnight
   c. Client must take *meds c̄* milk
   d. *OT* will perform *PROM qod*
   e. Record *I & O* and *wt qd*

Body Mechanics

11

Objectives

After you read this chapter, you will be able to:

1. Demonstrate good body mechanics when standing, sitting, lifting, and moving objects.

2. List three effects of immobility.

3. Describe the procedures for moving, positioning, and transferring clients.

4. Define the term *assistive devices* and give three examples.

5. List six rules to follow when assisting the client to walk.

6. Discuss 10 safety factors to consider when assisting clients to use walkers, canes, and wheelchairs.

7. Explain what you would do if the client begins to fall.

body mechanics
proper use of muscles to move and lift objects and maintain correct posture.

muscle tone
readiness of muscle to work.

fatigue
loss of strength and endurance.

Today is home care aide Lucy Wong's first visit to her client, Jorge, a 250-pound young adult who is partially paralyzed. The care plan requires that she give him a bed bath, change his position in bed, and prepare and feed him a noontime meal. When she introduces herself to him, his first remarks are, "You're too thin. You'll never be able to take care of me. You'll hurt yourself just trying to move me in bed." Lucy explains that she's been taught how to perform the tasks necessary to care for him. "It's not my size that counts but how I use my muscles that makes the difference." Jorge smiles and says, "Perhaps you're right. Let's see what happens." Jorge was pleased and surprised that Lucy performed her tasks efficiently and safely.

Body mechanics means the proper use of muscles to move and lift objects and maintain correct posture. It is a way of using your body so that the work is performed by several groups of muscles with the strongest ones being used.

Using Good Body Mechanics

The way you use your body to walk, sit, stand, lift, push, pull, or move objects is very important—not only at work but everywhere—every day. The body is like a finely tuned machine. When used properly, it performs very well. When misused, it performs poorly and eventually breaks down.

Benefits to the Home Care Aide

Practicing good body mechanics offers the following benefits:

- correct muscle groups are used for the task being performed
- muscle fatigue, strain, and body injury are reduced
- personal safety is maintained
- tasks are performed efficiently

Benefits to the Client

When the home care aide uses correct body mechanics, the client benefits in the following ways:

- anxiety and fears about moving are reduced
- position changes are made smoothly and without injury to the client
- concerns about falling are reduced
- confidence in the home care aide's ability to perform tasks correctly is increased

Steps to Good Body Mechanics

Using Correct Posture

The first step toward good body mechanics is correct posture. It helps promote proper balance, conserve energy, prevent muscle strain, and maintain the natural curves of the spine (Fig. 11-1). Tips for good posture include:

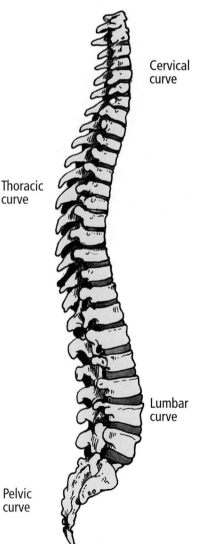

Cervical curve

Thoracic curve

Lumbar curve

Pelvic curve

11-1 Natural curves of the spine.

When Standing (Fig. 11-2)

- Head erect
- Shoulders back and at ease
- Chest up and forward
- Arms at sides
- Abdomen flat
- Buttocks tucked in
- Feet parallel to each other; one foot slightly forward
- When standing for a long time, put one foot on stool and change position every 20 minutes

When Sitting (Fig. 11-3)

- Head erect
- Shoulders back and at ease
- Chest up and forward
- Hips bent at right angles
- Weight supported by thighs
- Sit back in chair
- Rest both feet on floor

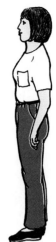

11-2 Correct posture when standing.

Maintaining Good Muscle Tone

Muscles work best when they are in good condition or tone. See Box 11-1 for a review of the muscular system. **Muscle tone** means the readiness of the muscle to work. Poor muscle tone occurs when muscles are not used frequently. They become weak, tire easily, and cause **fatigue.** Good muscle tone means that the muscle is strong and ready to work. Muscles that are in good condition do not tire easily. Therefore, fatigue is reduced.

Muscle tone can be improved by a program of regular exercise. Before starting such a program, always consult your physician. The program should begin gradually and be performed under the direction of a qualified person. Stretching large muscle groups, such as the arms and legs,

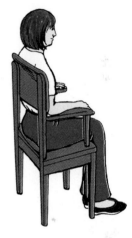

11-3 Correct posture when sitting.

Box 11-1

The Muscular System—A Review

- Muscles are attached to bones by means of tendons.
- Joints permit movement according to the type of joint— ball and socket, hinge, or pivot.
- The muscular system maintains the body's correct posture.
- Back and abdominal muscles help to provide correct posture.
- The large, strong muscles of the arms, legs, abdomen, and buttocks are used for lifting and moving objects.
- Back muscles are weak ones.
- Muscles are strengthened by use; proper exercise helps keep muscles in good working condition.

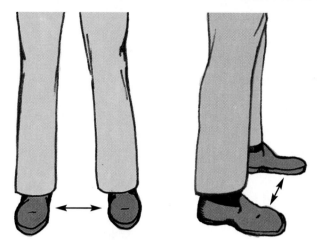

11-4 Good balance means keeping feet apart with one foot slightly forward.

is important before starting each exercise session because it prepares the muscles to work and helps prevent strains. One of the best exercises is walking briskly for 20 minutes at least three to four times a week. Exercising regularly should increase muscle tone and strength, reduce stress and fatigue, and strengthen the heart muscle, too.

Maintaining Balance

When standing, lifting or moving, it is important to keep your body in proper balance. Remember, when standing, keep your feet apart with one foot slightly forward. This will provide a wider base of support and better balance (Fig. 11-4).

Protecting Your Back

Back injuries usually occur because of a combination of many factors. Examples include: incorrect use of body mechanics; poor posture; maintaining one body position for too long; and lack of rest and relaxation to reduce the stresses of life. Developing poor habits at work and at home can contribute to back problems.

Being overweight places additional strain on the lower back. It is estimated that being overweight by 20 pounds equals 200 pounds of extra stress on the lower back. Therefore, it is important for the home care aide to maintain normal weight to avoid extra strain on the lower back.

Home care aides, who have previously injured their backs or require additional support for the back, may benefit from using a back belt when lifting or moving objects or clients (Fig. 11-5). It is important to have the belt specially fitted to the person's needs by a skilled professional. Consult your physician for further information.

assistive devices
equipment or other items to help clients perform activities of daily living more easily.

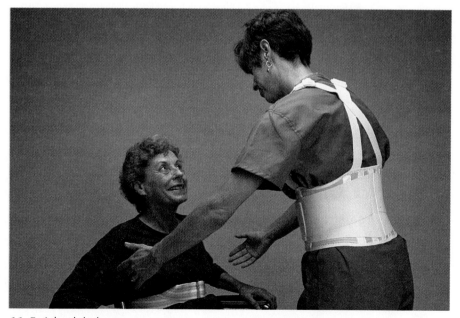

11-5 A back belt. *(Courtesy J. T. Posey Company, Arcadia, CA.)*

Most people have a maximum amount of weight that they can lift safely. Know your body. Know your limits. If unsure about whether you will be able to lift the weight, STOP and get help. Do not attempt to begin to lift the weight; you may injure yourself or your client.

Some clients may be able to assist when you are moving them in bed or when you are getting them out of bed. It is important to explain the steps they can take to help you and avoid strain on themselves or on you.

The following tips will help protect your back and practice good body mechanics. Make it a habit of following these guidelines each day, whether at work or at home.

Basic Rules for Protecting your Back and Practicing Good Body Mechanics

1. Wear Appropriate Clothing

   - Nonskid, comfortable shoes—low heeled or wedge
   - Back belt, if needed

2. Plan the Move and Prepare the Client

   - Go through the entire move mentally, before starting
   - Know where you are taking the client
     (chair, commode, etc.)
   - Tell the client what you are planning to do
   - Instruct the client about how he/she can assist you; make sure the client understands—get feedback before proceeding
   - Use **assistive devices,** if available
   - Get help, if necessary; instruct helper about the correct technique to use; remember, you are the leader; count 1–2–3 and MOVE TOGETHER

3. Move Objects Safely

   - Get help when lifting heavy objects
   - Push, slide, or roll object, when appropriate
   - Get as close to object as possible
   - Keep feet apart for wider base of support
   - Get on same level of the load—squat or get on one knee
   - Stagger feet and point them in the direction of the move
   - Keep back straight
   - NEVER BEND OVER FROM THE WAIST
   - Grasp object firmly and breathe in
   - Tighten abdominal muscles and lift slowly, by straightening the legs
   - Exhale as you perform the move
   - Avoid sudden jerking movements—lift smoothly
   - Turn your body as a unit, using your legs and feet:
     DO NOT TWIST YOUR UPPER TORSO
   - Adjust work heights to avoid reaching, twisting, or bending
   - Never lift a load that is overhead; use footstool to get as close to load as possible; test weight of load before lifting
   - Set object down slowly, bending knees and keeping back straight

The Client in Bed

Effects of Immobility

Clients who spend long periods of time in bed may experience the effects of immobility, which can include:

- **muscle atrophy** and/or **contractures**
- **decubitus ulcers**
- slowed circulation
- constipation
- reduced lung expansion, which could lead to **pneumonia**
- emotional effects of illness, as discussed in Chapter 5.
- generalized discomfort

Properly positioning and moving clients in bed helps reduce the effects of immobility by:

- encouraging effective moving and overall body function
- reducing excessive pressure on certain areas
- improving circulation and lung expansion
- promoting comfort and rest

Changing Positions in Bed

Many clients are able to move about in bed and should be encouraged to do so. However, if moving is difficult or impossible, the home care aide is expected to provide the necessary assistance. Explain what you are going to do and, if appropriate, how the client can help. For example, if the bed has side rails, you might ask the client to use them to help you make the move.

For those who are unable to help with the move, a useful device for moving and turning clients is the **lifting or turning sheet.** A regular draw sheet or a flat sheet that has been folded into fourths may be used. The turning sheet should be placed under the client and extend from the shoulders to the thighs. When you are ready to move the client, roll the edges of the turning sheet so you can hold it firmly as you move the client into a new position. The turning sheet provides ease in movement for both the client and the aide.

The care plan for a client who is unable to move will include a schedule for turning the client every two hours. A client's position MUST be changed at least every two hours in order to prevent complications that arise from immobility. Each time you turn your client, observe the skin for any changes. Immediately report redness, paleness, or white discoloration of the skin, particularly over **bony prominences,** as these signs may indicate a beginning decubitus ulcer.

Raising Client's Head and Shoulders

Sometimes it is necessary to raise the client's head and shoulders in order to readjust the pillows, bed linens, or clothing. Instruct the client to assist you (if appropriate), and follow Procedure 11-1.

muscle atrophy
wasting of muscle.

contracture
shortening of muscle whereby a joint becomes permanently immovable.

decubitus ulcer
sore on the skin caused by prolonged pressure on the part; also called "bed sore" or "pressure sore."

pneumonia
inflammation of the lung.

lifting or turning sheet
folded sheet placed under client from shoulders to thighs.

bony prominence
part of bone that is near the skin's surface.

Procedure 11-1

Raising Client's Head and Shoulders

1. Explain what you are going to do.

2. Wash your hands.

3. Provide privacy (close door, shut drapes, pull shades).

4. Raise bed to convenient working height.*

5. Lock wheels on bed, or push bed against wall if there are no brakes.

6. Lower rail on side of bed where you are working.*

7. Lower head of bed, remove pillows. Fold back top sheet.

8. Stand facing bed, feet about 12 inches apart.

9. Ask client to place near arm under your near arm and shoulder. Client's hand should reach to your shoulder (Fig. 11-6A).

10. Place your near arm under client's arm and shoulder. Your hand should reach to client's shoulder.

11. Slip your farthest arm under client's neck and shoulders (Fig. 11-6B).

12. On a count of three, shift your weight from foot nearest to head of the bed to your other foot. At the same time, rock client to a semi-sitting position (Fig. 11-6C).

13. Support client with arm locked under shoulder, use other arm to remove or readjust pillows.

14. Assist client to lie back on bed using locked arms and supporting neck and shoulders as before.

15. Make sure client is safe and comfortable. Replace top sheet.

16. Place bed in lowest position. (Raise side rail, if indicated.)*

17. Wash your hands.

Your client may not have an adjustable hospital bed; those steps marked with an asterisk (*) will not apply.

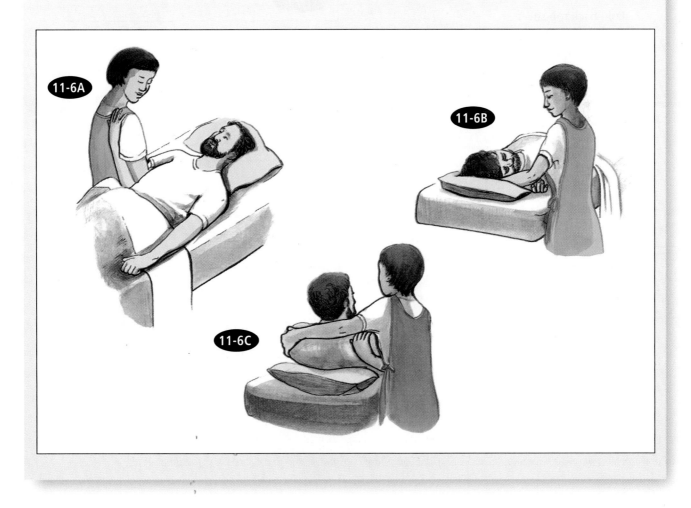

11-6A

11-6B

11-6C

Moving Client to Side of Bed

In order for you to perform certain procedures safely and properly, clients are positioned near the side of the bed. This is often one of the first few steps in a procedure, such as making an occupied bed, giving a bed bath, and placing clients in side-lying positions. See Procedure 11-2, Moving Client to Side of Bed. Some clients may not be moved in segments, as described in Procedure 11-2, because of back injuries or other problems. Check with your supervisor for the proper procedure to use with these clients.

Procedure 11-2

Moving Client to Side of Bed

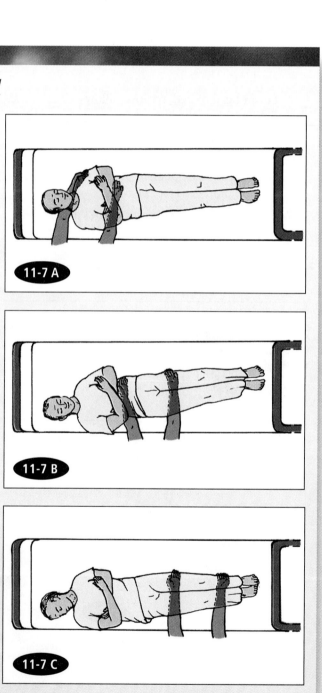

1. Explain what you are going to do.

2. Wash your hands.

3. Provide privacy (close door, shut drapes, pull shades).

4. Raise bed to convenient working height.*

5. Lock wheels on bed, or push bed against wall if there are no brakes.

6. Lower rail on side where you are working.*

7. Fold back top sheet.

8. Stand facing bed, feet about 12 inches apart, one foot in front of the other. As you perform each move, shift your weight from your front foot to your rear foot.

9. Slip one arm under client reaching across to the opposite shoulder. Place other arm under middle of client's back.

10. On a count of three, rock back and shift upper segment of client's body to edge of bed (Fig. 11-7A).

11. Place arms under client's waist and buttocks. Move to edge of bed in same manner (Fig. 11-7B).

12. Place arms under client's thighs and lower legs. Move to edge of bed in same manner (Fig. 11-7C).

13. Make sure client is in good body alignment. Replace top sheet.

14. Place bed in lowest position. (Raise side rail, if indicated.)*

15. Wash your hands.

11-7 A

11-7 B

11-7 C

Your client may not have an adjustable hospital bed; those steps marked with an asterisk (*) will not apply.

Moving Client Up in Bed

There are many reasons that a client will need to be moved up in bed. One of the most important is to help your client maintain proper body alignment. A client who is correctly positioned in bed will be more at ease and comfortable. In addition, moving a client up in the bed is the first step in many positioning and personal care procedures. Refer to Figs. 11-8 and 11-9 and Procedures 11-3A and 11-3B for the correct methods of moving a client up in bed.

Procedure 11-3 A

Moving Up in Bed When Client Can Help

1. Explain what you are going to do.

2. Wash your hands.

3. Provide privacy (close door, shut drapes, pull shades).

4. Raise bed to convenient working height.*

5. Lock wheels on bed, or push bed against wall if there are no brakes.

6. Lower rail on side where you are working.*

7. Fold back top sheet. Lower client's head; remove pillows.

8. Prop one pillow against headboard. This will protect the client from hitting his/her head when moving up.

9. Stand facing head of bed, feet 12 inches apart.

10. Slip one arm under client's shoulders, the other under client's thighs (Fig. 11-8A).

11. Instruct client to bend his/her knees, and firmly place feet against the mattress. On a signal from you, client will push with feet and hands to assist with move up in bed (Fig. 11-8B).

12. Help client move toward head of bed by shifting your body weight from your back leg to your front leg.

13. Several small upward moves may be used rather than one large move to reach head of bed.

14. Make sure client is in good body alignment. Replace top sheet and pillows.

15. Place bed in lowest position. (Raise side rail, if indicated.)*

16. Wash your hands.

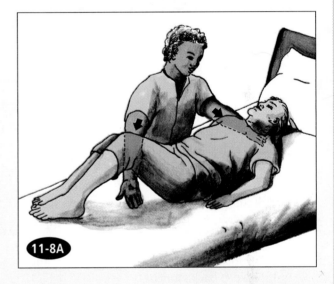

11-8A

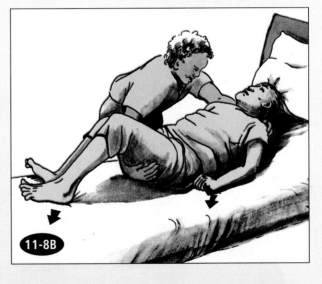

11-8B

Your client may not have an adjustable hospital bed; those steps marked with an asterisk (*) will not apply.

Moving Up in Bed When Client Cannot Help

1. Explain what you are going to do.

2. Wash your hands.

3. Provide privacy (close door, shut drapes, pull shades).

4. Raise bed to convenient working height.*

5. Lock wheels on bed, or push bed against wall if there are no brakes.

6. Lower rail on side where you are working.*

7. Fold back top sheet. Lower client's head; remove pillows.

8. Prop one pillow against headboard. This will protect the client from hitting his/her head when moving up.

9. Be sure turning sheet is in position under client's body.

10. *One person:*

    a. Keep side rails up.*

    b. Stand at head of bed, feet about 12 inches apart, one foot in front of the other, facing foot of bed.

    c. Roll top of turning sheet toward client's head.

    d. Firmly grasp top of turning sheet in both hands.

    e. Use good body mechanics—bend knees and hips, keep back straight.

    f. On count of "3," shift your weight from front leg to back leg, pulling turning sheet and client up toward head of bed (Fig. 11-9A).

    g. Several small moves may be necessary and are easier to do than one large upward move.

11. *Two persons:*

    a. Lower both side rails.*

    b. Each person stands at side of bed with feet 12 inches apart, one foot in front of the other facing head of bed.

    c. Roll sides of turning sheet close to client's body.

    d. Firmly grasp edges of turning sheet with both hands.

    e. Use good body mechanics—bend knees and hips, keep back straight.

    f. On a count of three, both persons shift their weight from rear leg to front leg, lifting turning sheet and moving client toward head of bed (Fig. 11-9B).

    g. Several small moves may be necessary and are easier to do than one large upward move.

12. Check lower sheets for wrinkles; smooth, if necessary.

13. Make sure client is in good body alignment. Replace top sheet and pillows.

14. Place bed in lowest position. (Raise side rail, if indicated.)*

15. Wash your hands.

---

*Your client may not have an adjustable hospital bed; those steps marked with an asterisk (*) will not apply.

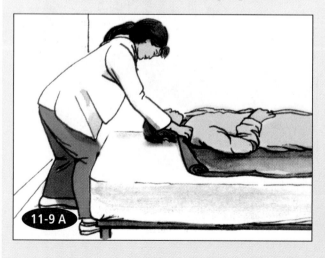

11-9 A

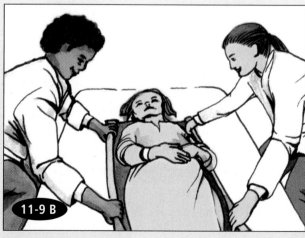

11-9 B

Positioning Clients in Bed

Positions Frequently Used

Proper positioning will provide comfort and relieve pressure on joints and bony prominences. Several positions are usually used, including:

Supine position is also known as the dorsal recumbent position (Fig. 11-10). The client lies on his/her back, with the bed flat. A small pillow is placed under the head and shoulders. Arms and hands are on the side, with the palms facing down. As an option, arms and hands may be elevated on pillows and a small pillow or folded towel may be placed under the small of the back as needed. Positioning devices, such as splints, hand rolls, or a footboard may be used. Supine position is used for sleeping and resting. (See Procedure 11-4, Positioning Client in Supine Position.)

Fowler's position is a sitting position. The head of the bed is elevated to a semi-sitting position, with the client's hips at the bend in the bed. A pillow is placed behind the head and neck. Support arms with pillows (Fig. 11-11). Positioning devices may be used as described earlier. Fowler's position is used when clients are eating, taking medications, reading, and watching TV. This position also provides comfort and easier breathing for clients who

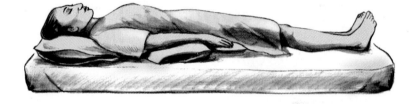

11-10 Supine position.

Positioning Client in Supine (Back-lying) Position
(See Fig. 11-10.)

1. Explain what you are going to do.
2. Wash your hands.
3. Provide privacy (close door, shut drapes, pull shades).
4. Raise bed to convenient working height.*
5. Lock wheels on bed, or push bed against wall if there are no brakes.
6. Lower rail on side where you are working.*
7. Fold back top sheet. Position client on back.
8. Adjust pillows properly:
   a. Small pillow under head and shoulders
   b. Support arms and hands with pillows
   c. Small pillow or folded towel under small of back, if your supervisor tells you to do so

9. Position other devices, such as footboard, trochanter rolls, bed cradle, as indicated in care plan.
10. Make sure client is in proper body alignment. Replace top sheet.
11. Place bed in lowest position. (Raise side rail, if indicated.)*
12. Wash your hands.
13. Record what you have done.

Your client may not have an adjustable hospital bed; those steps marked with an asterisk (*) will not apply.

have cardiac and respiratory conditions. If a hospital bed is not available, you will need to improvise a backrest for this position. Sofa pillows, a pillow armrest, or a wedge pillow can be used (Fig. 11-12). A straight chair can be used in the following manner:

- Turn the chair upside down with legs up in the air, braced against the back of the bed.

- Place pillows along the back of the chair that is behind the client's back. (See Procedure 11-5, Positioning Client in Fowler's Position.)

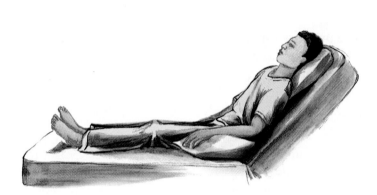

11-11 Fowler's position.

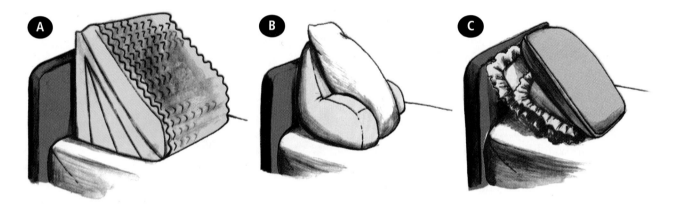

11-12 Types of backrests. **A,** Wedge pillow. **B,** Pillow armrests. **C,** Sofa pillows.

Procedure 11-5

Positioning Client in Fowler's (Semi-sitting) Position
(See Fig. 11-11.)

1. Explain what you are going to do.
2. Wash your hands.
3. Provide privacy (close door, shut drapes, pull shades).
4. Raise bed to convenient working height.*
5. Lock wheels on bed, or push bed against wall if there are no brakes.
6. Lower rail on side where you are working.*
7. Fold back top sheet. Position client on back.
8. Raise head of bed to 45° angle. If bed is not adjustable, use other devices to position client (see Fig. 11-12).

9. Adjust pillows properly:
   a. Small pillow under head and shoulders
   b. Support arms and hands with pillows
10. Position other devices such as foot board, trochanter rolls, bed cradle, as indicated in the care plan.
11. Make sure client is in good body alignment. Replace top sheet.
12. Place bed in lowest position. (Raise side rail, if indicated.)*
13. Wash your hands.
14. Record what you have done.

*Your client may not have an adjustable hospital bed; those steps marked with an asterisk (*) will not apply.

Lateral position is a side-lying position. The lower leg bears the weight, while the upper leg is positioned so that it does not rest on the one underneath. Pillows are placed under the client's head, between the legs, under the uppermost arm, and along the back (Fig. 11-13). The lower arm must be positioned properly to allow for movement and circulation. Watch lower arm for signs of impaired circulation, such as cool, discolored skin, and blue fingernails. If the client complains of numbness, tingling, and pain in the lower arm and hand, change the client's position immediately. Record observations. If the symptoms are not relieved within three to five minutes, call your supervisor. (See Procedure 11-6, Positioning Client in Lateral Position.)

Sim's position is also a side-lying position, but the client lies partially on the abdomen (Fig. 11-14). This position is used for taking rectal temperatures, administering enemas, and other types of treat-

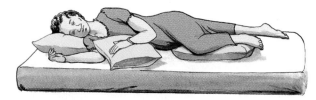

11-13 Lateral (side-lying) position.

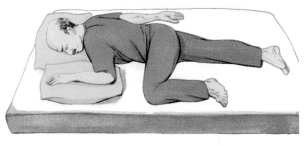

11-14 Sim's position..

Procedure 11-6

Positioning Client in Lateral (Side-lying) Position
(See Fig. 11-13.)

1. Explain what you are going to do.
2. Wash your hands.
3. Provide privacy (close door, shut drapes, pull shades).
4. Raise bed to convenient working height.*
5. Lock wheels on bed, or push bed against wall if there are no brakes.
6. Lower rail on side where your are working.*
7. Lower client's head; remove pillows. Fold back top sheet.
8. Ask client to move to side of bed nearest you. Assist client as needed. (See Procedure 11-2.)
9. Raise side rail.*
10. Go to other side of bed. Lower side rail.*
11. Place one hand around client's farthest shoulder and your other hand around farthest hip. Roll client toward you, turning on side facing toward center of bed. Bend upper leg. Both arms are slightly bent.

12. Adjust pillows properly:
    a. Small pillow under head and neck.
    b. Support upper arm and leg on pillows.
    c. A folded towel or pillow may be placed along the back to maintain the side-lying position. This is optional.
13. Position other devices as indicated in the care plan.
14. Make sure client is in good body alignment. Replace top sheet.
15. Place bed in lowest position. (Raise side rail, if indicated.)*
16. Wash your hands.
17. Record what you have done.

Your client may not have an adjustable hospital bed; those steps marked with an asterisk (*) will not apply.

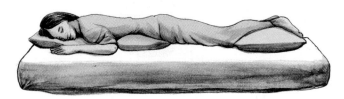

11-15 Prone position.

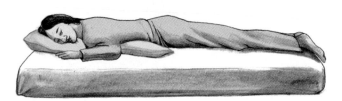

11-16 Prone position with client's toes hanging over mattress.

ments. However, some clients are comfortable in this position, and it can be used to relieve pressure on the bony prominences of the back. The upper leg is bent and rests on a pillow. The lower arm is behind the client. Pillows are positioned under the head and upper arm. The client's head is turned toward upper arm. Observe for proper circulation in lower arm and hand. (See Procedure 11-7, Positioning Client in Sims' Position.) *Prone position* places the client on his/her abdomen with the head turned to the side (Fig. 11-15). The feet may be elevated on a pillow or can hang over the end of the mattress to prevent pressure on the toes and ankle discomfort (Fig. 11-16). The arms are bent and a pillow is placed under the head. A small pillow or folded towel can be placed under the waist, if needed for comfort. The prone position is not for everyone; in fact, some people find it very uncomfortable and complain about feeling

---

Procedure 11-7

Positioning Client in Sims' Position
(See Fig. 11-14.)

1. Explain what you are going to do.

2. Wash your hands.

3. Provide privacy (close door, shut drapes, pull shades).

4. Raise bed to convenient working height.*

5. Lock wheels on bed, or push bed against wall if there are no brakes.

6. Lower rail on side where you are working.*

7. Lower client's head; remove pillows. Fold back top sheet.

8. Ask client to move to side of bed nearest you. Assist client as needed. (See Procedure 11-2.)

9. Raise side rail.*

10. Go to other side of bed. Lower side rail.*

11. Place one hand around client's farthest shoulder and your other hand around farthest hip. Roll client toward you, turning on side facing toward center of bed. Position the upper leg so it does not rest on the lower leg. Lower arm is behind client.

12. Adjust pillows properly:
    a. Small pillow under head and neck.
    b. Support upper arm and leg on pillows.

13. Position other devices as indicated in the care plan.

14. Make sure client is in good body alignment. Replace top sheet.

15. Place bed in lowest position. (Raise side rail, if indicated.)*

16. Wash your hands.

17. Record what you have done.

---

*Your client may not have an adjustable hospital bed; those steps marked with an asterisk (*) will not apply.

"stuck" and unable to move in this position. Make sure the client is able to breathe and that the pillows do not interfere with respiration, speech, and vision. This position is not usually used unless specified in the care plan. (See Procedure 11-8, Positioning Client in Prone Position.)

Positioning Devices

Devices are used to maintain proper positioning and good body alignment. These include:

- *Pillows*—placed under limbs and joints to prevent pressure, to keep skin surfaces separate, to promote comfort, to increase circulation, to provide support, and to maintain correct alignment.
- *Trochanter Rolls*—rolled towel, pillow, or blanket placed next to the hip to keep the leg from turning outward (Fig. 11-17A).
- **Footboard**—padded board attached to the mattress at the foot of the bed; this device keeps the client's feet in an upright position and helps to prevent **footdrop** (Fig. 11-17B).
- *High-top sneakers*—may be used instead of a footboard to maintain proper positioning of the feet. Remove the sneakers according to the schedule listed in the care plan. Inspect the skin; wash and dry the client's feet. Put on clean socks and replace the sneakers.
- **Bed cradle**—device used to keep the top bedding from resting on the client's feet and legs (Fig. 11-17C). Cradles are available from

footboard
a positioning device to keep client's feet in an upright position.

footdrop
inability to keep the foot in a normal walking position.

bed cradle
a device to keep the top bedding from resting on client's legs and feet.

Procedure 11-8

Positioning Client in Prone (Abdominal) Position
(See Fig. 11-15.)

1. Explain what you are going to do.
2. Wash your hands.
3. Provide privacy (close door, shut drapes, pull shades).
4. Raise bed to convenient working height.*
5. Lock wheels on bed, or push bed against wall if there are no brakes.
6. Lower rail on side where you are working.*
7. Lower client's head; remove pillows. Fold back top sheet.
8. Ask client to move to side of bed nearest you. Assist client as needed.
9. Raise side rail.*
10. Go to other side of bed. Lower side rail.*
11. Place one hand around client's farthest shoulder and your other hand around farthest hip.

Roll client toward you, turning on side and then onto the abdomen. Turn the client's head to the side for comfort and ease in breathing. Arms are flexed on each side of head.

12. Adjust pillows properly:
    a. Small pillow under head and neck.
    b. Optional small pillow under abdomen.
    c. Pillow under lower legs to relieve pressure on toes. Client may be positioned so that toes hang over mattress.
13. Make sure client is in good body alignment. Replace top sheet.
14. Place bed in lowest position. (Raise side rail, if indicated.)*
15. Wash your hands.
16. Record what you have done.

---

*Your client may not have an adjustable hospital bed; those steps marked with an asterisk (*) will not apply.

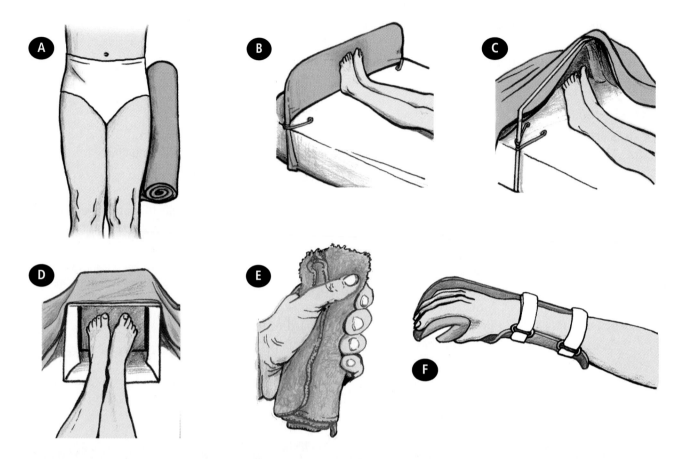

11-17 Positioning devices. **A,** Trochanter roll—rolled towel, pillow, or blanket next to hip to keep leg from turning outward. **B,** Footboard—keeps feet in an upright position and helps prevent footdrop. **C,** Bed cradle—keeps top bedding from resting on client's feet and legs. **D,** Carton bed cradle—a large carton can be used as a bed cradle. **E,** Hand rolls—rolled washed cloths can be used to keep client's hand in proper position. **F,** Splints—keep joints in proper position.

surgical supply stores, or you may improvise with a large carton (Fig. 11-17D).

- *Hand rolls*—padded rolls or rolled wash cloths that are placed in the client's hand to maintain a desired position as listed in the care plan (Fig. 11-17E). Remove during bathing. Wash and dry the hand before replacing the hand roll.
- *Splints*—devices of cloth, plastic, and metal used to keep joints in a desired position as listed in the care plan (Fig. 11-17F). Remove during bathing, wash and dry part, and replace splint according to the care plan.

Be sure that you understand the proper use of each device. If you have any questions, check with your supervisor.

Rules to Follow

Use the following principles of good body mechanics when positioning clients:

1. Encourage client to do as much as possible within physical limits.
2. Do not pull on client's arms or legs. Roll the client by placing your hands behind hips and shoulders or under shoulders or hips.

shearing
pressure against surface of skin and skin layers as client is being moved—one surface rubs against another surface.

transfer
moving client from one place to another.

3. As you move the client, shift your weight from one leg to the other. This assists in the moving process and allows you to use effective body mechanics.

4. Use a lifting or turning sheet or get a helper when necessary.

5. Whenever possible, completely lower the head of the bed, to prevent uphill movement.

6. Move client carefully to avoid any **shearing** motion that could damage the skin and cause a pressure sore.

7. Check the client's skin each time you change the position, at least every two hours. Observe skin over bony prominences and in areas where there may be pressure on soft tissue, such as ears, breasts, and buttocks.

Helping the Client to be Mobile

There are several methods to help clients to become mobile. Moving the client from one area to another is called a **transfer.** There are three main ways to transfer clients depending on their ability to perform the task.

1. *Standing transfer*—Client is able to bear weight on one or both legs.

2. *Sitting transfer*—Client is unable to support weight on both legs. A sliding board is used.

3. *Lifting transfer*—Client is unable to move or cannot be moved by one or more persons. A mechanical lift is used.

The transfer procedure is one that you will perform frequently. Getting the client out of bed to sit in a chair or wheelchair or to use the bedside commode are two common activities. Box 11-2 gives suggestions for preparing to safely transfer clients while using proper body mechanics. Follow these guidelines when performing the transfer procedures listed below.

Preparing the Client to Get Out of Bed

Most clients look forward to getting out of bed for the first time. For many, it is the first big step toward regaining independence. It is also a sign of improvement—of "getting better." Your supervisor will usually visit and evaluate the client's environment to assure that it is safe to get him/her out of bed. The care plan will indicate how frequently the client is to get out of bed, the activity when out of bed (sitting in a chair, walking, etc.), and the duration (10 minutes, a half hour, etc.).

Box 11-2

Preparing for Transfers

- Transfer across the shortest distance.
- Try to keep transfer heights the same.
- Obtain all necessary equipment (wheelchair, chair, assistive devices) BEFORE beginning the transfer.
- Make sure there is enough space for a safe transfer—remove obstacles.
- Position chair as close to client as possible.
- Lock brakes on hospital bed and wheelchair or make sure bed and chair are stable.
- Remove throw rugs or other hazards.
- Assist client to put on SAFE FOOTWEAR— no socks, floppy or slick-bottomed bedroom slippers.
- Check position of catheters or other tubing to be protected in the move.
- Obtain helper, if necessary.
- Place transfer belt on client, if needed.
- Put on your back belt, if needed.

Assisting Client to Sit on Side of Bed

Materials Needed

- Robe
- Sturdy footwear
- Chair, if needed

Procedure

1. Explain what you are going to do.
2. Wash your hands.
3. Obtain materials listed above.
4. Provide privacy (close door, shut drapes, pull shades).
5. Raise bed to convenient working height.*
6. Lock wheels on bed, or push bed against wall if there are no brakes.
7. Lower rail on side where you are working.*
8. Fold back top bedding.
9. Get as close to side of bed as possible—legs touching side of bed—so that you are level with client.
10. Position feet apart, with one foot staggered. Bend your hips and knees.
11. Ask client to move to side of bed nearest you. Assist client as needed (see Procedure 11-2).
12. Put up side rail and raise head of bed.*
13. Place client in Fowler's position without pillows (see Procedure 11-5).*
14. Lower bed and put side rail down.*
15. Place one arm around the shoulder area and the other arm under client's knees.
16. On count of 1–2–3, shift your weight to back leg, and slowly swing client's legs over edge of bed while pulling shoulders to sitting position (Fig. 11-18).
17. Place bed in lowest position so client's feet are touching the floor.*
18. Remain facing client with both hands supporting shoulders until client is stable.
19. Assist client to put on robe and footwear. Apply transfer or gait belt, if needed for transfer (Procedure 11-12).
20. Place back of chair next to bed, facing client. Have client hold back of chair to keep balance, if needed (Fig. 11-19).

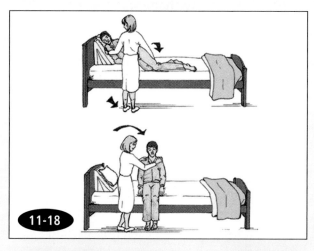

11-18

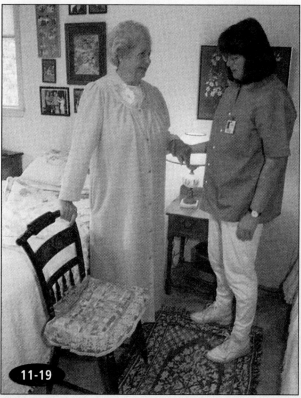

11-19

21. Remain with client.
22. Reverse procedure to return client to Fowler's position.
23. Wash your hands.
24. Record client's reaction to the procedure, amount of time spent sitting on side of bed, and any other observations.

---

*Your client may not have an adjustable hospital bed; those steps marked with an asterisk (*) will not apply.

Getting out of bed for the first time can produce some anxiety for the client. "Will I fall?" "Can I reach the chair?" Calm reassurance by the home care aide can help reduce some concerns. Explaining what you will do and how the client can assist you is a way to focus on the positive, not the negative.

Always use the same sequence of steps in the procedure each time you assist the client. Be consistent. Do not confuse the client by changing the procedure. Begin the procedure only when the client understands what you will do and how he/she can help. The first step is to have the client sit on the side of the bed with both feet on the floor. (See Procedure 11-9.) It is important that the circulatory system becomes accustomed to this position before the client begins to stand. It is not unusual for the client to experience some dizziness, which usually subsides in a few minutes. If the client remains dizzy, begins to sweat, becomes weak or pale, or there is a rapid increase in the pulse rate or change in the pulse rhythm, return him/her to a supine or Fowler's position in bed. Record your findings and report to your supervisor for further directions.

Transferring Client to a Chair/Wheelchair

Once the client has adjusted to sitting at the side of the bed, he/she is ready to transfer to a chair or wheelchair. The care plan should indicate the client's strong side. Be sure to place the chair or wheelchair parallel to this side so that the client can assist you with the transfer procedure (Box 11-3). (See Procedure 11-10 and Procedure 11-11). Explain what you are going to do and how your client can help. Encourage him/her to do as much as possible to foster independence.

Box 11-3

Safety Tips—Using the Wheelchair

- Place chair next to client's stronger side before making the transfer.

- Put footrests out of the way before client gets in or out of chair.

- Make sure BOTH wheel brakes are locked before client gets in or out of chair.

- Replace footrests in proper position, and assist client, as needed, to put feet on footrests after being seated.

- Make sure client is in a comfortable and safe sitting position before releasing the wheel brakes.

- Release both wheel brakes before attempting to move the chair.

- Make sure client's clothing or lap blanket does not trail on the floor or become caught in the wheels.

Transferring Client from Bed to Chair/Wheelchair—Standing Transfer

Materials Needed

- Chair or wheelchair
- Blanket, if needed
- Special chair cushion, if needed
- Robe
- Sturdy footwear

Procedure

1. Explain what you are going to do.
2. Wash your hands.
3. Obtain materials listed above.
4. Provide privacy (close door, shut drapes, pull shades).
5. Place chair parallel to bed and on client's strong side.
6. When using a wheelchair, lock brakes and move footrests out of the way (Fig. 11-20).
7. Lower bed, lock wheels, and lower rail on side where your are working.*
8. Assist client, as needed, to sit on side of bed (Procedure 11-9) and put on robe and footwear.
9. Stand directly in front of client, with your feet slightly apart. Bend hips and knees so that you are level with client.
10. Place your arms under client's arms and around client's back, locking fingers together or clasping one hand over the other wrist (Fig. 11–21). Have client hug your back or shoulders.
11. Lock your knees against client's to provide additional support and to prevent the knees from buckling (Fig. 11-22).
12. Bend your knees and ask client to rock with you as you count 1–2–3. Stand on count of "3".

Your client may not have an adjustable hospital bed; those steps marked with an asterisk (*) will not apply.

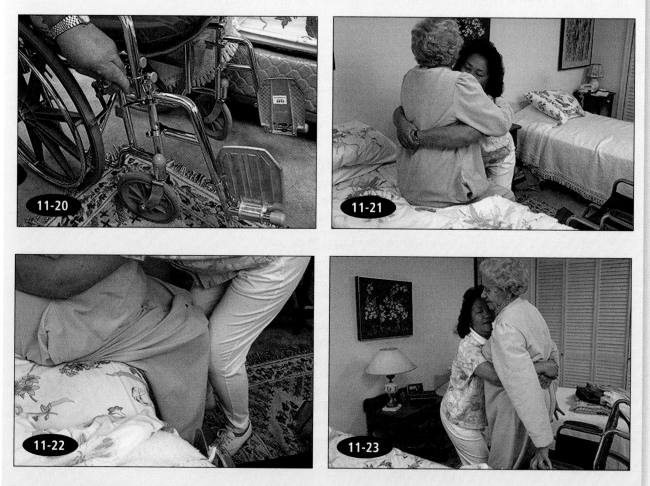

11-20

11-21

11-22

11-23

Procedure 11-10 cont'd.

13. Count to 10 before continuing. This allows time for the body to adjust to the standing position.
14. Walk with client to chair, taking small steps, while guiding client's back to chair. Continue until chair's sitting surface touches back of client's legs.
15. Have client reach back and grasp the farthest arm of the chair, then the nearest arm.
16. Bend your hips and knees while guiding client into chair (Fig. 11-23).

17. Make sure client is safe and comfortable.
    a. If in wheelchair, replace footrests and have client put feet on them
    b. Place necessary items within client's reach
18. Wash your hands.
19. Record client's reaction to the procedure, amount of time sitting in chair, and any other observations.

Procedure 11-11

Transferring Client from Bed to Chair/Wheelchair— Standing Transfer Using Transfer Belt

Materials Needed

- Chair or wheelchair
- Blanket, if needed
- Special chair cushion, if used
- Transfer belt
- Robe
- Sturdy footwear

Procedure

1. Explain what you are going to do and how the client can help you.
2. Wash your hands.
3. Obtain materials listed above.
4. Provide privacy (close door, shut drapes, pull shades).
5. Apply transfer belt. (See Procedure 11-13.)
6. Place chair parallel to bed and on client's strong side. If using a wheelchair, lock brakes and move footrests out of way. If bed has wheels, lock them.
7. Stand directly in front of client.
8. Make sure client's feet are firmly on the floor.
9. Have client place fists on bed next to thighs and lean forward.
10. Grasp transfer belt firmly at each side (Fig. 11-24).
11. Lock your knees against client's knees to provide additional support and to prevent client's knees from buckling.
12. Ask client to push fists down on bed and stand on count of "3."
13. Pull client into standing position as you straighten knees and legs.

14. Count to 10 before continuing to allow client's body to adjust to standing position.
15. Instruct client to:
    a. Take small steps while turning back to chair until legs touch the chair
    b. Reach back and grasp the farthest arm of the chair, then the nearest arm
    c. Lower buttocks into chair, leaning slightly forward while sitting down
    d. Slide hips back into chair and sit erect
16. Make sure client is safe and comfortable.
    a. If in wheelchair, replace footrests and have client put feet on them
    b. Place necessary items within client's reach
17. Wash your hands.
18. Record client's reaction to the procedure, amount of time sitting in chair, and any other observations.

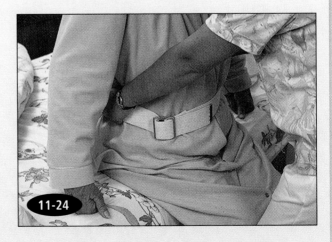

11-24

Returning the Client to Bed

Assist the client to return to bed according to the care plan. (See Procedure 11-12.)

Using Assistive Devices

Assistive devices are items used to help clients to perform activities of daily living more easily. In Chapter 8, devices such as plate guards and built-up utensils were described to help clients to eat. Likewise, there is equipment that can be obtained to assist and support the client to move more easily and safely. Assistive devices can be purchased or rented upon recommendation of the physician or the agency's physical therapist. Many community agencies loan this equipment on a temporary basis.

Transfer or Gait Belt

A transfer or gait belt is a belt worn by the client and used by the home care aide to hold on to the client during a transfer. It is used to help support a weak or unsteady client to move or walk. Apply the belt before beginning the transfer or before assisting the client to walk. (See Procedure 11-13, Applying a Transfer [Gait] Belt.)

Sliding Board

This board bridges two surfaces. For clients who have difficulty standing or are unable to bear weight on their legs, the sliding board can be used to move the client from one area to another. The client pushes himself/herself onto the board and scoots along the board to the other side. Keep hands on top of the board, not around the edges, to prevent injury to the fingers.

Procedure 11-12

Returning Client to Bed

1. Explain what you are going to do and how client can help you.
2. Wash your hands.
3. Provide privacy (close door, shut drapes, pull shades).
4. Prepare the bed; fold down top bedding.
5. Lower height of bed to lowest level.*
6. Place chair parallel to the bed—client moves toward strong side.
7. If wheelchair is used, lock brakes and place footrests out of the way. If bed has wheels, lock them.
8. Direct client to:
   a. Hold on to the armrests
   b. Slide to edge of chair
   c. Push down on armrests, straighten legs, and stand up
   d. Take small steps while turning back to bed until back of legs touch the bed
   e. Reach back and place hands on bed
   f. Lower buttocks into bed and slide back in bed
9. Assist client to remove robe and shoes; place in closet.
10. Make sure client is safe and comfortable.
11. Place bed in lowest position. (Raise side rails, if indicated.)*
12. Wash your hands.
13. Record what you have done.

Your client may not have an adjustable hospital bed; those steps marked with an asterisk (*) will not apply.

Procedure 11-13

Applying a Transfer (Gait) Belt

Materials Needed
- Transfer (gait) belt

Procedure

1. Explain what you are going to do.
2. Wash your hands.
3. Obtain transfer (gait) belt.
4. Assist client to a sitting position on side of bed.
5. Apply belt over clothing and around waist. Never apply over bare skin.
6. Place belt buckles off-center in the front or in the back, for client's comfort (Fig. 11-25).
7. Tighten belt, using buckles, until it is snug. Belt should not be uncomfortable, cause pain, or cause breathing difficulties.
8. Check that the female's breasts are not caught under the belt.
9. Prepare client for transfer.

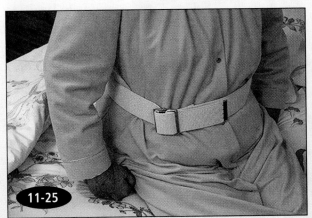

11-25

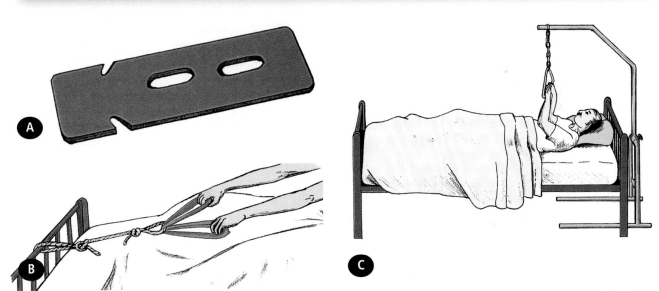

A

B

C

11-26 Assistive devices. *A,* Sliding board. *B,* Trapeze at the foot of the bed. *C,* Overhead trapeze.

Sliding boards are available from commercial home care supply companies. A leaf from the client's dining room table may also be used, but check first with the client's physician or physical therapist (Fig. 11-26A).

The Trapeze

A trapeze is a pull-up device attached to the bed. It can be used to help the client to raise himself/herself from a flat position in bed to a sitting position. The client grasps the handles of the trapeze and pulls up. Using this device requires strength in the arm muscles. The home care aide assists the client, as needed, to assume the sitting position (Fig. 11-26B and 11-26C).

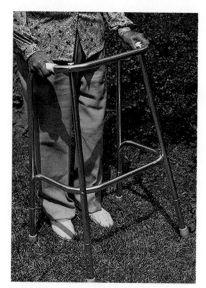

11-27 A walker helps this client to keep her balance.

Ambulation

The term **ambulate** means to move the body by walking with or without assistance. Once the client has tolerated sitting in a chair, the next step is to begin to walk. The physical therapist will instruct the client and caregiver about any special techniques required and will prepare a schedule for daily ambulation. Your role as the home care aide is to assist the client, as needed, making sure that the physical therapist's directions are followed. Sometimes the client may want to walk longer than the directions allow. Always follow the physical therapist's directions. Record your client's request and notify your supervisor for further instructions.

When assisting your client to walk, follow these general rules:

- Assist client to put on the gait belt, if needed
- Assist client to the standing position, then count to 10 before proceeding
- Stand by the client's weaker side and slightly behind
- Grasp gait belt in back with one hand while placing other hand in front of collarbone on the weaker side
- Do not rush the client—allow plenty of time
- Practice good body mechanics
- If client becomes tired, wait a few moments before proceeding
- Calmly encourage and reassure the client, as needed
- Record the distance walked, amount of time spent in walking, and how the client tolerated the activity
- Record and report any difficulty, such as dizziness, weakness, pain, or breathing difficulties

Using Walking Devices

Walking devices, such as walkers, canes, and crutches, may be needed to help support clients when walking. The physician determines the type(s) of assistive device according to the client's needs and abilities. The physical therapist fits the device to the client's size. Then, the client is instructed about the proper use and care of the device. It is your responsibility to make sure that the client follows these directions. Never change the directions given by the physical therapist. If the client is having difficulty using the device correctly, contact your supervisor for advice.

Walkers

Walkers are small metal stands that the client leans on when walking from place to place (Fig. 11-27). They are used for clients who have difficulty with balance or are weak and need additional support. Of all the types of assistive walking devices, walkers offer the greatest amount of stability because they provide four points of support. Some walkers have wheels and are pushed around; some are moved by lifting; and others have seats attached so that the client may rest when necessary. The type of walker is ordered by the doctor and usually obtained from a surgical supply house. The physical therapist will instruct the client and

ambulate
to move the body with or without assistance, to walk.

caregiver about the proper technique when using the walker. Listed below are some basic guidelines that the client should follow to use the walker correctly and safely.

The client is using the walker correctly and safely when:

- He/she stands BEFORE grasping the walker; walkers are not meant to support the client's full weight when rising from a sitting position. However, the client may use it to pull up to a standing position if you hold it steady; remind the client that, when unattended, the walker must never be grasped to rise from a sitting position or to lower self to a sitting position.
- All four legs of the walker are on the floor in a level position BEFORE taking a step; this technique will provide a solid base of support.
- The walker without wheels is advanced by picking it up and moving it forward while standing still; this technique will help keep the body in proper position and balance.
- The walker, with wheels, is advanced by pushing it forward
- One foot is moved and then the other into the walker, after the walker is in proper position.
- When getting into a chair from the walker, the client releases the walker, grasps the arms of the chair, and lowers self into the chair.

Canes

Canes are sticks that clients lean on for balance while walking. There are two types:

1. *Regular*—has a curved handle and provides one point of support (Fig. 11-28A).
2. *Broad-based*—has three or four prongs (tripod or quad cane) that provide a greater base of support than the regular cane (Fig. 11-28B).

Canes provide limited support to the client's weak side. Therefore, they should be used by those clients who are able to walk without much assistance. Like all assistive walking devices, canes must by properly fitted to the client. The physical therapist fits the cane and gives instructions about its proper use and care.

The client is using a cane correctly and safely when:

- It is held in the stronger hand with the elbow slightly bent.
- It is held in the hand opposite the weak leg.
- The rubber cap(s) is in place and replaced when worn.

Crutches

Crutches are walking aids that are held in place by the arms. The client must have strong shoulders, arms, wrists, and hands. At least one leg must be strong enough to bear weight. Other requirements include the ability to stand erect, have good balance, and be able to wear sturdy walking shoes.

There are three types of crutches:

1. *Axillary crutches*—made of wood or aluminum and fit under the axilla.

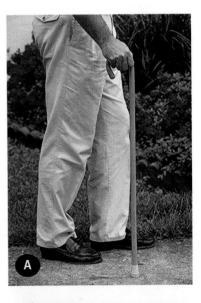

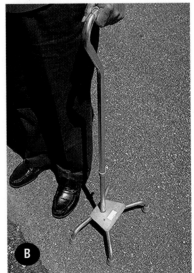

11-28 Common types of canes. *A,* Regular cane. *B,* Broad-based cane.

2. *Nonaxillary crutches (Canadian crutches)*—fit half way between the shoulder and elbow. They are held in place by a cuff that encircles the forearm.

3. *Adjustable ("Adjusto") or telescopic crutches*—can be adjusted to full length, elbow length, or can be used as a cane.

Before preparing to crutch walk, the doctor usually prescribes special exercises to strengthen the muscles of the upper body that will be used to bear weight. The physical therapist will instruct the client about how to do the exercises, when to practice, and for how long each day. When the client is strong enough, the therapist selects the type of crutch best suited to the client's physical condition. Measuring and fitting the crutch is also the responsibility of the therapist.

The client is using crutches correctly and safely when:

- Weight is placed on upper arms, wrists, and hands—NOT under the arms; nerves in the axillary area can be damaged if the client bears weight on the top of the crutches.
- Instructions given by the therapist are followed accurately.
- The rubber crutch caps are in place and replaced when worn (Box 11-4).

A Word of Caution

There may be situations where your client or family member has developed poor habits of positioning, lifting, moving, or using assistive devices incorrectly. When you observe this, explain, in a tactful manner,

---

Box 11-4

Safety Tips— Using Walkers, Canes, and Crutches

- Make sure that all bolts are tightened and tips have rubber safety protectors

- Place walkers, canes, or crutches, when not in use, near the client but out of traffic pattern of the room

- Assist client to put on walking shoes —no floppy slippers

- Remove obstacles from client's path

- Reinforce instructions of the physical therapist

- Do not rush the client—allow plenty of time to practice walking

- Practice using assistive devices when the client's energy level is high

the dangers to the client or the family member; why the action is incorrect; and demonstrate the correct method. Assist them to practice the activity until you are certain that they have learned the proper way. Usually, they are grateful for being instructed how to perform activities safely and correctly. If, however, they insist on continuing to perform activities incorrectly, report this to your supervisor and record your observations in the care record. Do not permit family members to assist you if they are unwilling to use the correct, safe procedure.

Assisting the Client to Fall

If you are with a client who becomes weak or dizzy during a transfer or ambulation, try to ease him or her down to the floor. Grasp the client firmly around the waist, using the gait belt if one is worn. Gently lower the client to the floor by bending your knees and keeping your back straight (Fig. 11-29). Do not try to stop a fall because both of you could be injured.

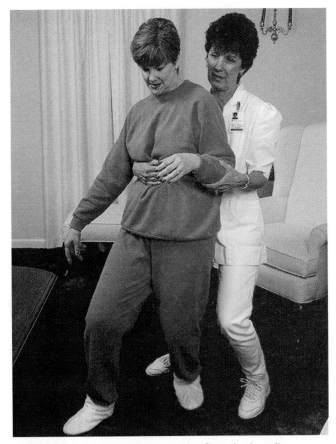

11-29 Ease the client down to the floor by bending your knees. Keep your back straight.

If there is another person in the home, call for help. Check for injuries, and telephone the Emergency Medical Service, if necessary. See Chapter 23 for additional information. If there are no obvious injuries, help the client into a comfortable position on the floor. Use pillows, blankets, etc. Allow the client to rest. You should take a few deep breaths and try to remain calm. Decide if you will be able to safely assist the client to get up, or if you will need additional help. If you do not feel confident about moving your client, do not be pressured into trying. Call your supervisor to report the incident and to get advice on how to proceed.

Report the following:

1. What happened. Did client have any complaints or symptoms prior to the fall?
2. Condition of the client after fall. Injuries? Complaints? Consciousness? Pulse? Color?
3. Did you call the Emergency Medical Service? Is client still on floor? Did you get client up to chair? Bed?
4. Assistance you will need to get client up from floor (if still there).

Record the fall on the client's record, including all the information above. Complete an Incident Report form as required by your agency.

CHAPTER SUMMARY

- Use good body mechanics to prevent injury to yourself or your client.

- Keep your body in good physical condition.

- Wear appropriate clothing and shoes.

- Follow rules for safe moving and lifting.

- Provide position changes in bed, transfers, and ambulation according to the care plan.

- Encourage clients to help as much as possible within their physical abilities. Instruct them how to help.

- If you are unsure about your ability to perform lifting, moving, and transfer activities, notify your supervisor. Do not take any chances that could result in injury to yourself or the client.

STUDY QUESTIONS

1. List three tips for maintaining good body mechanics when:
   a. standing
   b. sitting
   c. lifting

2. List three effects of immobility.

3. Define the following terms:
   a. muscle atrophy
   b. decubitus ulcer
   c. contracture
   d. bony prominence

4. Explain the use of the following devices:
   a. trochanter rolls
   b. bed cradle
   c. splints
   d. trapeze
   e. sliding board
   f. transfer belt
   g. turning or lifting sheet
   h. walker

5. Describe the following positions:
   a. Fowler's position
   b. Supine position
   c. Lateral position

6. List six rules to follow when assisting a client to walk.

7. List 10 safety factors to follow when assisting clients to use walkers, canes, and wheelchairs.

8. Explain how to assist a client who is falling.

Bedmaking

12

Objectives

After you read this chapter, you will be able to:

1. Discuss the importance of a correctly made bed.

2. List five rules for bedmaking.

3. Make an unoccupied bed and an occupied bed.

4. List five rules for infection control when handling linens during bedmaking.

Louise Sammons is a home care aide who cares for four clients in the same neighborhood. Each has different needs, and each has an individual care plan. Some clients receive daily care, and others are seen several times a week. But, in each home, Louise is responsible for making the client's bed. That task will be as varied as her clients:

Mrs. Santini is an 88-year-old widow who lives alone in a small house. She is recovering from heart failure and needs help with bathing, dressing, and simple housekeeping tasks. Mrs. Santini sleeps in her own double bed in her bedroom. The home care aide visits three times a week. Mrs. Santini's sister helps on the other days.

Mr. Morowski has a right leg amputation. He is 70 years old and lives with his wife and son. Mr. Morowski sleeps in a hospital bed in the living room. He can be transferred to a wheelchair. The small home has been equipped with a ramp so Mr. Morowski can go outdoors. The home care aide assists with bathing, dressing, and moving the client daily.

Mrs. Cullen is recovering from shoulder surgery. She needs help bathing, dressing, and simple household tasks. She is a 64-year-old widow who lives alone in a very small home. Mrs. Cullen hurt her back many years ago, and she sleeps in a reclining chair in the living room. Her son and daughter-in-law help out three days a week and on the weekend. The home care aide visits twice a week.

Mr. Tarrant, 50, is a hospice client who has cancer. He lives with his partner of many years. The hospice has provided a hospital bed with electrical controls, a trapeze, and a footboard. He requires a complete bed bath and linen change daily. His partner has a home-based business and has arranged his schedule to assist the home care aide in any way possible. The home care aide visits twice a week, and Mr. Tarrant says he will need more help as he gets sicker.

As you can see, Louise will be changing linens on several types of beds and one non-bed. Bedmaking is part of personal care and grooming for all clients. Making sure that the bed is clean and dry contributes to the client's comfort and relaxation and is an important part of the care plan.

Whenever possible, try to make the bed according to the household custom. If you are unable to follow the client's household custom, you must explain your reasons for the change to your client or family member. However, there will also be times when you need to be flexible. For example, there is no standard procedure for changing the linens on a reclining chair. Ask the client or family how this should be done. Once in a while you may find that a client's bed or sleeping arrangement isn't ideal, but there may be no other choice. Contact your supervisor if you are asked to make up a bed, chair, sofa, etc. that you think is unsafe or does not meet your client's need for care. Although the size and condition of the bed may vary, you must always be sure that the linens are clean and ready for the client when needed for rest or bedtime. Whenever possible, use sheets that fit the bed, and prepare it according to the care plan.

Types of Beds

The following beds are the types you are most likely to find in the home.

Regular Beds

Most of your clients will sleep in the bed they have always used in their homes. These beds usually do not have wheels and are not easily moved. If you think that the bed is not in a safe location for your client—near a large window or radiator, for example—discuss your concerns with your supervisor. Perhaps, with the client's or family's permission, it can be moved to another corner of the room for safety.

Water Beds

The mattress of this bed is filled with water and sits in a special frame. Special fitted sheets may be needed to make this type of bed. Although these waterproof mattresses are made of heavy duty plastic material, there is still risk of puncture. Do not use any sharp objects, such as scissors and straight pins or safety pins, near the water bed.

Hospital Beds

Hospital beds have wheels and can be raised and lowered horizontally. This makes it easier to transfer clients in and out of bed. This adjustable bed also permits the caregiver to work at a comfortable level and to use proper body mechanics. Always keep the hospital bed at its lowest position unless you are working at the bedside. When the bed is raised, there is great risk that the client could be injured trying to climb in or out of the bed. Also, since hospital beds are narrower than a regular single bed, it may be easier for the client to fall out of bed.

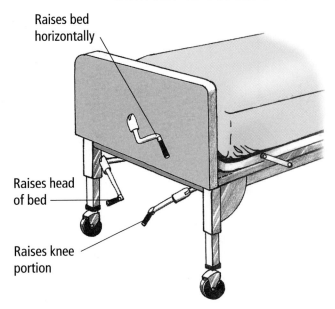

12-1 Controls for a manually operated hospital bed.

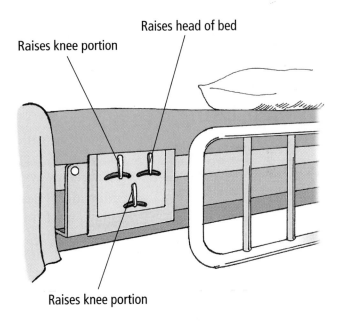

12-2 Controls for an electrically operated hospital bed.

The metal frame of the hospital bed is made up of three sections so that the head and foot of the bed can be raised or lowered. Some are operated manually, by turning a crank at the end of the bed (Fig. 12-1). Others are operated electrically by a control panel (Fig. 12-2). Many clients will be able to adjust their beds without assistance, but you should make sure they are able to safely operate the controls.

Safety Features of Hospital Beds

Wheel brakes Because hospital beds usually have wheels, brakes are needed to keep the beds from moving. Be sure to apply the wheel brakes during transfers, bedmaking, bathing, and other procedures where

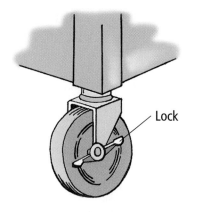

12-3 Brakes on bed wheel.

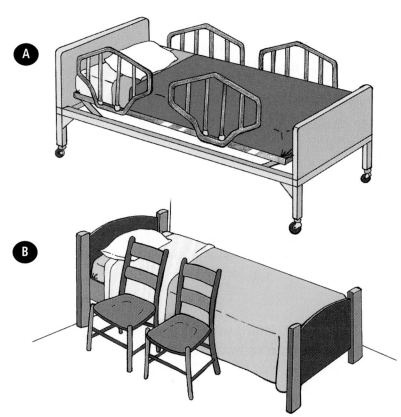

*12-4 **A,*** Side rails that attach to the side of the bed. ***B,*** Straight-backed chairs can be used if side rails are not available.

movement of the bed is not needed. In general, the brakes should be locked at all times and released only when movement of the bed is required. Always remember to relock the brakes (Fig. 12-3).

Side rails These are attached to the bed to prevent the client from falling out of the bed (Fig. 12-4A). Side rails are also used by clients to help in moving, turning, and transferring. Some clients prefer to keep the side rails down; others will like the safety and security provided by the raised rails. Follow the directions regarding the use of side rails in the care plan. See Box 12-1 for safety rules when using a hospital bed.

When side rails are not available, two or more straight-backed chairs may be used to provide protection for the client who is using a hospital or regular bed. Place the chairs at both sides of the bed with the back of each chair facing the bed (Fig. 12-4B).

Special Devices for Beds

Bed Boards

Bed boards are usually thin, flat pieces of wood cut to fit and placed under the mattress to add extra firmness for clients with back injuries or muscle disorders.

Footboards and Bed Cradles

Footboards and bed cradles are also used on beds, as discussed in Chapter 11. These devices are removed for bedmaking and are replaced after the bottom bed linens have been changed. Be sure that footboards and cradles are properly placed so they will not collapse and injure the client's ankles or feet.

Pressure Relieving Devices

A variety of devices are used in an effort to prevent pressure and the development of pressure sores. These are placed on top of the mattress. Here are some examples.

- *Flotation pads* contain a gel-like substance that acts as a layer of cushioning between the client's bony prominences and the surface of the bed. Cover the pad with a pillow case to keep the client's skin away from the plastic surface of the pad. Be certain that there are no wrinkles in the pillow case.

- *Foam mattresses* help to evenly distribute the client's weight in bed. They may have a flat surface, but the egg crate type is most often used (Fig. 12-5). Cover both the foam mattress and the regular mattress with a bottom sheet only. Do not use any other bottom linens that could interfere with the function of the egg crate. Foam mattresses are treated with a special chemical to retard fire. Washing removes this chemical and makes the mattress a fire hazard. Soiled egg crate mattresses and pads should be discarded and replaced.

- *Alternating pressure mattresses* to help distribute weight are also used. They are made of plastic and have several compartments that are alternately inflated and deflated by an electrical pump (Fig. 12-6). This reduces constant pressure on skin surfaces. These mattresses are used for clients who spend most of their time in bed. Always place a sheet between the client's skin and the plastic mattress. No other bottom linens are used. Do not use pins. Check with your supervisor for instructions about the operation of the air mattress.

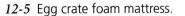
12-5 Egg crate foam mattress.

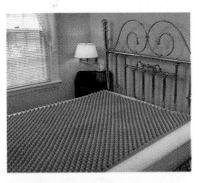

- *Sheepskin pads* are made of synthetic materials and look somewhat like lamb's wool (Fig. 12-7). These pads are very soft and comfortable to sit or lie on. They provide ease in moving and help to prevent shearing. Sheepskin pads can be washed in the regular laundry according to directions. Those that are too large will have to be washed in the large machines at the Laundromat.

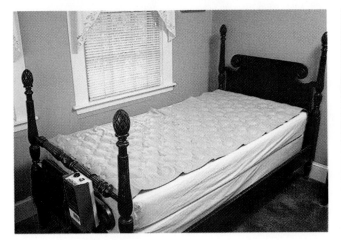
12-6 Alternating pressure mattress.

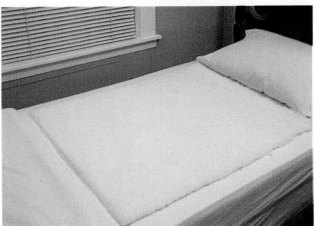
12-7 Sheepskin pad.

closed bed
made when the bed will remain empty for a period of time; may be made with or without a bedspread.

open bed
made when the bed will be occupied shortly; top linens are fan-folded to foot of bed.

occupied bed
made while the client is in the bed.

Always follow the care plan regarding the use of special devices for beds. Devices that relieve pressure do not take the place of turning and moving clients at least every two hours. Positioning, inspecting the skin and bony prominences, and keeping clients dry and clean are also needed to help prevent pressure sores.

Making the Bed

There are three ways to make a bed:
1. **Closed bed**—made when the bed will remain empty for a period of time; may be made with or without a bedspread (Fig. 12-8).
2. **Open bed**—made when the bed will become occupied shortly; top linens are fanfolded to the foot of the bed (Fig. 12-9).
3. **Occupied bed**—made while the client is in the bed.

Reasons for Bedmaking

There are several reasons for bedmaking and changing linens. These include:
1. providing comfort for the client
2. providing a clean, neat environment
3. preventing irritation and injury to the client's skin

For clients who spend most of their time in bed, the linens are almost like clothing and should be changed at least once daily. These clients may also be very sensitive to wrinkles in the linens or food crumbs, which may irritate the skin and cause pressure sores.

Other clients will spend little or no time in bed during the day. Their beds should be straightened and made each day. In this case, however, you may not need to use clean linens every time you make the bed. Before changing the bed linens, find out when they were last changed. Perhaps only the pillowcases need to be changed. Follow the directions in the care plan regarding bedmaking.

Regardless of how much time the client spends in bed, linens should be changed whenever they become wet or soiled. Remember to wear gloves if you will come in contact with urine or feces when changing the linens.

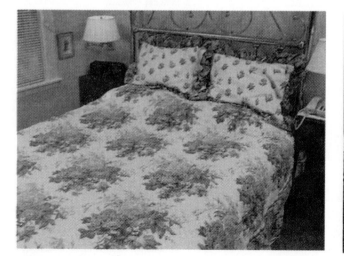
12-8 Closed bed.

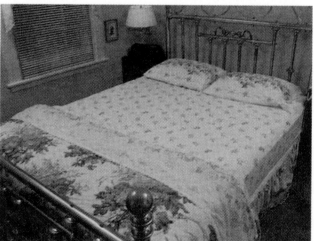
12-9 Open bed.

General Rules of Bedmaking

Whether you are changing linens or just making the bed, here are some general rules to follow when making a client's bed:

- Assemble all items needed before you start to make the bed.
- Practice good body mechanics while making the bed.
- Make bed according to client's custom.
- Make one side of bed as much as possible before going to other side, as this will save time and energy.
- Do not use torn linen.
- Keep bottom linens smooth and free of wrinkles.
- Remove crumbs and food particles from bed linens.
- Change linen when it becomes damp, wet, or soiled.
- Follow rules for infection control (Box 12-2).

Materials Needed for Bedmaking

Clients will usually want you to make their beds a certain way. This, of course, will vary from client to client. Some will want only sheets; others will want you to use both sheets and blankets. Some clients may have only one set of linens—those on the bed. You may have to launder these linens while the client is out of bed and then put them back on the bed. Follow the care plan regarding bedmaking. Other clients may have no linens at all; they may be lying on just a bare mattress. Contact your supervisor if your client has no linens or if you do not have enough linens to properly make the bed.

The following materials are usually used to make the client's bed:

- *Mattress pad or cover (optional)*—protects the mattress from being soiled. Made of cotton or plastic.
- *Bottom sheet (flat or fitted)*—provides additional protection for the mattress. Also provides comfort to the client when it is smooth and wrinkle free. Made of cotton, cotton blend, or flannel.

Box 12-2

Infection Control Reminders

- Keep all bed linens off the floor.
- Place used linens in laundry container immediately after removing from bed.
- Wash and dry soiled linens as soon as possible.
- Roll linens away from your clothing.
- Do not shake bed linens.
- Hold and fold linens away from your clothing.
- Wash hands before and after changing linens.
- Use gloves when handling linens soiled with body fluids.
- Follow rules in Chapters 7 and 9 for handling and washing soiled linens.

- *Draw sheet (optional)*—protects the mattress and bottom sheet. It is placed across the middle third of the bed and can serve as a turning or lifting sheet. It is about half the size of a regular sheet. To make a draw sheet, fold a regular sheet in half, lengthwise. If a plastic drawsheet is used, a cotton draw sheet **must** be placed completely over it to protect the client's skin. Plastic can be very uncomfortable because it retains the body's heat and moisture. Lying directly on a plastic sheet can cause damage to the skin's surface. Never use a plastic garbage bag or a dry cleaner's bag. They are not heavy enough to protect the bed. They can also cling to the nose or mouth and keep a client from breathing.
- *Bed protector/**incontinent** pad (optional)*—provides added protection to the bottom sheet. It is placed under the client's buttocks. Made of absorbent material, usually with a plastic underside. If the client soils the pad, it can be thrown away. This saves time and energy because bed linens do not have to be removed and replaced each time the client soils the bed. However, bed protectors can be costly. Use according to the wishes of the client/family.
- *Top sheet*—provides comfort for the client. Since it rests directly on the client, the sheet should not prevent a client from moving the feet or toes. To conserve linens, a clean top sheet can be used as a bottom sheet after the soiled bottom sheet is removed.
- *Blanket (optional)*—provides additional warmth and comfort for the client. Made of cotton, wool, and synthetic blends. When a blanket is used, the top sheet must always be placed between the client and the blanket.
- *Bedspread*—protects the bed linens when the bed is not in use. Bedspreads are used according to the preference of the client.
- *Pillow protector*—protects pillow from being soiled. Made of cotton or plastic.
- *Pillowcase*—provides comfort for the client. Made of cotton, cotton blend, or flannel.

Making a Closed Bed

This type of bed is easier to make than the occupied bed. Whenever possible, get your client out of bed before making the bed. You will save time and energy. Usually, the bed is made in the morning, after the client's bath. The procedure described applies to any size bed—hospital, twin, queen, or king size bed. The supplies you gather will depend on what is available in the home and the client's custom for making the bed. (See Procedure 12-1.)

When the client will return to bed shortly, an open bed is made using Procedure 12-2.

Making an Occupied Bed

This type of bed is made when the client is not able to get out of bed. Follow Procedure 12-3.

When making the bed it is important to:

- Explain what you are going to do before it is done
- Explain to your client how to help by rolling to one side of the bed at a time
- Keep the client fully covered with the blanket or top sheet during the procedure—do not expose the client

incontinent
the inability to control urination or bowel elimination.

Making a Closed Bed

Materials Needed

- Laundry container
- Mattress pad, if used
- Bottom sheet (flat or fitted)
- Plastic draw sheet, if used
- Cotton draw sheet, if used
- Top sheet
- Blanket, if used
- Bedspread, if used
- Pillowcase(s)

Procedure

1. Explain what you are going to do.
2. Wash your hands.
3. Obtain materials listed above and place them in order of use on chair near bed.
4. Place laundry container near bed.
5. Raise bed to convenient working height and lower both rails.*
6. Place bed in flat position.*
7. Remove pillow(s) and place on chair.
8. Loosen all bed linens—at head, sides, and bottom of bed.
9. Remove each piece of bed linen separately. Fold any linens to be reused (Fig. 12-10). Roll each

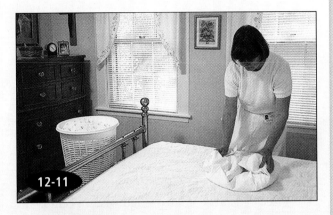

12-11

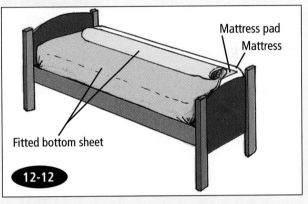

Mattress pad
Mattress
Fitted bottom sheet

12-12

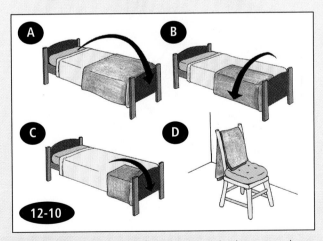

12-10

A, Fold top edge of blanket down to the bottom edge. **B,** Fold blanket over from far side of bed to the near side. **C,** Fold top edge of blanket down to bottom edge. **D,** Place folded blanket over back of chair.

remaining linen into a ball and discard in laundry container (Fig. 12-11).

10. Place clean mattress pad, folded lengthwise, in center of bed. Unfold one half and roll to center of bed.**
11. Place bottom sheet, folded lengthwise, in center of bed. Unfold one half and roll to center of bed.
    - Fitted sheet—place ends around corners— top and bottom (Fig. 12-12); tuck side of sheet under mattress
    - Flat sheet—place bottom hem of sheet even with edge of mattress at foot of bed; tuck top of sheet under mattress at head of bed
12. Miter corner at head end of mattress. (See Procedure 12-4, page 205.)
13. Tuck sheet under side of entire mattress. Work from head of bed to foot.
14. Place plastic draw sheet, folded in half, in center third of bed. Unfold and roll to center of bed.**

*Your client may not have an adjustable hospital bed; those steps marked with a single asterisk (*) will not apply.
**Optional—used according to client's needs and care plan.

Continued.

Making a Closed Bed

15. Place cotton draw sheet, folded in half, in center of bed, covering entire plastic draw-sheet (Fig. 12-13). Unfold and roll to center of bed.**
16. Tuck ends of plastic draw sheet and cotton draw sheet under mattress.**
17. Place top sheet, folded lengthwise, in center of bed, with top edge even with top of mattress. Unfold and roll to center of bed (Fig. 12-14).
18. Place blanket, folded lengthwise, in center of bed, with top edge even with top of mattress. Unfold and roll to center of bed.**
19. Place bedspread, folded lengthwise, in center of bed, with about 4 inches above top edge of mattress. Unfold and roll to center of bed.**
20. Tuck top sheet, blanket, and bedspread under foot of mattress. Miter corner.
21. Go to other side of bed.
22. Pull through mattress pad and straighten.
23. Pull through all lower linens. Straighten and tuck under mattress. Miter corner of sheet at head of bed. Or fit top and bottom corners of fitted sheet over mattress corners.
24. Pull through top sheet, blanket, and spread. Smooth out wrinkles (Fig. 12-15).
25. Tuck top sheet, blanket, and bedspread under foot of mattress.
26. Miter corner at foot of bed.
27. Make a cuff at top of bed and bring top sheet over blanket.
28. Place clean pillowcase on pillow, and place pillow at head of bed.
29. Cover pillow with bedspread.
30. Place bed in lowest position.*
31. Remove laundry container and bring to washing machine or other location as requested by client or family.
32. Wash your hands.

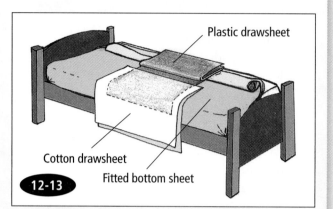

Plastic drawsheet
Cotton drawsheet
Fitted bottom sheet
12-13

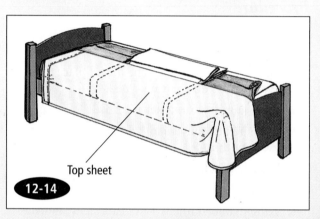

Top sheet
12-14

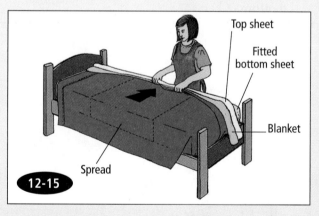

Top sheet
Fitted bottom sheet
Blanket
Spread
12-15

**Your client may not have an adjustable hospital bed; those steps marked with a single asterisk (*) will not apply.*
***Optional—used according to client's needs and care plan.*

Making an Open Bed

1. Wash your hands.
2. Obtain materials needed for making a closed bed.
3. Make a closed bed.
4. Fanfold top linens to foot of bed.
5. Wash your hands.

Procedure 12-3

Making an Occupied Bed

Materials Needed:

- Laundry container
- Mattress pad, if used
- Bottom sheet (flat or fitted)
- Plastic draw sheet, if used
- Cotton draw sheet, if used
- Top sheet
- Blanket, if used
- Bedspread, if used
- Pillow case(s)
- Disposable gloves, if needed

Procedure

1. Explain what you are going to do.
2. Wash your hands.
3. Obtain materials listed above, and place them in order of use on chair near bed.
4. Provide privacy (close door, shut drapes, pull shades).
5. Place laundry container near bed.
6. Raise bed to comfortable working height and lock wheels. Lower rail on side where you are working.*
7. Lower head of bed to level comfortable for client—as low as possible.*
8. Loosen top bedding at foot of bed.
9. Remove top bedding (bedspread, quilt), but leave client covered with one blanket or top sheet.
10. Instruct client to hold top sheet while you remove other top linens (Fig. 12-16).
11. Fold any linens to be reused, such as blanket or quilt. Roll each remaining linen into a ball and discard in laundry container.
12. Help client to roll to side of bed opposite to you and to grasp side rail for support.*
13. Roll each piece of bottom linen to center of bed and tuck along client's back (Fig. 12-17).
14. Smooth mattress pad, if used.**

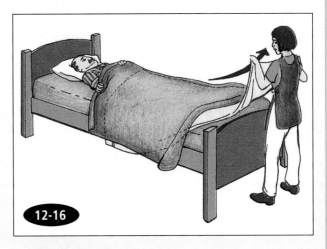

12-16

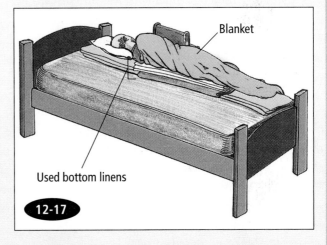

Blanket

Used bottom linens

12-17

15. Place clean bottom sheet, folded lengthwise, in center of bed. Unfold one half and roll to center of bed.
    - *Fitted sheet*—place ends around corners— top and bottom; tuck side of sheet under mattress
    - *Flat sheet*—place bottom hem of sheet even with edge of mattress at foot of bed; tuck top of sheet under mattress at head of bed
16. Miter corner at head end of mattress.
17. Tuck sheet under side of entire mattress. Work from head of bed to foot.
18. Place plastic draw sheet, folded in half, in center third of bed. Unfold and roll to center of bed. Tuck along client's back.**

*Your client may not have an adjustable hospital bed; those steps marked with a single asterisk (*) will not apply.
**Optional—used according to client's needs and care plan.

Continued.

Procedure 12-3—cont'd.

Making an Occupied Bed

19. Place cotton draw-sheet, folded in half, in center of bed, covering entire plastic drawsheet. Unfold and roll to center of bed. Tuck along client's back (Fig. 12-18).**

20. Tuck ends of plastic draw sheet and cotton draw sheet under mattress.**

21. Help client to roll toward you, over linens to clean side of bed.

22. Raise rail on side where you have been working.*

23. Go to other side of bed.

24. Lower side rail.*

25. Remove used bottom linens, roll, and discard in laundry container.

26. Pull through all bottom linens. Straighten and tuck under head of mattress. Miter corner of sheet at head of bed. Or fit top and bottom corners of fitted sheet over mattress corners.

27. Help client to roll back to center of bed.

28. Place clean top sheet entirely over the client and remove top linen. Discard in laundry container or fold for reuse.

29. Place blanket and bedspread over sheet.

30. Tuck top sheet, blanket, and bedspread under foot of mattress. Give "toe room" for client's feet. Make a mitered corner.

31. Raise side rail.*

32. Go to other side of bed. Lower side rail.*

33. Smooth and straighten top sheet, blanket, and bedspread. Tuck them under foot of mattress. Give "toe room" for client's feet (Fig. 12-19). Make mitered corner.

34. Make a cuff at top of bed and bring top sheet over bedspread.

35. Remove pillow from bed. Remove pillowcase and discard in laundry container.

36. Place clean pillowcase on pillow, and replace pillow under client's head.

37. Make sure client is safe and comfortable.

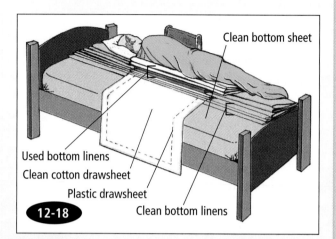

Clean bottom sheet

Used bottom linens
Clean cotton drawsheet
Plastic drawsheet
Clean bottom linens

12-18

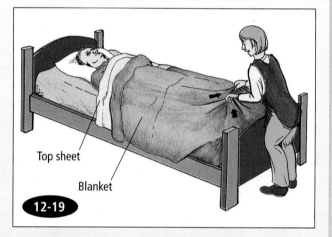

Top sheet

Blanket

12-19

38. Place bed in lowest position. (Raise side rail, if indicated.)*

39. Remove laundry container and bring to washing machine or other location as requested by client or family.

40. Wash your hands..

Your client may not have an adjustable hospital bed; those steps marked with a single asterisk (*) will not apply.
**Optional—used according to client's needs and care plan.*

Making a Mitered Corner

Bottom bedding

1. Tuck bottom sheet about 18 inches under the mattress at head of bed (Fig. 12-20).

2. Turn side of sheet up over the mattress in a triangle shape (Fig. 12-21).

3. Tuck the lower edge of the sheet (hanging down next to the mattress) under the side of the mattress (Fig. 12-22).

4. Turn the triangular area of sheet down over the mattress (Fig. 12-23).

5. Tuck sheet under the mattress (Fig. 12-24).

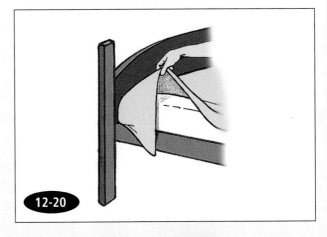
12-20

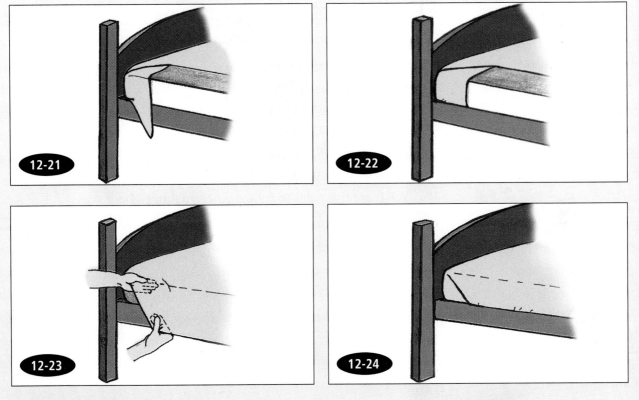
12-21

12-22

12-23

12-24

Upper bedding

Follow the procedure for mitered corners for bottom bedding, omitting the fifth step. The upper sheet hangs freely over the mattress (Fig. 12-25).

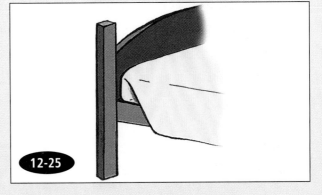
12-25

CHAPTER SUMMARY

- Bedmaking provides comfort and a clean environment for the client.
- There are several types of beds.
- Make sure the bed is neat, clean, dry, and free of wrinkles and crumbs.
- Procedures for bedmaking may have to be adjusted according to the needs of the client, type of bed, and materials available.
- Practice good body mechanics when bedmaking to avoid the possibility of injury.
- Handle bed linens correctly to avoid the spread of microorganisms. Observe universal precautions at all times.

STUDY QUESTIONS

1. List three reasons for bedmaking.
2. Describe a hospital bed.
3. Explain the use of the following:
   Egg crate mattress
   Sheepskin pad
   Bed cradle
4. List five items used in bedmaking.
5. What are five rules to follow when making a bed?
6. List five rules for infection control when handling linens during bedmaking.

Personal Care

13

Objectives

After you read this chapter, you will be able to:

1. List five reasons why clients may be unable to perform personal care activities.

2. List four purposes of bathing.

3. Discuss six principles to follow when bathing clients.

4. Explain the difference between the following types of baths:
   a. complete bed bath
   b. partial bath
   c. tub bath
   d. shower bath

5. Discuss safety factors to be considered while giving personal care.

6. Give two examples of the use of universal precautions during personal care of clients.

7. List three benefits of range of motion exercises and four points to remember when assisting with these exercises.

8. Demonstrate procedures for oral hygiene, bathing, grooming, and range of motion exercises.

Part 3 Home Care Procedures

ersonal care and grooming are important services provided by the home care aide. Clients are often unable to perform self-care, such as bathing, shampooing, oral hygiene, and skin and nail care. There are many reasons for clients' inability to care for themselves, including:

- the effects of illness
- lack of energy and strength
- pain and discomfort
- not being able to reach body parts
- not being able to obtain, carry, or use supplies needed for personal care
- anxiety and fear of injury
- confusion, inability to understand, forgetting what to do and how to do it

A client's inability to perform self-care may be described by using the following terms:

- *temporary*—will improve with time, performing self-care will return
- *permanent*—will not change, the client will always need assistance
- *progressive*—will continue and increase with time.

The care plan lists the personal care to be given to your client. If you have any questions, check with your supervisor. Remember to encourage clients to be as independent as possible according to their abilities and limitations. Give as much personal care as needed. Establish a communication system so that the client can call you when needed (Fig. 13-1).

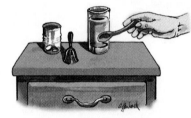

13-1 Communication systems. Client may call aide using a bell, tapping partially filled water glass with a spoon, or shaking a small can with a few coins inside.

Oral Hygiene (Mouth Care)

Oral hygiene means cleaning the mouth, teeth, gums, and tongue to remove pieces of food and bacteria. This helps prevent tooth decay, gum disease, and mouth odor. Oral hygiene also gives the mouth a clean feeling and a good taste. Since the mouth is the first organ of the digestive system, a clean and healthy mouth is important for good nutrition.

Follow the care plan regarding the type of mouth care and the amount of assistance needed. Observe the client's mouth, gums, lips, and teeth for any signs of irritation, loose teeth, or sores. Report abnormal findings to your supervisor. Oral hygiene is usually given in the morning upon awakening, after meals, and at bedtime.

Brushing Teeth

Important points to remember when giving mouth care include:

1. Wash hands before and after procedure. Wear gloves. Practice universal precautions.
2. Encourage self-care according to the client's ability and the care plan.
3. Get all the supplies ready and let the client perform self-care at the bedside, in the bathroom, or at the kitchen sink.
4. Use a soft-bristled toothbrush.
5. Have client balloon cheeks in and out to distribute water or mouthwash throughout mouth and between teeth.

lubricant
a fluid, ointment, or other substance for reducing friction between parts that rub together and for making a surface slippery; it protects skin and prevents drying.

aspiration
breathing in or inhaling a substance into the bronchial tubes and lungs.

6. Clients who can not balloon or swish rinse water and/or mouthwash can turn their heads from side to side (as if to signal "no") to distribute fluid throughout mouth.

7. Gently brush all surfaces of teeth, mouth, and gums.

8. Apply **lubricant** to prevent dry, cracked lips.

9. Assist client to use adaptive toothbrushes (Fig. 13-2), if needed.

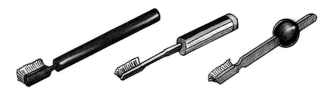

13-2 Examples of adaptive toothbrushes.

Follow Procedure 13-1, Brushing Teeth (page 210).

Flossing Teeth

Flossing between the surfaces of the teeth helps to remove food particles and other materials that may cause decay, gum disease, and mouth odor. Teeth are usually flossed before brushing, but dentists recommend that flossing be done immediately after breakfast and at bedtime.

There are two types of dental floss, waxed or unwaxed. The waxed floss is smoother, does not fray easily, and glides between the teeth smoothly. The unwaxed floss is thinner and may be more effective in removing food particles where teeth are very close together. Both types of floss are also available with flavoring, such as mint.

Some clients will use tiny toothbrushes to clean between the teeth. These are used after regular brushing and usually after each meal. You will need to floss for clients who are unable to do this for themselves. Always wear gloves as there is risk of bleeding from the gums. Follow Procedure 13-2, Flossing Teeth, on page 211.

Mouth Care for the Unconscious Client

Unconscious patients require frequent mouth care—about every two hours. They usually breathe through the mouth and, as a result, have a very dry mouth, tongue, and lips. Because they are unable to drink or swallow, secretions may dry and become crusted, causing odor and providing a place for bacterial growth.

Since these clients cannot swallow, there is a danger of choking and **aspiration** of fluids into the lungs. To prevent aspiration, place the client in a side-lying position so fluids drain out of the mouth instead of down the throat.

Always explain what you are going to do, and talk to the unconscious clients when giving personal care. Most clients are able to hear and understand what is happening, even though they are unable to respond to your communication.

Unconscious clients cannot hold their mouths open during the cleaning procedure. You will need to hold the mouth open by using a padded tongue depressor or a spoon wrapped in gauze. Do not use your fingers because the client may accidentally bite you. Remember, any break in the surface of your skin could permit the entrance of pathogenic organisms and lead to an infection. Wear gloves and practice universal precautions.

Procedure 13-1

Brushing Teeth

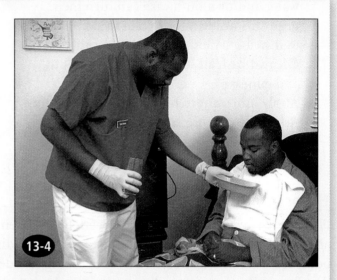

13-4

Materials Needed

- Toothbrush
- Toothpaste
- Glass of cool water
- Mouthwash
- Emesis basin or small plastic bowl
- Face towel
- Paper towel
- Disposable gloves

Procedure

1. Explain what you are going to do.
2. Wash hands.
3. Obtain materials listed above.
4. Provide privacy (close door, shut drapes, pull shades).
5. Spread paper towel on work area. Arrange supplies on paper towel.
6. Raise bed to convenient working height. Lower rail on side where you are working.*
7. Assist client to an upright position, or turn on side if unable to sit up.
8. Place face towel under client's chin and over chest.
9. Put on gloves.
10. Assist client with self-care as necessary.
11. Hold toothbrush over emesis basin and pour a little water over the brush to moisten. Apply toothpaste.
12. Brush client's teeth (if he/she is unable to do so) (Fig. 13-3A–D).

13. Have client rinse mouth with water. Hold emesis basin so client can spit into it (Fig. 13-4).
14. Have client rinse with mouthwash. Hold emesis basin so client can spit into it.
15. Wipe client's mouth with face towel.
16. Remove face towel.
17. Remove and discard gloves.
18. Make sure client is safe and comfortable.
19. Place bed in lowest position. (Raise side rail, if indicated.)*
20. Clean equipment and store in proper location.
21. Wipe work surface with paper towel and discard.
22. Place soiled face towel in laundry container to be washed.
23. Wash your hands.
24. Record what you have done. Report any unusual conditions to your supervisor.

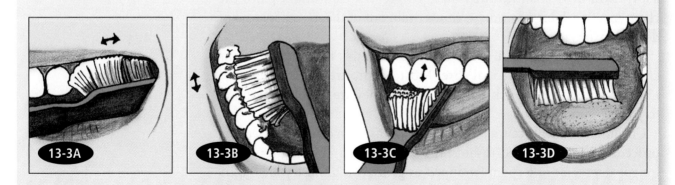

13-3A   13-3B   13-3C   13-3D

*Your client may not have an adjustable hospital bed; those steps marked with an asterisk (*) will not apply.

Procedure 13-2

Flossing Teeth

Materials Needed

- Dental floss dispenser
- Glass of cool water
- Emesis basin or small plastic bowl
- Face towel
- Paper towel
- Disposable gloves

Procedure

1. Explain what you are going to do.
2. Wash your hands.
3. Obtain materials listed above.
4. Provide privacy (close door, shut drapes, pull shades).
5. Spread paper towel on work area. Arrange supplies on paper towel.
6. Raise bed to convenient working height. Lower rail on side where you are working.*
7. Assist client to an upright position, or turn on side if unable to sit up.
8. Place face towel under client's chin and over chest.
9. Put on gloves.
10. Remove 18 inches (44–46 cm) of floss from dispenser.
11. Wrap floss around the middle finger of each hand to clean upper teeth (Fig. 13-5).
12. Hold floss with index fingers to clean lower teeth (Fig. 13-6).
13. Insert floss between teeth and use up and down, back and forth motions to remove any materials between teeth. Proceed from tooth to tooth:
    a Upper teeth, left to right (Fig. 13-7)
    b. Lower teeth, left to right.
14. Have client rinse mouth with water. Hold emesis basin so client can spit into it.
15. Wipe client's mouth with face towel.
16. Remove face towel.
17. Remove and discard gloves.
18. Make sure client is safe and comfortable.
19. Place bed in lowest position. (Raise side rail, if indicated.)*
20. Clean equipment and store in proper location.
21. Wipe work surface with paper towel and discard.
22. Place soiled face towel in laundry container to be washed.
23. Wash your hands.
24. Record what you have done. Report any unusual conditions to your supervisor.

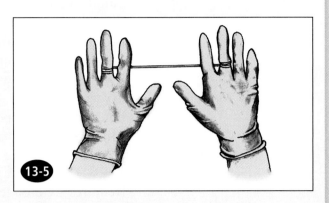

13-5

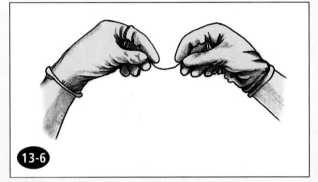

13-6

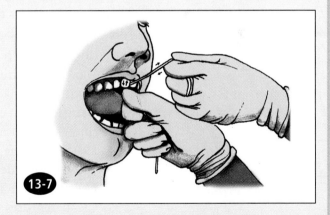

13-7

*Your client may not have an adjustable hospital bed; those steps marked with an asterisk (*) will not apply.

Cotton-tipped applicators may be used to clean the surfaces of the mouth. Glycerine swabs are also used, but they can make the mouth feel dry. Toothettes (foam-tipped applicators) can also be used. Clean the mouth and the oral surfaces with mouth wash or a **normal saline solution.** To make a normal saline solution, use one teaspoon of table salt in two cups (500 ml) of warm water. Stir to dissolve salt.

After cleaning, apply a little petroleum jelly or other lubricant to the lips to prevent drying, cracking, and discomfort. If client is receiving oxygen, do not use petroleum jelly. Follow the care plan and instructions from your supervisor regarding any special mouth care needed by your client. See Procedure 13-3, Mouth Care for Unconscious Clients.

Denture Care

Dentures are false teeth that are worn to replace missing natural teeth. A client may have a complete set of false teeth or a partial set. They must be removed from the mouth for thorough cleaning. Any remaining natural teeth are cleaned as usual following Procedure 13-1. Many clients will be able to clean their own dentures. Gather the supplies needed and provide assistance as necessary. Dentures are cleaned in the morning and at bedtime and, if necessary, after meals.

Some clients are not able to clean their own dentures. Ask them to remove the dentures and place them in an **emesis basin.** Sometimes it may be necessary for you to remove the dentures. Wear gloves and follow the steps listed in the Procedure 13-4, Caring for Dentures, on page 214.

Important points to remember about denture care include:

1. Practice universal precautions. (See Box 13-1, on page 215, Infection Control Reminders.) Wear gloves when handling dentures.
2. Handle dentures very carefully. They are easily broken. Replacement is costly and inconvenient.
3. Use gauze or a clean washcloth to grasp dentures. They are very slippery when wet.
4. Partially fill the sink with warm water to act as a cushion in case you drop the dentures during cleaning.
5. Use warm water to clean dentures. Hot water may damage them.
6. Clean dentures with a toothbrush and toothpaste.
7. Have client rinse mouth with mouthwash or other solution before replacing the dentures in the mouth.
8. Apply denture adhesive to the false teeth if the client uses this product.
9. Place unworn dentures in a covered denture cup or box, either dry or with solution, according to client's preference. Store in a safe location. Never place dentures in tissues or paper towels because they may be accidentally thrown in the trash.
10. Observe the condition of the client's mouth and report any abnormal findings. Observe the condition of the dentures and report any cracks, sharp edges, loose teeth, or broken areas.

See Procedure 13-4, Caring for Dentures.

normal saline solution
a solution of table salt and water in the same concentration as in the body tissue.

emesis basin
a kidney-shaped basin that fits against the neck to collect vomitus.

Procedure 13-3

Mouth Care for Unconscious Clients

Materials Needed

- Toothettes or applicators
- Padded tongue depressor
- Glycerine swabs (optional)
- Petroleum jelly or mineral oil for lips (optional)
- Mouthwash
- Glass of cool water
- Emesis basin or small plastic bowl
- Face towel
- Paper towel
- Disposable gloves

Procedure

1. Explain what you are going to do.
2. Wash your hands.
3. Obtain materials listed above.
4. Provide privacy (close door, shut drapes, pull shades).
5. Spread paper towel on work area. Arrange supplies on paper towel.
6. Raise bed to convenient working height. Lower rail on side where you are working.*
7. Place client in a side-lying position.
8. Place face towel and emesis basin under client's chin.
9. Put on gloves.
10. Gently open client's mouth with padded tongue depressor (Fig. 13-8).
11. Moisten Toothette and clean all surfaces of mouth: roof of mouth, tongue, gums, lips, inside

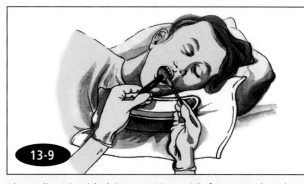

Place client in side-lying position with face towel and emesis basin under chin. Open mouth with padded tongue depressor. Clean all surfaces with toothette.

of cheeks. Rinse and re-wet Toothette as necessary. Clean teeth with Toothette (Fig. 13-9).

12. Wipe client's mouth with face towel.
13. Remove face towel.
14. Apply lubricant to lips.
15. Remove and discard gloves.
16. Make sure client is safe and comfortable.
17. Place bed in lowest position. (Raise side rail, if indicated.)*
18. Clean equipment and store in proper location.
19. Wipe work surface with paper towel and discard.
20. Place soiled face towel in laundry container to be washed.
21. Wash your hands.
22. Record what you have done. Report any unusual conditions to your supervisor.

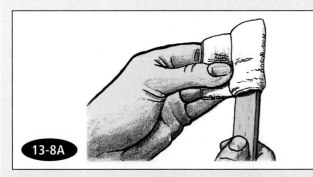
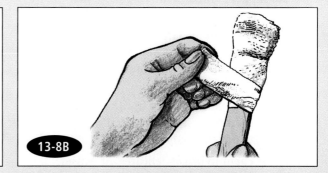

Making a padded tongue depressor.
A, Place two wooden tongue depressors together and wrap gauze around top half. **B,** Tape gauze in place.

Your client may not have an adjustable hospital bed; those steps marked with an asterisk (*) will not apply.

Caring for Dentures

Materials Needed

- Toothpaste
- Toothbrush
- Tissues or gauze
- Denture cup or box
- Mouthwash or saline solution
- Glass of cool water
- Emesis basin or small plastic bowl
- Paper towel
- Disposable gloves

Procedure

1. Explain what you are going to do.

2. Wash your hands.

3. Obtain materials listed above.

4. Provide privacy (close door, shut drapes, pull shades).

5. Spread paper towel on work area. Arrange supplies on paper towel if procedure will be done at bedside. Otherwise, take supplies for cleaning dentures to sink.

6. Raise bed to convenient working height. Lower rail on side where you are working.*

7. Assist client to an upright position or turn on side, if unable to sit up.

8. Put on gloves.

9. Ask client to remove dentures and place in emesis basin. If you must remove dentures, grasp them with gauze or a tissue (wet dentures are slippery and difficult to grasp). Remove in this manner:

   a. *Upper dentures.* Grasp between thumb and index finger and move up and down gently until you feel the suction release. Pull down and remove.

   b. *Lower dentures.* Grasp in the same manner and gently twist sideways and up, lifting them out of the mouth.

10. Assist client to brush dentures. At bedside, client uses water in cup, toothbrush, paste, etc. At sink, same materials are used.

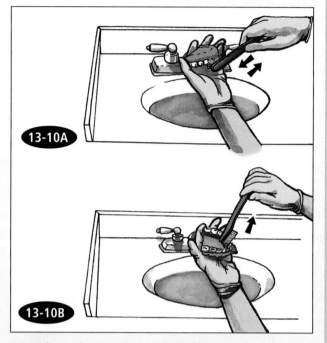

A, With toothpaste on brush, hold dentures over sink and brush outside of teeth from side to side and then up and down. **B,** Turn over dentures and brush insides with an up-and-down motion.

11. Aide cleans dentures at sink:

    a. Partially fill sink with warm water to act as a cushion, should dentures be accidentally dropped (Fig. 13-10A).

    b. Brush with warm water and toothpaste in an up and down motion. Rinse thoroughly (Fig. 13-10B).

12. Return dentures to the client for replacement in the mouth or store in denture cup or box, dry or in solution, according to client's wishes.

13. Remove and discard gloves.

14. Make sure client is safe and comfortable.

15. Place bed in lowest position. (Raise side rail, if indicated.)*

16. Clean equipment and store in proper location.

17. Wipe work surface with paper towel and discard.

18. Wash your hands.

19. Record what you have done. Report any unusual conditions to your supervisor.

Your client may not have an adjustable hospital bed; those steps marked with an asterisk (*) will not apply.

Box 13-1

Infection Control Reminders

- Use gloves when:
  - giving personal care to clients with open sores in mouth or on skin
  - giving perineal care
  - handling clothing, towels, or washcloths soiled with blood or body fluids
  - removing, cleaning, or inserting dentures
  - giving mouth care
  - shaving client with a blade razor
- Keep client's clothing, towels, and washcloths off the floor, even when soiled
- Place soiled clothing in container and bring to laundry area immediately to be washed
- Keep client's personal grooming items (comb, toothbrush, denture box, etc.) separate from other family members' items

Bathing

Some cultures believe that bathing is a very important part of the healing process. In ancient times, people went to the "baths" to be cured by the warm, soothing waters. Even today, people seek out the soothing, relaxing waters of the spas and mineral baths for relaxation and tension relief. All cultures do not view bathing as particularly helpful during sickness. Some believe that a bath may cause the sick person to become chilled, and, as a result, they may become sicker. If your clients do not want to bathe, try to find out why. They may be afraid of falling in the bathroom, they may have pain, or they may be too tired. Discuss the situation with your supervisor.

Purposes

The bath has many purposes, including:

- cleansing the skin
- removing bacteria
- preventing body odor
- stimulating circulation
- moving joints and muscles
- observing client's skin (Box 13-2)
- communicating with client
- preventing pressure sores
- providing comfort and a sense of well-being.

Box 13-2

Observing Client's Skin— Check For

C Cuts, changes in color (pale, red, blue), cracked
H Hot to the touch
E Edema (swelling)
C Contusions (bruises)
K Krusty areas, knobby lumps
F Flaky skin
O Open sores
R Redness, rash

The frequency of the bath depends on the care plan and the needs of the client. For example, some clients may take a tub bath or shower only twice a week. This includes older adults with very dry skin and clients who are very weak and tire easily. Others with limitations, such as those with casts, recent **surgical incisions,** and **traction,** will not follow a pattern of daily bathing. Incontinent clients will need to be bathed each time the skin becomes soiled to prevent irritation and breakdown.

General Principles for Bathing Clients

General principles for bathing clients or assisting them to bathe include:

1. Be organized. Have the necessary supplies at hand.
2. Provide privacy. Do not expose the client's body unnecessarily.
3. Prevent chilling. Keep client covered as much as possible and avoid drafts.
4. Work efficiently.
5. Wash from clean to dirty areas.
6. Change bath water when it gets too soapy, or cool, or becomes contaminated with body secretions.
7. Prevent falls by following rules of safety.
8. Use good body mechanics.
9. Keep soap in dish, not in bath water.
10. Encourage client to help to do as much as possible according to care plan and physical condition.
11. Rinse skin thoroughly. Wash off soap, which can be drying and irritating.
12. Pat the skin dry. Be gentle.
13. Practice universal precautions when feces and urine are present. Wear gloves.

Skin Care Products

Many products are available for use on the skin. They include:

- *Soap* is used to clean the skin. It may be plain, medicated, perfumed, or moisturizing. Plain soap is drying to the skin and is not necessary for every bath. Many older adults have dry skin from aging. They may prefer a soap that contains a lubricant. Use the soap preferred by your client, unless the care plan lists a special product to be used.
- *Bath oil* is placed in the bath water to soften the skin and prevent drying. However, this product can make the tub and client's skin very slippery, increasing the risk of falls. In addition, it is very difficult to clean bath oil from the tub surfaces. Avoid the use of bath oil for your client. Instead, apply a lubricant to the skin after the bath.
- *Creams and lotions* are applied to soften the skin and prevent drying. Encourage clients to put on the lotion or cream themselves. Assist them by applying the product to areas they can not reach. Warm the lotion between your hands before applying to the skin. Gently apply lotion to the surface of the skin. Do not mas-

surgical incision
a cut produced surgically by a sharp instrument creating an opening into an organ or space.

traction
to put under tension by means of weights and pulleys to straighten or immobilize a body part or to relieve pressure on it.

genitalia (genitals)
organs of reproduction, usually external organs.

sage or rub in vigorously. Use a small amount, remove any excess cream or lotion with a towel. Too much lotion makes the skin feel hot and sticky. This is uncomfortable for the client. It may also provide a place for bacteria to live and grow. Use the lotion preferred by your client, unless the care plan lists a special product to be used.

- *Powder* is used to soothe and cool the skin and to prevent friction between two skin surfaces. Do not use a lot of powder but just enough to have a thin layer on the skin. Do not combine powder with creams and lotion. This will cause the powder to crust and cake on the skin, causing irritation and risk of infection. Do not shake powder in the air, as inhaled particles may irritate the respiratory tract and cause sneezing.
- *Deodorant* is used to prevent body odor. Antiperspirants help stop sweating and reduce body odor. They are applied to the armpits after bathing. Do not apply to irritated or broken skin.

Types of Baths

Complete Bed Bath The complete bed bath is given to clients who are not able to get out of bed to bathe themselves. Unconscious, paralyzed, or very weak clients may need to be bathed in bed. Those with casts will not be able to use the tub or shower and may need a bed bath.

Encourage clients to do as much as they can to care for themselves during the bed bath. Check the care plan with your supervisor to determine the level of activity permitted for the client. The complete bed bath may be embarrassing to the client and increase his/her feelings of dependence. Provide privacy, work quickly and efficiently, and talk to the client as you perform the bed bath. Follow the general principles for bathing clients listed earlier and in Procedure 13-5, Giving a Complete Bed Bath.

Partial Bath In a partial bath, the face, hands, underarms, back, buttocks, and **genitalia** are washed. This may be done in bed or at the bedside. A partial bath may also be given in the bathroom, at the sink, if this is listed in the care plan. Assemble all of the materials needed for bathing. Oral hygiene may also be done at this time. Place a straight chair in front of the sink so the client can sit while bathing. Help the client as needed. Dressing and grooming are usually done at the bedside.

Tub Bath A tub bath is relaxing and soothing. But it can also be a risky procedure because of the danger of burns, falls, and chills. Always make sure there is a rubber mat or non-slip surface in the tub. (See Box 13-3, Bath and Shower Safety.) Tub baths can also cause clients to become weak and tired. The bath should not be any longer than 20 minutes. Tub baths are drying to the skin and are usually given once or twice a week, with partial bathing in between. NEVER GIVE A TUB BATH UNLESS IT IS WRITTEN IN THE CARE PLAN. Follow Procedure 13-6, Giving a Tub Bath. Remember to use good body mechanics and be extremely careful when transferring clients into and out of the bath tub.

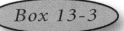

Box 13-3

Bath and Shower Safety

- Always place rubber or non-skid mat in tub before client enters.
- Be sure bathroom floor is dry to help prevent slips and falls.
- Do not add oil to bathtub water; apply oil to client's skin following the bath.
- Be sure bath water is the proper temperature; adjust water pressure before giving a shower.
- Stay near bathroom while client is bathing.
- Use good body mechanics.
- Bath or shower chairs should have rubber suction cups at ends of legs; these will steady the chair and prevent it from sliding.
- Have client use grab bars, if present; do not permit client to use towel bar or tile soap dish as an aid in moving.

Giving a Complete Bed Bath

Materials Needed

- Wash basin
- Soap dish and soap
- Orangewood stick, optional
- Bath blanket, optional
- Washcloth
- Face towel
- Bath towels (2)
- Paper towels
- Clean clothing (gown, pajamas, or other clothing)
- Oral hygiene materials
- Brush and/or comb
- Other articles used by client (deodorant, body powder or lotion, etc.)
- Disposable gloves

Procedure

1. Explain what you are going to do.
2. Wash your hands.
3. Obtain materials listed above.
4. Provide privacy (close door, shut drapes, pull shades).
5. Raise bed to convenient working height and lock wheels. Lower rail on side where you are working.*
6. Offer bed pan or urinal. (See Procedures 14-1 and 14-2.)
7. Lower head of bed to a level comfortable for client—as low as possible.
8. Remove top bedding and cover client with bath blanket or top sheet.
9. Help client to remove clothing, if needed.
10. Help client to move to side of bed near you.
11. Help client with oral hygiene, if needed.
12. Fill wash basin two-thirds full with warm water (110°–115° F) (43°–46° C)
13. Place towel under client's head and a towel over client's chest.
14. Make a mitt with washcloth (Fig. 13-11) to be used throughout procedure.
15. Wash eye areas gently with clean water only. Start from inner corner of eye to outer corner of eye. Use opposite corners of washcloth for each eye (Fig. 13-12).
16. Ask client if you should use soap or cleansing cream for cleansing the face.

Your client may not have an adjustable hospital bed; those steps marked with an asterisk (*) will not apply.

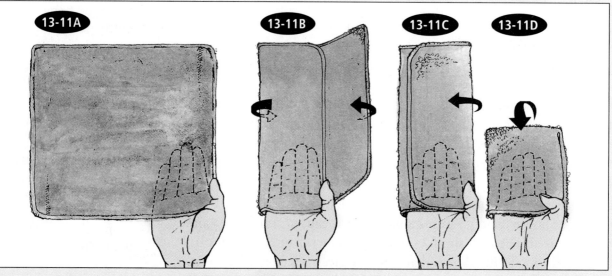

Making a washcloth mitt. **A,** Place hand under lower right hand corner of washcloth.
B, Secure washcloth with thumb and wrap around back of hand. **C,** Continue to fold washcloth over palm of hand and secure with thumb. **D,** Fold top of washcloth down and tuck it under the bottom.

17. Wash face from center outward. Use firm, gentle movements.

18. Wash ears and neck. Rinse and dry using towel on client's chest.

19. Put a towel, lengthwise, under the arm and a towel near hand on which to place the wash basin.

20. Put client's hand in basin (Fig. 13-13); allow it to soak. Wash the arm and armpit (Fig. 13-14).

21. Wash, rinse, and dry arm, armpit, and hand. Apply deodorant under arm, if requested. Push back cuticles; clean under nails with orange-wood stick. Dry between fingers thoroughly.

22. Follow steps 19–21 for the other arm and hand.

23. Place basin back on bedside table or chair.

24. Put towel over chest and abdomen. Pull bath blanket (top sheet) to thighs (Fig. 13-15). Do not expose client when washing chest and abdomen.

25. Wash, rinse, and dry chest and abdomen. Cover chest and abdomen with bath blanket (top sheet). Remove towel.

26. Uncover leg. Do not expose genital area. Place towel under the leg and foot. Place another towel near foot and put basin on towel.

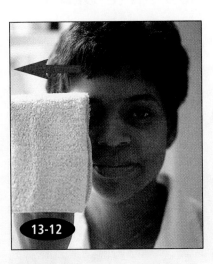

13-12

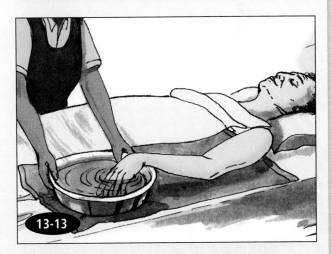

13-13

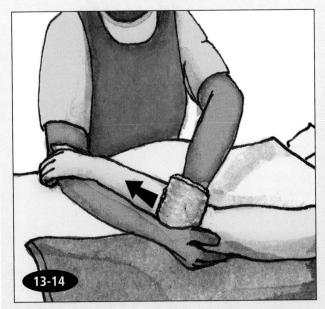

13-14

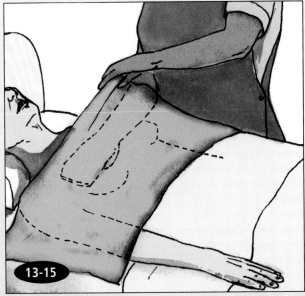

13-15

Continued.

Giving a Complete Bed Bath

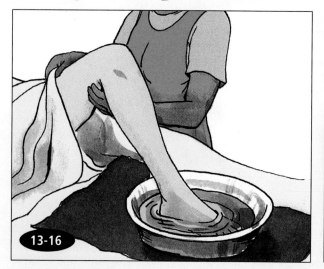

13-16

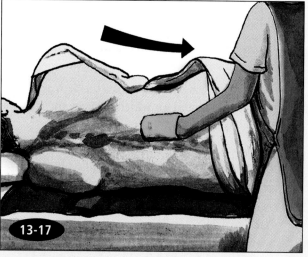

13-17

27. Bend client's knee and put foot in basin; allow it to soak. Wash and dry leg while foot is soaking (Fig. 13-16).

28. Wash and dry foot. Clean under toenails. Dry between toes thoroughly.

29. Repeat steps 26–28 for other leg and foot.

30. Place basin back on bedside table or chair.

31. Turn client on side: drape bath blanket (top sheet) to expose back and buttocks.

32. Place towel on bed, tucked lengthwise along neck and shoulders to buttocks.

33. Wash, rinse, and dry neck, shoulders, back, and buttocks. Work from neck to buttocks. Use long strokes for washing the back (Fig. 13-17).

34. Give back rub (Procedure 13-7).

35. Change bath water.

36. Turn client on to back.

37. Place towel under buttocks. Place basin, soap, and towels within reach. Have client wash genital and rectal areas. Ask client to tell you when finished. If client is unable to wash these areas, complete this part of the bath wearing disposable gloves (Procedure 13-8).

38. Help client to put on gown, pajamas, or other clothing.

39. Comb or brush client's hair (Procedure 13-10).

40. Make sure client is safe and comfortable.

41. Place bed in lowest position. (Raise side rails, if indicated.)*

42. Empty and clean wash basin. Wipe off work area with paper towels and discard them. Place soiled towels and washcloth in laundry container to be washed. Return other supplies to their proper place.

43. Wash your hands.

44. Record what you have done. Report any unusual conditions to your supervisor.

*Your client may not have an adjustable hospital bed; those steps marked with an asterisk (*) will not apply.

Giving a Tub Bath

Materials Needed

- Soap
- Washcloth
- Bath towels (2)
- Straight chair, optional
- Bath chair or bath stool, optional
- Slide board, optional
- Skid-proof bath mat
- Other articles used by client (deodorant, body powder or lotion, etc.)
- Clean clothing

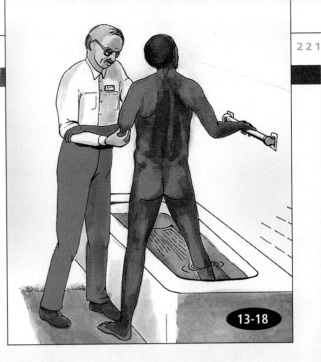

13-18

Procedure

1. Explain what you are going to do.
2. Wash your hands.
3. Obtain materials listed above.
4. Prepare bathroom by: placing skid-proof mat on bottom of tub; making sure room is warm and free of drafts; placing straight chair in bathroom; placing bath chair in tub; and bringing slide board, if used, to tub.
5. Provide privacy (close door, shut drapes, pull shades).
6. Help client to undress, put on bathrobe and footwear. Place client in wheelchair, if used. Lock brakes and put footrests in place.
7. Fill tub one-third full of warm water (110°–115° F) (43°–46° C)
8. Help client to bathroom and close door.
9. Place client in chair facing tub. If using wheelchair, lock brakes and place footrests out of the way.
10. Help client to lift one foot, then the other, over the side of the tub (Fig. 13-18).
11. When bath chair is used: have client hold onto grab bars while sliding off the chair to side of tub. If a slide board is used: help client to slide from surface of wheelchair to surface of bath chair in tub (Fig. 13-19). When bath chair is NOT used: have client hold onto grab bars while sliding off the chair to side of tub. Help client to lower into water, using grab bars for support.
12. Help client to bathe as needed.
13. Drain water from tub before getting client out of tub.

14. Help client to dry body. Assist client to put on bathrobe or cover with dry towel.
15. Place straight chair or wheelchair facing tub and place dry towel on side of tub.
16. Help client to sit on towel on side of tub using grab bars. (Reverse steps 10 and 11.)
17. Help client to stand, get out of tub into straight chair or wheelchair, and put on footwear.
18. Help client to room.
19. Give back rub.
20. Help client to put on clean clothing and return to bed, sofa, etc. Place in comfortable position.
21. Make sure client is safe and comfortable.
22. Return to bathroom. Clean tub and straighten area.
23. Place soiled towels and washcloth in laundry container to be washed.
24. Wash your hands.
25. Record what you have done. Report any unusual conditions to your supervisor.

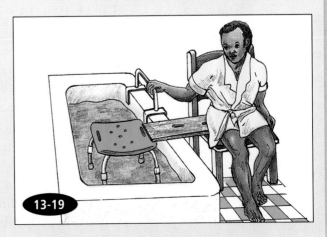

13-19

Shower Some clients will prefer a shower to a tub bath. Some homes have bathrooms with shower stalls and/or hand-held shower attachments. It will be easier for the client to step into the shower stall than a bathtub. Some important points to keep in mind when helping the client with the shower include:

- Obtain necessary materials as listed in Procedure 13-6, Giving a Tub Bath.
- Check to be sure shower chair, if one will be used, is secure and steady.
- Place non-skid mat on shower floor without blocking the drain.
- Turn on water; test and adjust water temperature (109° F or 43° C) and water pressure before client enters the shower.
- Encourage client to use grab bars, if installed, when getting in and out of the shower or tub.
- If required, assist client to get wet, then turn off water before applying soap to skin; turn on water again to rinse off.
- Avoid chilling; keep the bathroom door and shower curtains closed as much as possible.
- Encourage client to bathe self as much as possible, but give help when needed.
- Use aids to showering, such as soap-on-a-rope and long-handled back brushes or sponges, if available.
- Stay with client during entire procedure, if necessary.
- Even if client is able to bathe self, remain close to bathroom so that you will hear if the client calls for help.
- Help client to slowly get out of shower. Do not rush. The risk of falling on wet surfaces is great.
- Help client to completely dry off and put on robe or wrap up in bath sheet or large towel. Dressing and grooming may be done at the bedside.

NEVER GIVE A SHOWER UNLESS IT IS WRITTEN IN THE CARE PLAN.

Back Rub

The back rub involves applying lotion to the client's back in long, firm strokes from the buttocks to the shoulders. The back rub has several purposes:

- stimulates circulation
- provides relaxation and comfort
- prevents decubitus ulcers

Back rubs are given after the bath and at bedtime. Lotion is used to prevent friction and to soften the skin. Do not use too much. Wipe off any excess with a towel. Do not use alcohol because it is drying and can cause the client to become chilled. Warm lotion between your hands. When giving the back rub, be sure to observe the back and buttocks for any abnormal findings. Report them to your supervisor.

The care plan will tell you if there is a reason not to give a back rub. Follow Procedure 13-7, Giving a Back Rub.

Procedure 13-7

Giving a Back Rub

Materials Needed

- Small towel
- Lotion

Procedure

1. Explain what you are going to do.
2. Wash your hands.
3. Obtain materials listed above.
4. Provide privacy (close door, shut drapes, pull shades).
5. Raise bed to convenient working height and lock wheels. Lower rail on side where you are working.*
6. Lower head of bed to a level comfortable for client—as low as possible.
7. Remove clothing from upper body.
8. Place client on side or abdomen to expose entire back.
9. Put small amount of lotion on your hands. Rub hands together to warm lotion.
10. Use correct body mechanics. Face head of bed, one foot slightly forward, knees bent.
11. Start at the lower back moving upward toward the shoulders. Apply pressure using palms of both hands. Use long, firm but gentle strokes—up—out—and down. Repeat several times (Fig. 13-20).
12. Remove excess lotion with towel.
13. Help client to put on clothes.
14. Make sure client is safe and comfortable.
15. Place bed in lowest position. (Raise side rail, if indicated.)*
16. Wash your hands.
17. Record what you have done. Report location and size of any reddened areas or other unusual conditions to your supervisor.

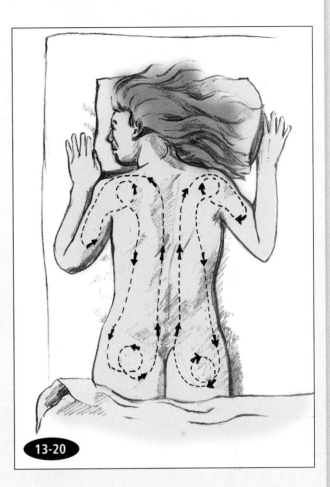

13-20

Your client may not have an adjustable hospital bed; those steps marked with an asterisk (*) will not apply.

Perineal Care

Perineal care refers to cleaning the perineum, the area between the legs. Sometimes the client will refer to this as "washing the privates," "the crotch," or "between the legs." In medical terms, this procedure is also known as "pericare."

Perineal care is done at least once daily, usually during the bath. Some clients will require more frequent perineal care. These clients include mothers who have just had a baby and those who are incontinent. Check the care plan to be sure about the frequency.

Most clients will be able to perform their own perineal care. If not, it is the responsibility of the home care aide. This can be embarrassing for both the client and the aide, since it is a very personal and intimate procedure. Protect the client's privacy, work quickly, efficiently, and as calmly as possible.

Wear disposable gloves, and always practice universal precautions. Wash from the cleanest area to the dirtiest area. The urinary meatus is a clean area. Wipe away from this structure toward the anus. The perineal area is very sensitive and easily injured. Be gentle. Rinse thoroughly because any remaining soap is extremely irritating to the perineum. Follow Procedure 13-8, Giving Perineal Care.

Grooming

Caring for Hands and Feet

Hands and feet need special attention to prevent infection, skin breakdown, odor, and injury. Hand and foot care can be given as part of the bath, or the care plan will give directions for giving care at another time. Some clients have foot problems that require special attention. In these cases, a podiatrist, a doctor trained in the treatment of nail or foot problems, will give the care.

Caring for the hands and feet gives the home care aide a chance to observe the condition of the skin and nails. Record and report the following conditions:

- sores, swelling, bruises, or reddened areas on hands and feet and between fingers and toes
- changes in coloring of skin and nails
- change in temperature of hands and feet— hot or cold to touch

It is not usually the home care aide's responsibility to cut the client's nails. Cutting thick nails may cause the nail clipper to slip and accidentally cut the skin around the nail. This can be very serious for clients who heal very slowly or are prone to infection. Check with your supervisor about the agency's policy about cutting nails. Follow Procedure 13-9, Caring for Nails and Feet.

perineal (perineum)
pertaining to the perineum, the area between the legs; in women, the area between the vagina and anus; in men, the area between the scrotum and anus.

Giving Perineal Care

Materials Needed

- Wash basin
- Soap dish and soap
- 5–6 washcloths or package of cotton balls
- Bath towel
- Waterproof protector pad
- Paper or plastic bag
- Paper towels
- Toilet tissue
- Disposable gloves

Procedure

1. Explain what you are going to do.
2. Wash your hands.
3. Obtain materials listed above.
4. Spread paper towel on work area. Arrange supplies on paper towel.
5. Provide privacy (close door, shut drapes, pull shades).
6. Raise bed to convenient working height. Lower rail on side where you are working.*
7. Fold top bedding to foot of bed and cover client with sheet or blanket.
8. Help client into supine position and remove clothing from waist down.
9. Position waterproof protector pads under buttocks.
10. Drape the client (Fig. 13-21A and B).
11. Raise side rail.*
12. Fill wash basin two-thirds full with warm water (105°–109° F) (41°–43° C).
13. Place basin on work area on top of paper towels.
14. Lower rail on side where you are working.*
15. Fold back the corner of blanket or sheet between client's legs and onto abdomen.
16. Help client to bend knees and spread legs.
17. Put on disposable gloves.
18. Apply soap and water to the washcloth or cotton balls.

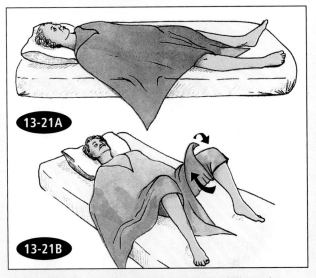

A, Position bath blanket or sheet like a diamond.
B, Wrap blanket around leg by bringing the corner around under leg and over the top. Tuck corner under the hip.

19. Give female perineal care
    a. Separate labia.
    b. Clean downward, with one stroke, from front to back. Use clean washcloth or cotton ball for each stroke. Put used cotton balls in bag or set aside used washcloths. Repeat this step until area is clean (Fig. 13-22).
    c. Rinse area, using same procedure as in steps 19a and 19b.
    d. Dry area thoroughly.
    e. Fold blanket back between client's legs.
    f. Help client to straighten legs and turn on side away from you.

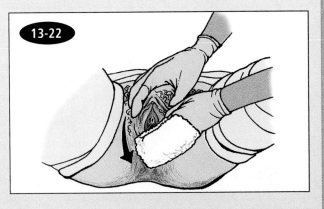

*Your client may not have an adjustable hospital bed; those steps marked with an asterisk (*) will not apply.

Continued.

Giving Perineal Care

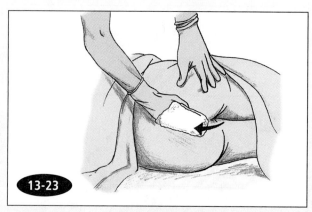

13-23

g. Separate buttocks and clean rectal area with toilet tissue, if needed (Fig. 13-23). Wash area from vagina to anus, using clean washcloth for each stroke. Repeat this step until area is clean.

h. Rinse area, using same procedure as in step 19g.

i. Dry area.

20. Give male perineal care

a. Gently pull back the foreskin, if client is uncircumcised (Fig. 13-24).

b. While holding penis, clean tip, using circular motion. Start at the urethral opening and work outward. Repeat this step, using a clean washcloth or cotton ball, until the area is clean (Fig. 13-25). Put used cotton balls in bag or set aside used washcloths.

c. Rinse and dry area thoroughly, using same procedure as steps 20a and b.

d. Return foreskin to natural position if client is uncircumcised.

e. Clean shaft of penis using a wash cloth with firm but gentle downward strokes. Rinse and dry area thoroughly.

f. Help client to bend knees and spread legs.

g. Gently clean scrotum. Wash skin folds carefully. Rinse and dry area thoroughly.

h. Help client to straighten legs and turn on side away from you.

i. Separate buttocks and clean rectal area with toilet tissue, if needed. Wash from scrotum to anus using clean washcloth for each stroke. Repeat this step until area is clean.

j. Rinse area using same procedure as in step 20i.

k. Dry area.

21. Remove soiled bedding, washcloths, and waterproof protector pad and place in laundry container to be washed.

22. Remove gloves and discard into bag.

23. Straighten bedding; remove sheet or blanket.

24. Make sure client is safe and comfortable.

25. Place bed in lowest position. (Raise side rail, if indicated.)*

26. Empty and clean wash basin. Wipe off work area with paper towels and discard into bag. Return other materials to their proper place.

27. Wash your hands.

28. Record what you have done. Report any unusual conditions to your supervisor.

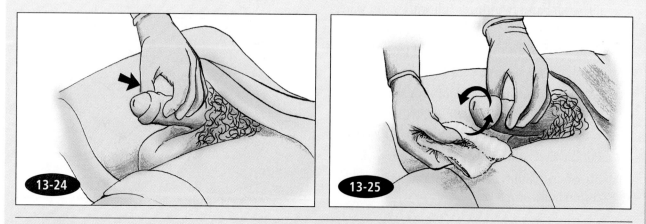

13-24   13-25

*Your client may not have an adjustable hospital bed; those steps marked with an asterisk (*) will not apply.

Procedure 13-9

Caring for Nails and Feet

Materials Needed

- Paper towels
- Wash basin
- Emesis basin or small plastic bowl
- Washcloth
- Small towel
- Emery board or nail file
- Bath mat or newspapers
- Orangewood stick, optional
- Pumice stone, optional
- Disposable gloves, optional
- Hand lotion, optional

Procedure

1. Explain what you are going to do.
2. Wash your hands.
3. Obtain materials listed above.
4. Spread paper towel on work area. Arrange materials on paper towel.
5. Provide privacy (close door, shut drapes, pull shades).
6. Help client into chair or to side of bed.
7. Assist client to remove footwear, if appropriate.
8. Put bath mat, towel, or newspapers under feet.
9. Fill basin with water 100°–110° F (43°–44° C).
10. Place basin on bath mat. Put on gloves (optional). Help client put feet in basin.
11. Allow feet to soak for 10 minutes. Add warm water as needed.
12. Place table or ironing board in front of client at convenient height and close to client. Cover table with hand towel or paper towels (Fig. 13-26).
13. Fill emesis basin or small bowel with water 100°–110° F (43°–44° C). Put client's fingers in basin and soak for 2–3 minutes.
14. Clean under fingernails with orangewood stick. Dry fingers thoroughly and set basin aside.
15. Shape fingernails with emery board or nail file. Push back cuticles gently with washcloth or orangewood stick. Apply hand lotion (optional).

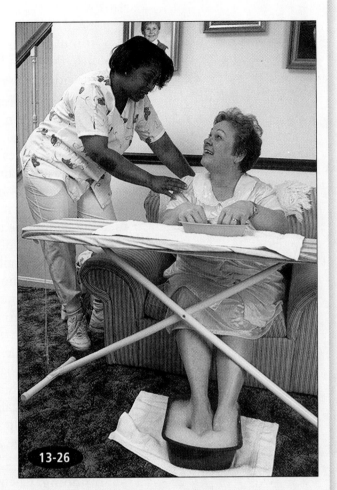

13-26

16. Remove table.
17. Remove one foot from basin. Smooth any calloused areas using washcloth or pumice stone. Dry foot and between the toes thoroughly. Repeat procedure for other foot. Apply lotion, as needed.
18. Remove gloves, if worn, and discard in paper bag.
19. Help client to put on footwear or help back to bed.
20. Clean equipment and store in proper location. Discard disposable supplies.
21. Place soiled towels in laundry container to be washed.
22. Wash your hands.
23. Record what you have done. Report any unusual conditions to your supervisor.

Hair Care

Some clients may not be able to do hair care themselves. They will need assistance to brush, comb, wash, and style hair. Hair care is done to:

- clean the hair and scalp
- stimulate circulation to the scalp
- help the client look attractive
- provide a sense of well-being and comfort.

Brushing and Combing Part the hair, dividing it into at least four sections. Brush from root to end, one section at a time. Follow by combing hair. Encourage clients to do as much of their own hair care as possible. This provides good exercise for the shoulders and upper arms. Follow the care plan and assist when necessary. Never cut clients' hair, even if there are tangles. Long hair may be braided. Some barbers and beauticians make home visits to groom, cut, and style hair. A family member should be able to arrange for this service. If not, notify your supervisor about your client's wishes.

Hair care is usually done twice daily, once in the morning (usually with the bath or shower) and again at bedtime. However, hair care can be done at any time convenient for aide and client. Curly, kinky hair may be very dry. You may need to apply oil to the hair before you can brush and comb it. Always ask clients how they care for their hair and what they would like you to do. Some women will have elaborate braids that are left in the hair for several months. In this case, you will need to learn how to wash and care for the scalp from your client and/or a family member. Again, follow the care plan.

Observe the scalp for any scaling, crusting, irritation, bruises, bleeding, lumps, or large areas of missing hair. Report these observations to your supervisor. See Procedure 13-10, Assisting Clients with Hair Care.

Shampooing Clients may wish to have their hair washed two or three times a week. Some people wash their hair daily. Hair can be washed in bed, at the sink in the kitchen or bathroom, or as part of the shower. Check the care plan to see where and how often the shampoo is to be done. If you are giving a shampoo in the tub, wash the hair last so the client does not have dripping wet hair while bathing. If you are shampooing at the sink, have the client sit in a chair with his/her back to the sink. For a bed shampoo, you will need a plastic trough that drains the water away from the bed. See Procedure 13-11, Giving a Shampoo. A dry shampoo may also be used. Follow instructions on the container.

Shaving

Men usually shave their beards daily. Women may shave their legs and underarms when necessary. Most clients will shave themselves. This provides good exercise for the shoulders and upper arms. Assist clients, as necessary, according to the care plan.

Electric or blade razors may be used. Electric razors should not be used when the client is receiving oxygen because there is danger that an electrical spark could cause a fire. Blade razors should not be used when the client is taking certain types of medications because of danger of bleeding or infection. Wear disposable gloves when using a blade razor to shave a client.

Assisting Clients with Hair Care

Materials Needed

- Brush
- Comb
- Bath towel
- Other grooming supplies—
  hair spray, oil, hair tonic (optional)
- Hair pins, barrettes, etc. (optional)
- Mirror (optional)

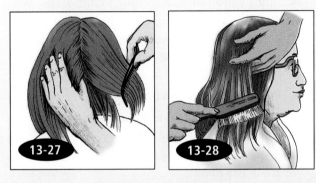

13-27   13-28

Procedure

1. Explain what you are going to do.

2. Wash your hands.

3. Obtain materials listed above.

4. Provide privacy (close door, shut drapes, pull shades).

5. Raise bed to convenient working height. Lower rail on side where you are working.*

6. Place client in upright position in bed or in chair, if possible.

7. Place bath towel around client's shoulders. If the client is in bed, place towel under head to cover the pillow.

8. Part hair and separate into sections (Fig. 13-27).

9. Brush hair, section by section, working from the root to end of hair (Fig. 13-28).

10. Arrange hair according to client's wishes.

11. Remove towel.

12. Make sure client is safe and comfortable.

13. Place bed in lowest position.*

14. Clean supplies and store in proper location.

15. Place soiled bath towel in laundry container to be washed.

16. Wash your hands.

17. Record what you have done. Report any unusual conditions to your supervisor.

*Your client may not have an adjustable hospital bed; those steps marked with an asterisk (*) will not apply.

Soften facial hairs with warm water before shaving. Beards and moustaches should be washed with soap and water, dried, and brushed. Check with the client regarding any special care for facial hair. Trimming may be done by the client with special clippers, or the barber may visit.

Shaving may be done at the sink, bedside, or in bed. Gather all of the materials needed and place within the client's reach. Follow Procedure 13-12, Assisting Clients to Shave.

Giving a Shampoo

Materials Needed

- Shampoo
- Conditioner, optional
- Comb
- Brush
- Bath towel
- Washcloth (folded)
- Hand-held shower attachment
- Hair dryer
- For bed shampoo:
  - Waterproof bed protector
  - Trough
  - Basin or bucket
  - Pitcher of warm water

Procedure

1. Explain what you are going to do.
2. Wash your hands.
3. Obtain materials listed above.
4. Provide privacy (close door, shut drapes, pull shades). Remove glasses, hearing aides. Store properly.
5. Raise bed to convenient working height. Lower rail on side where you are working.*
6. Position client for shampoo—at sink, in tub or shower, or in bed with trough under head and neck (Fig. 13-29A and B).
7. Brush and comb hair.
8. Have client hold folded washcloth over eyes to protect from shampoo.

9. Wet hair, from front to back, with warm water (100;dg F) (43° C)
10. Put a small amount of shampoo in palm of your hand.
11. Apply shampoo to scalp; lather from front to back, rubbing gently.
12. Rinse thoroughly with warm water.
13. Repeat steps 10 through 12.
14. Apply conditioner, according to directions, as desired.

    (CAUTION: Conditioner can make the bottom of the tub slippery. Rinse conditioner down drain before assisting client to step out of tub.)

15. Wrap client's head in bath towel.
16. Bath/shower stall—Help client out and assist with drying body and hair.
17. Bed shampoo—Remove trough from bed. Towel dry hair.
18. Dry hair using dryer, if available. Arrange hair according to client's wishes.
19. Make sure client is safe and comfortable. Replace eye glasses, hearing aids, if appropriate.
20. Place bed in lowest position. (Raise side rail, if indicated.)*
21. Clean materials and store in proper location.
22. Place soiled bath towel in laundry container to be washed.
23. Wash your hands.
24. Record what you have done. Report any unusual conditions to your supervisor.

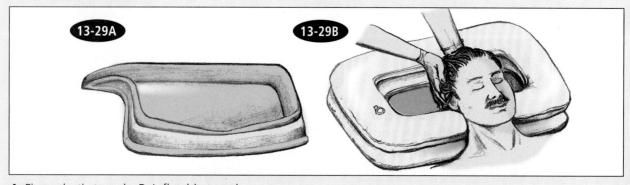

A, Firm, plastic trough. **B,** Inflatable trough.

Your client may not have an adjustable hospital bed; those steps marked with an asterisk (*) will not apply.

Shaving the Male Client

Materials Needed

- Razor—blade or electric
- Shaving cream or soap (for blade razor)
- Shaving brush, optional
- Mirror
- Aftershave lotion
- Tissues
- Bath towel
- Face towel
- Washcloth
- Wash basin or sink
- Warm water (for blade razor)
- Disposable gloves

Procedure

1. Explain what you are going to do.

2. Wash your hands.

3. Obtain materials listed above.

4. Provide privacy (close door, shut drapes, pull shades).

5. Raise bed to convenient working height. Lower rail on side where you are working.*

6. Place client in an upright position in bed (or assist to sit by bathroom sink, if possible).

7. Shaving with a blade razor:

    a. Put on disposable gloves.

    b. Wet washcloth with warm water (115° F) (46° C). Place on client's face for a few minutes. Remove.

    c. Apply shaving cream and lather the face.

    d. Hold the skin taut and shave in the direction of hair growth (Fig. 13-30).

    e. Rinse the blade razor when necessary.

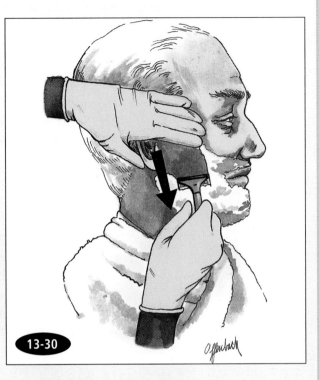

13-30

8. Shaving with an electric razor:

    a. Put on disposable gloves (optional).

    b. Make sure face is clean and dry. Do not apply shaving cream or water to the face.

    c. Turn on razor.

    d. Hold skin taut and shave in the direction of hair growth.

    e. Turn off razor.

9. Remove towel.

10. Remove and discard gloves.

11. Make sure client is safe and comfortable.

12. Place bed in lowest position. (Raise side rail, if indicated.)*

13. Clean materials and store in proper location.

14. Place soiled bath towel in laundry container to be washed.

15. Wash your hands.

16. Record what you have done. Report any unusual conditions to your supervisor.

*Your client may not have an adjustable hospital bed; those steps marked with an asterisk (*) will not apply.

Caring for Eyeglasses, Contact Lenses, and Hearing Aids

Eyeglasses   Some people need glasses to read; others need them every minute of the day in order to see. Be careful when handling glasses; they are very expensive and break easily. Clean glasses with water, and dry with a soft tissue. Unworn glasses should be stored in an eyeglass case that is always kept in the same location.

Contact Lenses   Contact lenses are worn directly on the surface of the eye. Some lenses require special cleaning and storage. Other lenses are disposable and need no special care. Clients usually care for their own lenses.

Hearing Aids   These devices make sounds louder. However, all sound is increased, even background noise, and clients may find this very distracting and irritating. Hearing aids operate on batteries that must be replaced as needed. Also, hearing aids must be turned on in order to work. Very tiny aids are worn in the ear canal. Others have two parts, an ear mold and a behind-the-ear battery and control portion (Fig. 13-31 A–D). Remove earwax from the ear piece with an applicator dampened with water and a little soap. Do not let the battery section get wet. This will cause serious damage to the hearing aid.

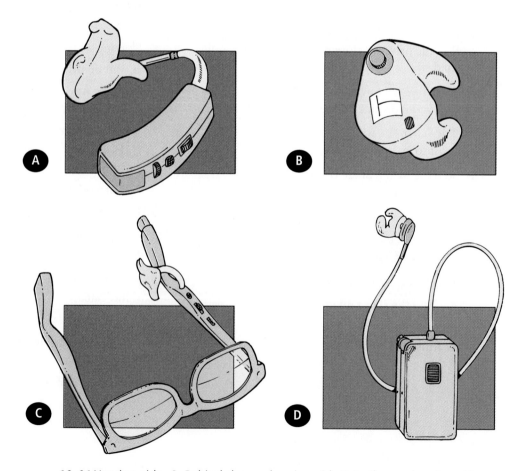

13-31 Hearing aids. **A,** Behind-the-ear hearing aid. **B,** In-the-ear hearing aid. **C,** Eyeglass aid. **D,** Body-worn aid. *(From Sorrentino S:* Mosby's Textbook for Nursing Assistants, *ed. 4, 1996, St. Louis, Mosby-Year Book, Inc.)*

Hearing aids are very expensive and difficult to fit. Handle carefully and do not drop. Store in the special container provided and keep in the same location.

Helping the Client to Dress and Undress

When clients dress in regular clothing, rather than in bedclothes, during the day, they usually feel better. Being dressed and well groomed contributes to one's self-esteem. To some, it is a sign of getting back to the normal routines of daily life. Most clients will need some help with dressing and undressing. Some will only need their clothing placed within easy reach, so that they can dress themselves without any further help. Others will need more help. Clothing for clients who need help to dress should be easy to put on and take off, for example, shirts or dresses with zippers or snaps, instead of buttons.

Special Aids to Help with Dressing There are special aids that can be used to help make dressing easier. A long-handled shoehorn (Fig. 13-32A) allows the person to put on shoes without bending over. Elastic shoelaces make it easier to slip the foot into or out of the shoe without tying or untying the shoelaces. Velcro strips sewn on garment closures eliminate the need to button and unbutton shirts, pants, and trousers (Fig. 13-32B). The occupational therapist may teach the client ways to make dressing easier with the use of these and other special aids.

Preparing to Dress the Client It is important to ask the client what he/she wants to wear, whenever possible. Choosing what to wear gives the client a sense of being in control. Clothes should be:

- easy to put on and take off
- comfortable, not too tight or binding
- the correct size (or one size larger) for ease in dressing
- suitable for the home environment
- suitable for weather conditions, if client is going outdoors

The following guidelines should be followed when helping the client to dress:

- Lay out clothing in proper order according to client's dressing practices (underwear first, then outer wear, socks, and shoes).
- Follow client's dressing practices when helping to put on clothing.
- Encourage client to dress himself/herself, as much as possible.
- Do not rush; getting dressed can be hard work; muscles stretch and joints bend with each movement.
- Put clothing on weak side first.
- Remove clothing from strong side first.

Follow Procedure 13-13, Helping Client to Dress and Undress, and Procedure 13-14, Helping Client with an IV to Dress.

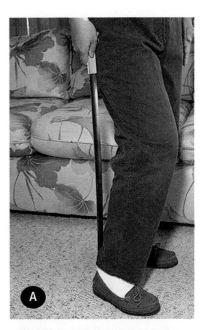
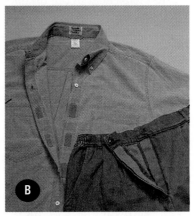

13-32 A, Long-handled shoe horn reduces bending and discomfort. *B,* Velcro clothing makes it easy to dress and undress.

Procedure 13-13

Helping Client to Dress

Materials Needed

- Outer clothing
- Underwear
- Socks
- Shoes

Procedure

1. Explain what you are going to do.

2. Wash your hands.

3. Obtain materials listed above.

4. Arrange clothing in order of use.

5. Provide privacy (close door, shut drapes, pull shades).

6. Lower bed to lowest position. Lower rail on side where you are working.*

7. Help client to sit on side of bed, if possible. If client must stay in bed, place in supine position.

8. Help client to put on undershirt or bra, shirt, or pajama top.

   a. Over-the-head-type garment—Place injured arm into garment first (Fig. 13-33). Pull neck of garment over client's head. Guide other arm into garment.

   b. Front-button or zipping type garment— Place injured arm through sleeve first. Bring shirt to the back of client and guide the other arm into the sleeve (Fig. 13–34).

9. Help client to put on underwear, slacks, shorts, or pajama bottoms. If leg is injured, place into garment first, then the other leg. Help client to stand at side of bed and pull up clothing to the waist. If client is in bed, help client to lift buttocks while you pull up the garments.

10. Help client to put on socks or stockings and footwear.

11. Make sure client is safe and comfortable.

12. Place bed in lowest position. (Raise side rail, if indicated.)*

13. Wash your hands.

14. Record what you have done. Report any unusual conditions to your supervisor.

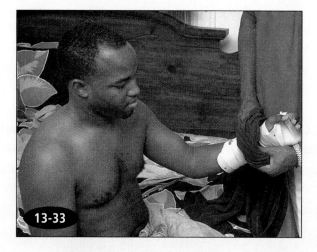

13-33

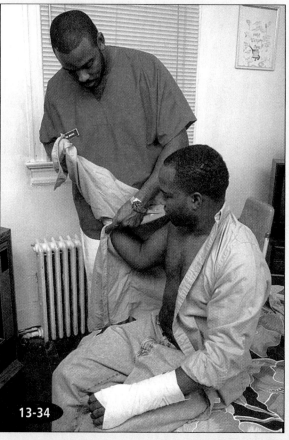

13-34

NOTE: To help client to undress, reverse the procedure. Injured arm or leg is removed from garment last.

Your client may not have an adjustable hospital bed; those steps marked with an asterisk (*) will not apply.

Procedure 13-14

Helping Client with an IV to Remove Used Clothing and Apply Clean Clothing

Materials Needed

- Clean clothing

Procedure

1. Explain what you are going to do.

2. Wash your hands.

3. Obtain clean clothing.

4. Arrange clothing in order of use.

5. Provide privacy (close door, shut drapes, pull shades).

6. Lower bed to lowest position. Lower rail on side where you are working.*

7. Help client to sit on side of bed, if possible. If client must stay in bed, place in supine position.

8. Help client to remove used garment from arm without the IV.

9. Gather up sleeve of garment on arm with IV. Slide sleeve over the IV site and tubing. Remove client's arm and hand from the sleeve.

10. Slide your hand along tubing to IV bag, keeping sleeve gathered.

11. Remove IV from pole. Slide bag and tubing through the sleeve. Keep bag above client's arm. Do not pull on the tubing. Place used clothing on chair (Fig. 13-35).

Your client may not have an adjustable hospital bed; those steps marked with an asterisk (*) will not apply.

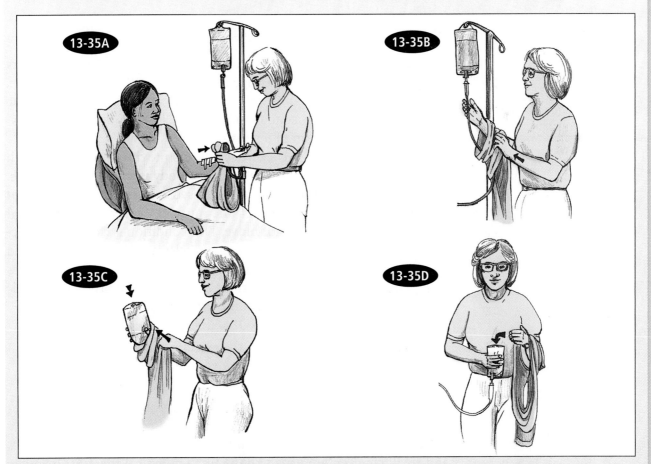

A, Pajama top is removed from arm without IV. Other sleeve is gathered up, slipped over IV site and tubing.
B, Gathered sleeve is slipped over tubing and up to IV bag. **C,** Remove IV bag from pole and pass through sleeve.
D, To dress client, start with IV first. Gather sleeve of shirt, slip over IV bag and back up to shoulder.

Continued.

Helping Client with an IV to Remove Used Clothing and Apply Clean Clothing

12. Hang bag back on the pole.

13. Gather the sleeve of clean garment that is to be put on the arm with the IV.

14. Remove the IV bag from the pole. Make sure the bag is above the client's arm.

15. Slip sleeve and garment shoulder over the bag. Place bag back on the pole.

16. Slide the gathered sleeve over the tubing, hand, arm, and IV site.

17. Adjust garment over client's shoulders and help client to put other arm through other sleeve.

18. Check that IV is working properly. (See Chapter 17.)

19. Assist client to remove other garments and put on clean garments, as needed.

20. Make sure client is safe and comfortable.

21. Place soiled garments in laundry container.

22. Place bed in lowest position. (Raise side rail, if indicated.)*

23. Record what you have done. Report any abnormal conditions to your supervisor.

Your client may not have an adjustable hospital bed; those steps marked with an asterisk (*) will not apply.

Range of Motion Exercises

In Chapter 4, the types of body joints were described. Each joint performs a certain movement. Hinge joints, such as the elbow and knee, cause movement back and forth. Ball and socket joints, such as the shoulder and hip, cause a circular movement. Joints move because muscles are attached by mean of tendons.

Range of motion (ROM) exercises means moving the joint through the desired motion. During an illness, the body is usually not as active, so the muscles and joints may not be used as much. If a joint is not moved through its normal ROM, the muscles weaken. Then the joint stiffens and, with time, cannot move. This condition is called a **contracture.** To prevent this from happening, muscles need to be exercised, and joints need to be moved through their normal ROM. ROM exercises help to improve muscle tone, increase circulation, and prevent deformities. An excellent time to perform these exercises is during bathing.

There are two main types of ROM exercises:

1. Active—the client performs the exercise without help.
2. Passive—the home care aide moves the body part without help from the client.

The care plan will indicate the exercises to be done and how frequently each exercise is to repeated. Head and neck exercises are usually not performed by the home care aide. Also, hip exercises for older adults and small children are usually done by the physical therapist or nurse because of the danger of injury to the client. The following are important points to remember when helping with ROM exercises:

• Support the body part being moved above and below the joint.
• Move the part in a slow, steady manner.

contracture
a shortening or permanent contraction of muscle tissue as a result of spasm, scar, or paralysis.

- Move the joint through as complete a range as possible.
- Stop the exercise if the client complains of pain or shows signs of severe discomfort; report these findings to your supervisor.
- Stop if you feel resistance or tightness in the joint.

Follow Procedure 13-15, Helping with Range of Motion Exercises in Bed—General Procedure.

Procedure 13-15

Helping with Range of Motion Exercises in Bed— General Procedure

1. Explain what you are going to do and how the client can help.

2. Wash your hands.

3. Provide privacy (close door, shut drapes, pull shades).

4. Raise bed to convenient working height. Lower rail on side where you are working.*

5. Fold top bedding to foot of bed. Cover client with sheet or blanket.

6. Help client to move to side of bed near you. Make sure client is in correct supine position.

7. Repeat each exercise as listed in the care plan.

8. Exercise upper body, both sides. Then exercise lower body, both sides.

9. Help client to center of bed; replace top bedding; and remove sheet or blanket covering client.

10. Make sure client is safe and comfortable.

11. Place bed in lowest position. (Raise side rail, if indicated.)*

12. Wash your hands.

13. Record what you have done. Report any unusual conditions to your supervisor or physical therapist.

Your client may not have an adjustable hospital bed; those steps marked with an asterisk (*) will not apply.

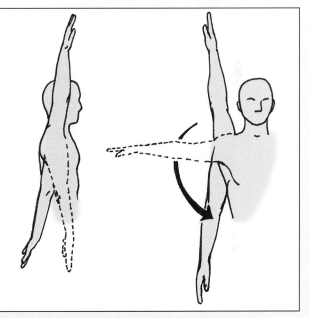

Shoulder/Arm Exercises

Directions: hold client's wrist and hand with one hand. With the other hand, grasp client's arm above the elbow.

Movement:

a. Move arm, with palm down, forward and upward along side of head and downward to the side. Repeat with palm up.

b. Move arm with palm down, away from body, sideways, to above the head and return. Repeat with palm up.

Continued.

Helping with Range of Motion Exercises in Bed— General Procedure

Forearm and Elbow Exercises

Directions: Rest client's upper arm on bed with forearm raised upright and elbow bent. Support client's wrist and hand.

Movement: Move lower arm down, then up, with palm down. Repeat with palm up.

Directions: Rest client's upper arm on bed with forearm upright. Support client's wrist with one hand and the client's hand with the other.

Movement: Twist palm toward client, then away.

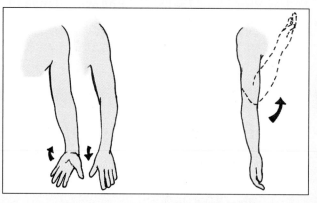

Wrist Exercises

Directions: Hold client's wrist with one hand. Use other hand to:

Movement:

a. Move hand forward, then backward.

b. Move hand from one side to the other.

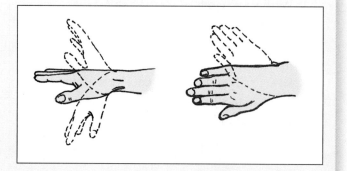

Finger Exercises

Directions: Hold client's wrist with one hand. With other hand:

Movement:

a. Bend fingers (make a fist), then straighten.

b. Spread finger and thumb apart, then bring together.

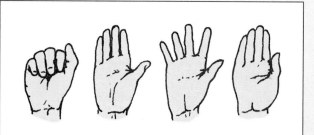

Thumb Exercises

Directions: Hold client's hand and fingers with one hand. With other hand grasp thumb:

Movement:

a. Move thumb across palm of hand and straighten, then return to side.

b. Touch each finger tip with thumb.

c. Bend thumb into palm and return to straightened position.

d. Move thumb using wide, circular motion.

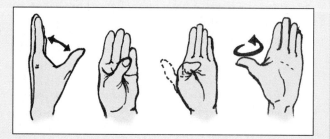

Hip, Leg, and Knee Exercises

Directions: Support client's leg with one hand under knee and other at the heel.

Movement:

a. Bend knee and raise toward chest, then lower.

b. Raise leg straight up as high as possible, then lower leg gently.

*Directions: Support client's leg with one hand under knee and other hand under the ankle.

Movement:

a. Move leg outward, away from body as far as possible. Return to starting position.

b. Move leg across the other leg as far as possible and return to starting position.

*Directions: Place one hand over top of knee and grasp. Place other hand over top of ankle and grasp.

Movement: Turn leg so toes are pointed inward, then outward.

Directions: Support client's leg with one hand just above the knee and the other hand at the ankle.

Movement: Bend the knee and slide the heel toward the buttocks as far as possible. Then straighten knee to starting position.

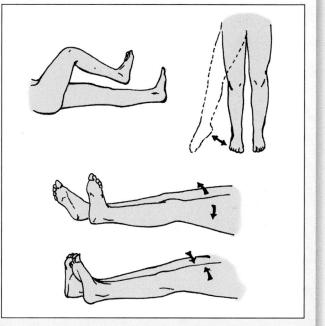

---

*These exercises cause the ball and socket joint of the hip to rotate. Do not perform these exercises unless indicated in the client's care plan. Older adults and young children may be severely injured by these exercises.

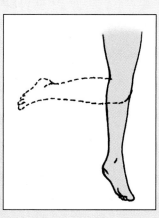

Foot and Ankle Exercises

Directions: Support ankle by placing client's heel in palm of one hand with other hand just above the ankle.

Movement:

a. Bend foot up toward the leg, then down, away from leg.

b. Turn foot outward, sole facing away from body, then turn foot inward toward body.

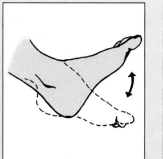

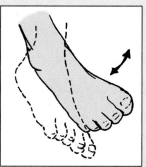

Continued.

Helping with Range of Motion Exercises in Bed— General Procedure

Toe Exercise

Directions: Hold client's foot with one hand. Use the other hand to do the following:

Movement: Bend toes down toward the ball of the foot, then bend toes back to front of foot.

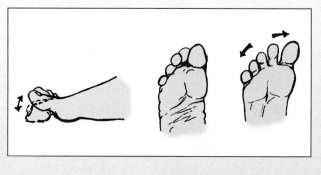

CHAPTER SUMMARY

- Clients may be unable to perform self-care because of: the effects of illness, pain and discomfort, lack of strength and energy, fear of injury, anxiety, or confusion.
- The home care aide may assist the client to perform the following personal care activities:
  - oral hygiene (brushing and flossing teeth, denture care)
  - bathing
  - grooming (caring for hands and feet, hair care, shampooing, and shaving)
  - dressing and undressing
  - care of eyeglasses, contact lenses, and hearing aids
- Bathing is done to cleanse the skin, remove bacteria, prevent body odor, stimulate circulation, move joints and muscles, prevent pressure sores, and provide comfort and a sense of well-being.
- Bathing provides the opportunity to communicate with the client, observe his/her skin, and perform range of motion (ROM) exercises.
- It is important to be aware of safety hazards that may arise when performing personal care activities.
- The home care aide needs to be alert to possible safety hazards (to client and self) when performing personal care activities. Be sure to practice safety principles discussed in this chapter and Chapter 6.
- Always use universal precautions when giving personal care to clients.
- Respect the client's need for privacy when performing personal care activities. Some of these procedures can cause embarrassment for the client.
- Range of motion exercises to improve muscle tone, increase circulation, and prevent deformities.

STUDY QUESTIONS

1. List five reasons why clients may not be able to perform personal care activities.

2. Describe how you would care for the following:
   a. false teeth
   b. eye glasses
   c. hearing aids

3. List four purposes of bathing.

4. List six principles to follow when bathing clients.

5. Explain the difference between the following:
   a. complete bed bath
   b. partial bath
   c. tub bath
   d. shower bath

6. List three safety practices to follow for each of the following procedures:
   a. tub bath
   b. shower
   c. denture care

7. Describe three personal care procedures where universal precautions must be followed.

8. List five important points to remember when performing range of motion exercises.

14

Elimination

Objectives

After you read this chapter, you will be able to:

1. Describe the normal characteristics of urine and feces.

2. List six ways to promote normal urinary and bowel elimination.

3. Discuss the care needed for clients with urinary incontinence.

4. Describe the care needed for clients with catheters.

5. Discuss common bowel problems.

6. Discuss the care of clients with a colostomy or ileostomy.

7. Give five examples of the use of universal precautions when handling body waste.

8. Demonstrate the procedures in this chapter.

Elimination of body wastes takes place in a number of ways:

- Perspiration, through the skin
- Carbon dioxide and moisture from the lungs
- Urine from the kidneys
- Bowel movements from the digestive system

Normal elimination is usually so automatic that we do not even think about it. Clients, however, may have problems with elimination for many reasons: for example,

- Clients who are physically limited and cannot walk to the bathroom because it is upstairs, outside, or down the hall
- Clients with diseases that affect elimination
- Clients who take medications that influence elimination

Urinary Elimination

Urinary System Review

- The kidneys filter blood, remove waste and impurities, regulate the salt and water in the body, and manufacture urine.
- The ureters are tubes that connect the kidneys to the urinary bladder.
- The bladder is a muscular organ that stores urine until it is eliminated from the body.
- The urethra is a tube from the bladder to outside of the body.
- The urinary meatus is the external opening of the urethra, located in the perineum.
- The process of urination is a complex one that involves several body systems: nervous, muscular, and urinary.

Urine is the liquid waste produced by the kidneys. The amount of urine a person produces differs according to age, illness, activity, medications taken, fluid intake, body temperature, and the amount of other types of **output.** However, the amount of urine produced by the kidneys is usually about the same as the amount of fluid intake each day.

The medical terms for passing urine are: void, voiding, urinate, urinating, urination, and micturition. Most English-speaking adults are familiar with the words *urine* and *urinate,* although many people will use the term *pass water* for emptying the urinary bladder. If your client speaks another language, try to find out the term used for the elimination of urine. Children, too, will often have their own terms to describe urination. Again, try to find out what term the client uses, and use it whenever possible.

In some cultures, health matters regarding elimination are considered very private and are not discussed with strangers. Sometimes clients may refuse care because it makes them feel so uncomfortable or because such intimate contact with strangers is not acceptable in their culture. Respect differences among cultures and be willing to learn about the reasons for your client's behavior. You may find that some of your male clients object to having a female aide assist with procedures involving elimination. Some women, too, may be embarrassed by the type of personal care involved with elimination. However, helping your client to use the bathroom, commode, bedpan, or urinal as needed is part of

elimination
the process of removing waste products from the body.

output
all fluids lost from the body that can be measured.

Box 14-1

Helping Clients Maintain Normal Urination

- Make sure the path to the bathroom is direct and free of clutter
- Place a commode, urinal, or bedpan at the bedside
- Offer toileting at times when the person usually needs to void
- Keep walker or crutches nearby so they can be used when needed
- Attend to client's need to void immediately; do not make client wait.
- Give clients adequate amounts of fluids— eight glasses of fluid a day.

- Reduce intake of fluids and foods that irritate urinary bladder and increase urinary frequency, such as coffee, tea, colas, alcohol, chocolate, and large amounts of sugar.
- Provide privacy.
- Give clients enough time to urinate, but don't let them sit on the bedpan, toilet, or commode for too long.
- Position client in normal voiding position— standing for men; sitting for women— whenever possible.

your job. Discuss any embarrassing situations with your supervisor and be sure to report any problems your client may have with elimination.

Characteristics of Normal Urine/Urination

- Urine is clear and has a light yellow color; a high fluid intake will make urine a very pale yellow color; a low fluid intake will make a darker, concentrated urine.
- Normal urine may have a slight acidic odor or none at all; certain foods and drugs may produce other odors.
- Amount of urine will vary, but the normal adult will produce and eliminate about 1000 milliliters (ml) to 1500 ml daily.
- Frequency of urination will also vary; some adults will urinate every two to three hours during the day; others will not void as often; the bladder is able to hold urine for longer periods when we sleep.
- Urination is done with ease and without pain or discomfort; see Box 14-1 for suggestions to help clients maintain normal urination.

Characteristics of Abnormal Urine/Urination

- Urine is dark, cloudy; it may appear to contain blood, shreds of mucus, or other substances.
- Odor may be present; it may have a strong smell.
- Amount of urine may be much greater or much less than what is considered normal (1000 ml to 1500 ml); report right away anything above what is normal or anything less than 600 ml in a 24-hour period.
- Frequency may increase or decrease; observe, record, and report changes in voiding patterns and the presence of any **dysuria**; frequent voiding of small quantities of urine may indicate abnormal emptying of the bladder; be sure to let your supervisor know the frequency of the voiding and the amount voided.

dysuria
difficulty urinating.

diagnose(d)
to determine the type and cause of an illness or condition based on a variety of information.

diuretic(s)
a drug or other substance that causes urine to be produced or excreted.

sedative(s)
a substance, procedure, or measure that has a calming effect.

impaction
the presence of a large, hard mass of feces in the rectum or colon.

Urinary Elimination Problems

Urinary Retention

The inability to urinate or to completely empty the bladder is called urinary retention. This may occur after perineal surgery, childbirth, and with some diseases of the nervous system. If your client is unable to void, or frequently voids small quantities of urine, report this to your supervisor *immediately*.

Urinary Incontinence

The inability to control the release of urine from the bladder is called urinary incontinence. Although it is not a disease, it can be a symptom of other problems. For example, illness may cause some clients to become incontinent. It is estimated that about 10 million Americans (mostly women) experience incontinence at some time in their lives. Many are too ashamed or embarrassed to discuss this with a health care professional. Instead, they will use pads or absorbent undergarments without having their conditions properly **diagnosed** and treated.

There are several types of urinary incontinence. (See Box 14-2.) Incontinence may be caused by many factors, including:

- inability to get to the bathroom fast enough
- inability to remove clothing fast enough to use the commode or toilet due to injury or disability
- having to wait too long for the bedpan or urinal
- urinary tract infection
- disease conditions of the nervous system and other disorders
- medications, for example, **diuretics** and **sedatives**
- immobility, being confined to bed or wheelchair
- emotional disorders, including depression
- confusion, forgetting to void, forgetting how to void
- stool **impaction**
- weakening of pelvic floor muscles resulting from birth of several children
- urinary retention may cause overflow.

Managing Urinary Incontinence   If the client has been incontinent for some time, the care plan will tell you what to do. If this is a new symptom, you must report it *immediately*. The client's condition will be assessed by the nurse and doctor, and a plan to treat, or manage, the symptoms will be developed. The treatment is based on the cause of the incontinence. Sometimes surgery or medications may be necessary to correct the problem. However, there are several treatments frequently used in home care: bladder training, habit training, pelvic muscle exercise, absorbent products, and catheters.

The incontinent client is at great risk for skin breakdown caused by irritation from the urine and bacterial growth in the warm, moist environment. Check the skin for rash and redness at least every two hours. Record and report abnormal findings to your supervisor.

Give perineal care each time the client is incontinent. Wash all the skin that has been in contact with the urine using mild soap, warm

---

Box 14-2

Types of Urinary Incontinence

Stress Incontinence— leakage of small amounts of urine during "stressful" activities, such as laughing, sneezing, coughing, lifting heavy objects, or certain types of exercise.

Urge Incontinence— involuntary loss of urine when the "urge" to void occurs. The person is "unable to make it to the toilet in time."

Overflow Incontinence (dribbling)— involuntary loss of urine that occurs when urine is being retained and the bladder is overfilled.

water, and soft washcloths. Dry the skin gently and apply cream or ointment according to the care plan. Since you will be coming in contact with body fluids, you must wear gloves when giving skin care and when changing and washing contaminated linens.

Bladder training Bladder training is a program of education, scheduled voiding, praise, and encouragement. The nurse or physical therapist, together with the client, establishes the schedule of voiding. This causes the bladder to be "trained" to hold more urine for a longer amount of time. Fluid intake, output, and voiding patterns are recorded daily, usually by the client. This information is used to evaluate the success of the training program and to make changes as necessary. The home care aide helps clients to carry out the program according to the care plan by:

- encouraging the client to follow the schedule
- teaching clients or family members to record intake and output accurately
- following suggestions to help clients to maintain normal urination (see Box 14-1)
- providing privacy and following procedures for use of bedpan, urinal, and commode
- praising clients for success in the program
- encouraging clients not to give up or become discouraged if incontinence occurs.

Bladder training may take several months, with repeated visits from the therapist or nurse to provide continuing instruction. Be sure to record progress, or lack of progress, and notify your supervisor.

Habit training Habit training is a program of timed voiding. Both the client and nurse develop the schedule for voiding. This should be as close to the person's natural pattern of urination as possible. Clients void at specific times, for example, upon awakening, before and after meals, and at bedtime. The bladder is not trained to hold more urine, rather the client is encouraged to void at times when he/she would usually use the bathroom. Assist the client by following the care plan and the above suggestions for bladder training.

Pelvic muscle exercises Also called Kegel exercises, they strengthen the muscles of the pelvic floor. Urine leakage can be improved and often prevented by the use of these exercises. They are easy to do and are taught by a nurse or therapist. These are resistance exercises used mostly by women (also by men after prostate surgery). The exercises are performed by "drawing in" the muscles of the perineum as if to control voiding and moving the bowels. Encourage the client to practice the exercises according to the care plan. Report any problems to your supervisor.

Absorbent products They include pads, briefs, diapers, and underpads (placed under the client's hips to keep the bed dry). These products often give a false sense of security because the client no longer worries about having an "accident." This may delay diagnosis and effective treatment of incontinence. Protective absorbent products, when used improperly, may lead to skin breakdown and urinary tract infection. Odor control is another problem. Absorbent products should be changed every two to three hours. Perineal care is given, and all soiled skin areas are cleansed. For clients in bed, the changing schedule is every two hours. Observe the skin and report any abnormal findings to your supervisor. Underpads and diapers are available in a disposable form and in a washable, reusable form. Disposable products are convenient, but they are expensive. Reusable products (Fig. 14-1A and B) must be laundered according to the directions in Chapter 7, pages 97–98. Always wear gloves when handling soiled absorbent products.

Catheters Catheters are tubes used to remove and/or insert fluids into a body cavity. Some clients will be taught by the professional nurse to perform intermittent self-catheterization to remove urine.

Indwelling catheters remain in the body and are used for the management of incontinence. They carry great risk of urinary tract infection. External collecting devices (condom catheters) are used by men. Care of the client with an indwelling catheter and external collecting devices is discussed later in this chapter and in Procedures 14-4 and 14-5.

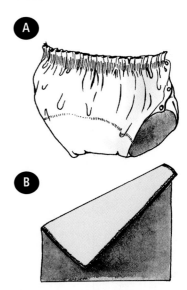

*14-1 **A,** Reusable undergarment. **B,** Reusable underpants for use in bed.*

Caring for the Client

Assisting with the Bedpan and Urinal

Bedpans and urinals are used by clients who are unable to get to the toilet to eliminate body wastes. Men will use a urinal for voiding (Fig. 14-2). There are two types of bedpans—the regular, large pan and the fracture pan (Fig. 14-3A and B), a smaller version used for clients with problems of mobility in bed. Bedpans and urinals can be made of metal or plastic. Metal bedpans are very cold, so warm them by rinsing with warm tap water. Wear gloves when removing and emptying the bedpan. You need to wear gloves when giving the bedpan if there is any risk of contact with body fluids. Check to see if the client or linens are soiled with urine or feces before providing the bedpan or urinal. Cover the bedpan with newspaper or a washable cloth when carrying it to the client and then into the bathroom to be emptied.

Be sure to give clients privacy when using the bedpan or urinal. Do not let them sit on the bedpan too long, as this causes pressure and damage to the tissues of the hips and buttocks. Empty bedpans and urinals immediately after use to avoid odors and growth of bacteria. Rinse with cold water, clean thoroughly, and disinfect according to Chapter 9, page 144. Store properly when not in use. Do not keep on the table or under the bed.

See Procedure 14-1, Giving and Removing a Bedpan, and Procedure 14-2, Giving and Removing a Urinal.

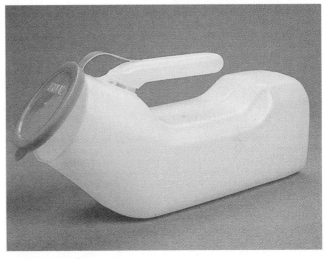

14-2 A urinal.

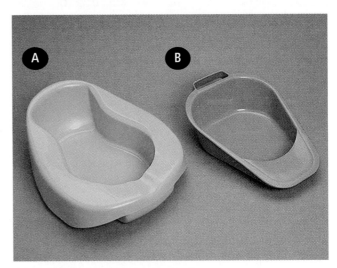

*14-3 **A,** Regular bedpan. **B,** Fracture pan.*

Giving and Removing a Bedpan

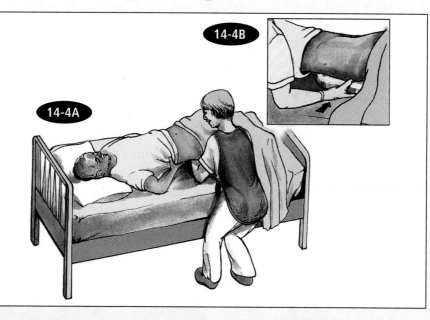

14-4B

14-4A

Materials Needed

- Bedpan
- Bedpan cover
- Toilet tissue
- 2 pairs disposable gloves

Procedure

1. Explain what you are going to do.
2. Wash your hands.
3. Obtain materials listed above.
4. Provide privacy (close door, shut drapes, pull shades).
5. Raise bed to convenient working height.*
6. Warm bedpan with warm tap water. Dry with paper towels.
7. Take bedpan to bedside and place on chair or bed.
8. Lower rail on side where you are working.*
9. Assist client to lie on back. Elevate head of bed slightly.
10. Fold back upper linens.
11. Instruct client to bend knees and raise buttocks. Assist as needed (Fig. 14-4A). If bed or client is soiled, put on gloves.
12. Slide the bedpan under the client (Fig. 14-4B).
13. When the client cannot raise the hips to get onto the bedpan, do the following:
    a. Turn the client on his/her side, facing away from you.
    b. Position the bedpan firmly against the buttocks.
    c. Turn the client on to his/her back, while holding the bedpan in place under the buttocks.
14. Cover client with top sheet to avoid chilling and exposure.
15. Raise side rail and place bed in sitting position.*
16. Prop up client with pillows if the bed is not adjustable.
17. Make sure bedpan is in correct position.
18. Give toilet paper and ask client to call when finished.
19. Leave room. Remove gloves, if using. Discard gloves.
20. Wash your hands.
21. Return to room when client calls.
22. Lower rail on side where you are working.*

---

*Your client may not have an adjustable hospital bed; those steps marked with an asterisk (*) will not apply.

23. Put on gloves.

24. Place client in flat position and remove bedpan in same manner used to give the bedpan.

25. Cleanse perineal area with toilet tissue if necessary, wiping from front to back.

26. Raise side rail.*

27. Cover bedpan, take to bathroom, and empty contents. Measure output if necessary. Observe contents.

28. Rinse bedpan with cold water, clean, and disinfect following instructions in Chapter 9, page 144.

29. Remove and discard gloves.

30. Wash your hands.

31. Put bedpan away.

32. Lower rail on side where you are working.*

33. Help client to wash his/her hands.

34. Make sure client is safe and comfortable.

35. Place bed in lowest position. (Raise side rail, if indicated.)*

36. Wash your hands.

37. Record what you have done. Report any abnormal elimination.

Your client may not have an adjustable hospital bed; those steps marked with an asterisk (*) will not apply.

Procedure 14-2

Giving and Removing a Urinal

Materials Needed
- Urinal
- Cover
- Disposable gloves

Procedure

1. Explain what you are going to do.

2. Wash your hands.

3. Obtain materials listed above.

4. Provide privacy (close door, shut drapes, pull shades).

5. Take urinal to bedside and place on chair or bed.

6. Assist client to stand. If client can not stand, place client on his back.

7. Fold back upper linens.

8. Give urinal to client so he can position it properly.

9. If client is unable to position urinal, put on gloves and position for him.

10. Cover client with top sheet to avoid chilling and exposure.

11. Leave room. Remove gloves, if using. Discard gloves.

12. Wash your hands.

13. Return to room when client calls.

14. Put on gloves.

15. Remove the urinal in the same manner you gave it to the client.

16. Cover urinal, take to bathroom, and empty contents. Measure output if necessary. Observe urine.

17. Rinse urinal with cold water, clean, and disinfect following instructions in Chapter 9, page 144.

18. Remove and discard gloves.

19. Wash your hands.

20. Put urinal away.

21. Help client to wash his hands.

22. Make sure client is safe and comfortable.

23. Wash your hands.

24. Record what you have done. Report any abnormal urine or urination.

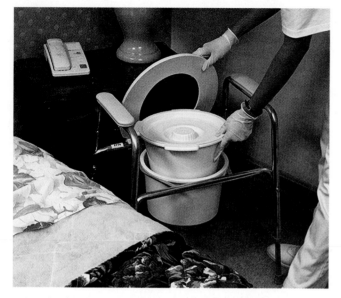

14-5 The bedside commode has a toilet seat and a removable pail.

Assisting Clients to Use the Commode

Commodes are placed near the bedside to be used by clients who are very weak; are unable to get to the bathroom because it is inaccessible; or because they are too slow to "make it in time." These commode chairs should be stable and be wide enough for large clients to sit comfortably (Fig. 14-5). If the commode has wheel brakes, lock them before transferring the client to the commode chair using transfer techniques in Chapter 11. Provide privacy. Place toilet tissue within reach. Instruct the client to call you when finished. Return the client to bed, wash his/her hands, and provide perineal care (Procedure 13-8) as needed. Empty the commode in the toilet. Clean according to directions in Chapter 7 to avoid the presence of bacteria and offensive odor.

Intake and Output (I and O)

Measuring the client's fluid intake and output is an important part of the care plan and helps to determine the effectiveness of treatment. For example, clients with kidney, heart, and liver disease may retain fluid in the tissues (edema). Some may take diuretics to increase the production of urine and promote fluid loss from the tissues. The loss of too much fluid can cause dehydration, a serious medical problem that may lead to death.

Occasionally, the doctor may restrict the fluid intake to a specific amount. All fluid intake must be measured to make sure the client does not go over the restricted amount.

Fluid Intake Intake of the following is to be measured and recorded when the care plan calls for I and O (measuring and recording of fluid intake and output):

- *All liquids taken in by mouth:* water, tea, coffee, milk, juice, soda, and soup
- *Semi-solid foods:* ice cream, sherbet, ice pops, pudding, Jello, custard, creamed soups, and creamed cereals
- *Intravenous fluids*
- *Tube feedings*

Fluid Output Measure and record the amount of the following:

- *Urine* that is voided and from catheter drainage
- *Feces;* only liquid feces can be measured; for formed stool, the quantity is described as large, medium, or small amount.
- *Vomitus;* if the client vomits into an emesis basin, it can be measured, otherwise describe the amount as large, medium, or small quantity; in addition to measuring the vomitus, describe its appearance; report vomiting to your supervisor.
- *Drainage from wounds;* this is reported according to the care plan; follow instructions from your supervisor; large amounts of drainage must be reported.

Remember: the fluids listed are body fluids. You must wear gloves when handling these materials and when changing and washing the client and soiled linens. Review Chapters 7 and 9.

Measuring Intake and Output Intake and output is measured in milliliters (ml) or cubic centimeters (cc). These are metric system measurements. One fluid ounce equals about 30 ml. One pint is about 500 ml, and a quart is 1000 ml. Fluids are measured in a special pitcher called a "graduate" that has markings to show the amount being measured. A graduate is like a measuring cup and is marked in both the metric system and the household system. Most plastic emesis basins, urinals, and commode pails have these markings for measuring output.

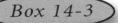

Box 14-3

Examples of the Capacity of Serving Containers

Tea cup	6 ounces	180 ml
Juice glass	4 ounces	120 ml
Water glass	8 ounces	240 ml
Iced tea glass	12 ounces	360 ml

You will need to know much fluid is held by containers in which liquids are served to your client. Fill serving containers—and cups, glasses, and bowls—with water to measure their contents. For example: Fill a drinking glass with water. Pour the water into a graduate or measuring cup. Measure the amount. Prepare a list of the contents of various containers used for fluid intake. Box 14-3 lists some examples of container contents. The sizes of bowls, cups, glasses, and mugs vary greatly, so always measure to be sure of the exact capacity of each container. NEVER USE THE SAME GRADUATE TO MEASURE BOTH INTAKE AND OUTPUT. The graduate for measuring output should be left in the bathroom.

When output is to be measured, clients cannot use the toilet as usual for elimination. They use the urinal, bedpan, and/or commode. A special insert known as specimen collector, or a "hat," may be placed under the toilet seat to collect the urine. These containers are usually marked for ease in measuring urinary output. Tell your client not to put toilet tissue into the bedpan, commode, or "hat" since it can interfere with accurate measurement of urine.

Clients and family members may need to be taught to measure and record intake and output. Follow the care plan and make sure they know how to do this properly.

Recording Intake and Output Record the amount of the intake and output immediately after measuring it. Use the I and O form provided by your agency. Put it in a convenient place as a reminder to measure intake and output. A total is added up for each day (Fig. 14-6). Procedure 14-3 (page 253) lists the steps for measuring and recording intake and output.

Care of a Client With an Indwelling Catheter

An indwelling or retention catheter remains in the bladder and provides constant drainage of urine. The catheter is inserted by the nurse. It is not the responsibility of the home care aide to insert or remove indwelling catheters. A balloon, inflated with sterile solution, holds the

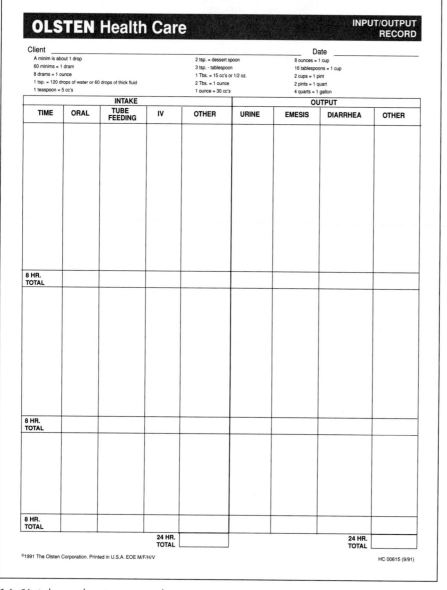

OLSTEN Health Care

INPUT/OUTPUT RECORD

Client _____   Date _____

A minim is about 1 drop
60 minims = 1 dram
8 drams = 1 ounce
1 tsp. = 120 drops of water or 60 drops of thick fluid
1 teaspoon = 5 cc's

2 tsp. = dessert spoon
3 tsp. - tablespoon
1 Tbs. = 15 cc's or 1/2 oz.
2 Tbs. = 1 ounce
1 ounce = 30 cc's

8 ounces = 1 cup
16 tablespoons = 1 cup
2 cups = 1 pint
2 pints = 1 quart
4 quarts = 1 gallon

| INTAKE | | | | | OUTPUT | | | |
TIME	ORAL	TUBE FEEDING	IV	OTHER	URINE	EMESIS	DIARRHEA	OTHER
8 HR. TOTAL								
8 HR. TOTAL								
8 HR. TOTAL								
			24 HR. TOTAL				24 HR. TOTAL	

©1991 The Olsten Corporation. Printed in U.S.A. EOE M/F/H/V   HC 00615 (9/91)

14-6 Intake and output record. *(Courtesy Olsten Kimberly QualityCare, Melville, NY.)*

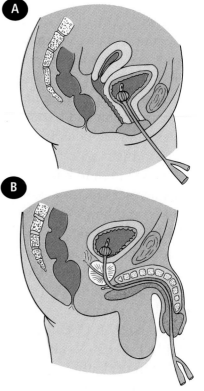

*14-7 **A,*** An indwelling catheter in the female bladder. An inflated balloon prevents the catheter from slipping out of place. ***B,*** An indwelling catheter in the male bladder.

catheter in place and prevents it from slipping out of the bladder (Fig. 14-7A and B). The catheter is connected to a drainage tube and collection bag.

Long-term use (more than two to four weeks) of indwelling catheters can lead to urinary tract infection and damage to the bladder and urethra. Therefore, catheters are used only when absolutely necessary.

The inside of the catheter and drainage system is sterile and should never come in contact with any other objects. Do not insert anything into the catheter or drainage tubing or let any part of the system come in contact with the floor. Keep the collection bag below the level of the urinary bladder to prevent backflow of urine into the bladder. Attach the collection bag to the bed frame; keep it free from linens and side rails. Clients are often ashamed and embarrassed when visitors see the urine collection bag. Try to cover it with bed linens or a lap robe when the client has visitors.

Procedure 14-3

Measuring and Recording Intake and Output

Materials Needed

- Measuring cups or graduates—separate measuring containers are needed for intake and output
- List of serving containers, which you measured earlier (see page 251)
- Pencil
- Paper
- Intake and output (I and O) form
- Disposable gloves

Procedure

Intake

1. Wash your hands.
2. Obtain materials listed above.
3. Measure each remaining liquid separately after client finishes eating or drinking. Pour into measuring cup.
4. Hold at eye level and measure the amount left.
5. Subtract the remaining amount from the amount of the original full serving.
6. Repeat for each liquid and record.

7. Rinse, clean, dry, and store container used to measure intake.
8. Wash your hands.
9. Record the amount of fluid intake and the time on the I and O form.

Output

1. Wash your hands.
2. Put on gloves.
3. Empty bedpan, urinal, commode pail, "hat," or emesis basin into a graduate if original container is not marked for measuring.
4. Measure amount of liquid and discard into toilet.
5. Rinse, clean, disinfect, dry, and store container used to measure output.
6. Remove and discard gloves.
7. Wash your hands.
8. Record the amount of fluid output and the time on the I&O form.

Some guidelines to remember when caring for clients with catheters include:

1. Always practice universal precautions. Wear gloves when there is a chance of coming in contact with body fluids.
2. Make sure urine is draining freely into the collection bag. Check for kinks in the tubing.
3. Tape the catheter to the thigh. Be sure it is connected to the drainage tubing and collection bag or leg bag (Fig. 14-8).
4. Pin connecting tubing to lower bed linen. Arrange in a coil to prevent dangling and drainage problems as seen in Fig. 14-8.
5. Empty the collection bag according to the care plan. Record the amount, color, odor, and clarity of the urine.
6. Provide perineal and catheter care daily, or more frequently if indicated in the care plan. Keep catheter and tubing clean.
7. Record and report the following to your supervisor:
   a. leakage of urine around the catheter
   b. client complaints of pain, burning, irritation, and feeling the urge to void

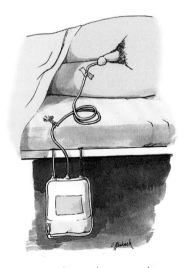

14-8 Tape the catheter to the thigh. Be sure the catheter is connected to the drainage bag.

   c. discharge from the urinary meatus or vagina

   d. abnormal quantity or appearance of urine

   e. leaks in the drainage tubing or collection bag

8. When moving client, move the tubing and bag apparatus also.

9. Leg bags are not used when clients are laying in bed because of the possibility of backflow of urine into the bladder and the risk of urinary tract infection. At bedtime the leg bag is removed and the regular drainage system is connected.

10. Whenever the catheter is separated from the drainage tube, it must be handled in a manner that will prevent it from being contaminated. Follow Procedure 14-4, Care of the Client with an Indwelling Catheter, and Procedure 14-5, Emptying a Catheter Drainage Bag.

Procedure 14-4

Care of the Client with an Indwelling Catheter

Materials Needed

- Materials for perineal care
- Cotton balls or gauze
- Disposable gloves
- Waterproof protector pad
- Plastic or paper bag

Procedure

1. Explain what you are going to do.

2. Wash your hands.

3. Obtain materials listed above.

4. Provide privacy (close door, shut drapes, pull shades).

5. Put on gloves.

6. Perform perineal care, Procedure 13-8, page 225.

7. Female client: separate labia to visualize the urinary meatus. Male client: retract foreskin (if uncircumcised).

8. Moisten cotton balls or gauze with soap and water.

9. Wash catheter tube in a downward motion away from the urinary meatus for approximately 4 inches (20 cm.) (Fig. 14-9). Use one cotton ball or gauze pad for each stroke. Rinse with water in the same manner. Discard used cotton balls or gauze into bag.

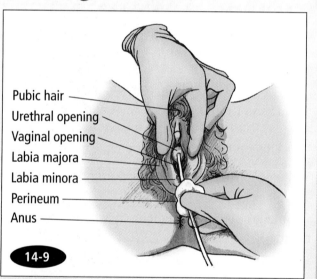

Pubic hair
Urethral opening
Vaginal opening
Labia majora
Labia minora
Perineum
Anus

14-9

10. Tape and position catheter properly (see Fig. 14-8).

11. Remove waterproof protector pad. Replace top linens.

12. Make sure client is safe and comfortable.

13. Clean materials and store in proper location.

14. Remove and discard gloves.

15. Wash your hands.

16. Record what you have done. Report any abnormal conditions to your supervisor.

Care of a Client with a Condom Catheter

Condom catheters are used in place of indwelling catheters to reduce the risk of urinary tract infections. The catheter goes over the penis and is connected to a drainage system, usually a leg bag (See Fig. 14-8). Velcro or self-adhesive holds the condom in place. The catheter is changed daily and perineal care is given.

In some states the home care aide may perform this procedure, while in others it is the responsibility of the nurse. Follow your agency policy and the rules that apply in your state. See Procedure 14-6, Applying a Condom Catheter. This procedure can be extremely embarrassing for the client. Do not expose him any more than necessary. Provide privacy and have a professional, matter-of-fact attitude when giving this care.

Procedure 14-5

Emptying a Catheter Drainage Bag

Materials Needed

- Disposable gloves
- Measuring container or graduate

Procedure

1. Explain what you are going to do.

2. Wash your hands.

3. Obtain materials listed above.

4. Provide privacy (close door, shut drapes, pull shades).

5. Put on gloves.

6. Place measuring container under drainage tube of collection bag.

7. Open clamp on drainage tube so urine can empty into graduate (Fig. 14-10). The drainage tube must not touch the insides of graduate.

8. Close clamp and replace drainage tube in the holder on collecting bag.

9. Measure urine, then discard in toilet.

10. Rinse, clean, disinfect, and store graduate.

11. Remove and discard gloves.

12. Wash your hands.

13. Record what you have done. Note the amount, color, and clarity of the urine. Report any abnormal conditions to your supervisor.

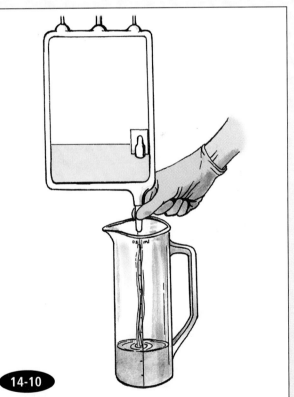

14-10

Applying a Condom Catheter

Materials Needed

- Condom catheter and collection bag
- Velcro band
- Materials to give perineal care
- Disposable gloves
- Small plastic bag

Procedure

1. Explain what you are going to do.

2. Wash your hands.

3. Obtain materials listed above.

4. Provide privacy (close door, shut drapes, pull shades).

5. Help client to lie on back.

6. Put on gloves.

7. Cover client with sheet or bath blanket as for perineal care.

8. If condom catheter is present, remove gently and place in plastic bag.

9. Give perineal care. (See Procedure 13-8)

10. Attach collection bag to leg or bed frame.

11. Apply protective coating to the skin of the penis, if using a self-adhesive catheter.

12. Hold penis firmly. Roll the condom catheter onto penis with drainage opening at the urinary meatus.

13. Secure edge of condom catheter in place with Velcro band. Be careful not to constrict the penis.

14. Connect catheter tip to drainage tubing (Fig. 14-11).

15. Make sure tubing is in correct position and that tip of catheter is not twisted.

16. Make sure client is safe and comfortable.

17. Discard used supplies in plastic bag.

18. Remove and discard gloves.

19. Wash your hands.

20. Record what you have done. Report any abnormal findings to your supervisor.

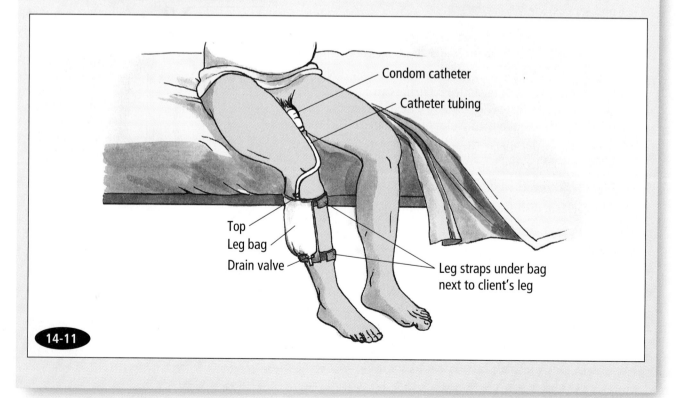

Condom catheter

Catheter tubing

Top
Leg bag
Drain valve

Leg straps under bag next to client's leg

14-11

Bowel Elimination

There are many terms used to describe the process of eliminating solid waste (feces) from the body. The correct term, defecation, may not be familiar to your client. The terms *bowel movement* or "*BM*" are more commonly understood. Another word for feces is stool. It is important that you understand the words your client uses for defecation and feces. However, use the correct terms, not slang, when discussing elimination with your client.

Digestive System Review

In Chapter 4, information about the organs of the digestive system and how they function were discussed. From this material you know that:

- The digestion of food is completed in the small intestine.
- The substances not absorbed in the small intestine (seed, food fiber, other waste products, water) pass into the large intestine.
- The large intestine absorbs water and stores semi-solid waste materials (feces) until they are eliminated.
- The powerful action of muscles (peristalsis) in the lower part of the large intestine helps to move the feces during defecation.
- The anal sphincter muscles control the opening and closing of the anus during the process of defecation.
- The process of defecation is a complex one that involves several body systems: nervous, muscular, and digestive.

Maintaining Healthy Bowel Habits

Eliminating waste products helps to keep the body functioning properly. Principles of maintaining healthy bowel habits include:

Maintaining an Established Routine   Some clients have well-established bowel habits. Knowing your client's habits is very important. For example, Lucille has a BM every day after breakfast. As Lucille's home care aide, you plan to provide the time for her to maintain this habit.

Maintaining Privacy   Defecation is a very private act. Some clients will resist the urge to defecate if they think their privacy is at risk. It is the home care aide's responsibility to be sensitive to clients' concerns and provide the privacy needed to carry out this body function.

Encouraging Fluids and a Well-Balanced Diet   Fluids are essential to keep the body functioning properly. The large intestine absorbs water as waste products pass through. With sufficient amounts of water, feces are soft and easy to eliminate. In Chapter 8, the importance of a well-balanced diet was discussed. Foods high in natural fiber, such as fruits, vegetables, and whole grains, provide bulk. Bulk helps to stimulate peristaltic action of the muscles of the digestive system, and defecation occurs more easily. When the amounts of fluids, fruits, vegetables, and whole grains in the diet are limited, problems with defecation can occur. Feces become hardened and difficult to eliminate. Encourage your client to drink fluids and eat foods high in fiber content, according to the diet ordered by the doctor.

Encouraging Activity and Exercise Activity and exercise help the body systems work more efficiently, including the digestive system. Inactivity, due to illness, usually makes the digestive system sluggish. The large intestine is not as active, and the process of defecation may be slowed. Help your client to be as active as possible.

Bowel Elimination Problems

Some clients spend most of their time in bed or have limited exercise and activity. Others may be taking a variety of medication or have poor appetites. All of these situations will make eating well-balanced meals with fiber and bulk more difficult. As a home care aide, you will need to recognize and report the following problems

Diarrhea

Diarrhea occurs when feces move through the intestines so fast that the water is not absorbed. The stool in diarrhea is not formed but is watery. The client may have frequent urges to defecate. These urges may be so strong that the client is unable to control the release of the stool. Complaints of cramping and soreness around the anus from the frequent bowel movements are not unusual.

Bowel (Fecal) Incontinence

The inability to control the release of feces and **flatus** (gas) from the anus is called bowel incontinence. There are many causes, such as disease, nervous system disorders, weakness of the anal sphincters, or the inability to get to the bathroom or commode quickly enough when the urge to defecate comes. No matter what the cause, this condition is usually very embarrassing for the client.

Constipation

Constipation occurs when feces remains in the large intestine for long periods of time. Water from the feces continues to be absorbed, and the stool becomes dry and hard. Elimination is painful because the stool is hard to pass. The stool may be large or in small, marblelike pieces.

Fecal Impaction

This condition occurs when feces are held in the rectum for so long that they become too hard and dry to pass without help. Small amounts of liquid feces may pass around the hardened feces and leak out of the anus. The client may complain of abdominal discomfort or pain; of a full feeling in the rectum; or even rectal pain. Treatment may include the use of medications or enemas. Sometimes a nurse must remove the impacted stool with a gloved finger. Fecal impaction can be avoided by reporting the lack of bowel movements to your supervisor. It is much easier to treat constipation than a fecal impaction.

flatus
air or gas in the intestine that passes through the rectum.

Caring for the Client

Helping the Client to Reestablish Bowel Routine

A member of the home care team, such as the nurse or physical therapist, may perform procedures and assist with exercises to help the client with bowel elimination. The home care aide also plays an important role in helping the client to return to normal bowel function. These activities include:

- giving the bedpan or helping the client to the commode or bathroom as soon as the client requests—do not delay
- recording each time the client defecates; after several days of recording the frequency and time of bowel movements, you may see that your client has a regular pattern of bowel movements. For example, many clients will have the urge to defecate after a meal; be sure to offer the bedpan or help the client to the commode based on this pattern.
- providing adequate time to defecate; do not rush your client or give the impression that you are in a hurry for the client to finish.
- encouraging the client to drink water and other fluids and to eat high fiber foods
- reporting changes in bowel habits to your supervisor, such as diarrhea, constipation, or other signs of problems

Observing and Recording Feces

It is important to carefully observe feces eliminated by the client. This waste product can tell a lot about the health of the entire digestive system. The following should be recorded:

- *Frequency*—the amount of bowel movements (once daily; two to three times daily; every two to three days); the frequency varies with each client; find out what is normal for your client.
- *Amount of each bowel movement*—large amount, small amount; the amount varies with each client because of food and fluids consumed.
- *Consistency*—normal feces are formed, soft, and shaped like the rectum.
- *Color*—normal feces are light to dark brown; this color may vary according to the foods eaten.
- *Odor*—feces have a characteristic odor; foods eaten can also affect the odor.
- *Flatus*—during defecation, flatus may be passed with feces; eating gas-forming foods, such as cabbage, onions, beans, or brussel sprouts, can increase the amount of flatus.

In addition to the above, notice the behavior of your client. Defecation should be easy and should not cause pain or discomfort.

Other factors can affect the frequency, consistency, color, and odor of feces. These include:

- *Medications*—some types of vitamins can cause the feces to become darker in color; other medications may cause more frequent or fewer bowel movements.

- *Other treatments*—cancer treatments, such as chemotherapy and radiation, may affect one or more characteristics of bowel movements.
- *Emotions*—worry, anxiety, and fear can affect the bowel and cause changes in the frequency of bowel movements.

ALWAYS CHECK WITH YOUR SUPERVISOR IF YOU NOTICE CHANGES IN YOUR CLIENT'S BOWEL MOVEMENTS.

The Client With an Ostomy

Ostomy is a suffix that means "to form a new opening." This is performed by making a surgical opening in the bladder or small or large intestine. You may care for clients who have had surgery where part of the intestine is brought out through the abdominal wall. An artificial opening, called a "stoma," is made so that fecal material, flatus, and urine can be expelled through the stoma rather than the anus or urethra. This surgical procedure may be performed when there is cancer, other diseases, or severe injury to the intestines or bladder. Ostomies may be temporary, meaning that the bowel will be reconnected when healing takes place. Or, the ostomy may be permanent, meaning that the diseased or injured part of the bowel was removed.

When part of the large intestine is brought out through the abdominal wall, the surgical opening is called a "colostomy." When part of the small intestine is brought out through the abdominal wall, the surgical opening is called an "ileostomy."

The care needed for an ostomy depends on the location of the surgical opening. If the surgery has been performed on the small intestine (ileostomy), less water can be absorbed by the intestines. Therefore, the bowel contents will have a more liquid appearance. If the surgery has been performed farther down in the large intestine (colostomy), more water can be absorbed from the feces. The feces' appearance will be more formed and normal.

An appliance, usually called a pouch, will be attached to the stoma to collect fecal material. There are two types of pouches: a *closed pouch*, which must be changed after each use (Fig. 14-12); and a *drainable pouch*, which has a removable clamp to empty the contents of the pouch (Fig. 14-13). This type of pouch is usually changed every three to five days. However, the pouch should be changed more often if it becomes loose around the stoma or if the skin around the area becomes irritated. Some

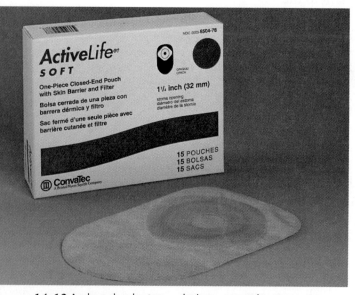

14-12 A closed colostomy drainage pouch. *(Courtesy ConvaTech, a Bristol-Myers Squibb Company, Princeton, NJ.)*

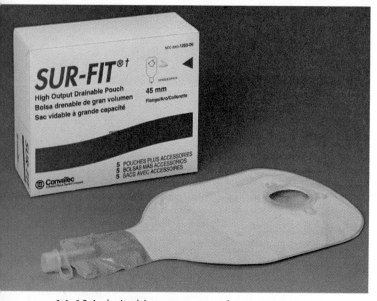

14-13 A drainable ostomy pouch. *(Courtesy ConvaTech, a Bristol-Myers Squibb Company, Princeton, NJ.)*

clients, who have had a colostomy for some time, will not wear any pouch around the stoma. The colostomy is regulated to eliminate feces like a normal bowel movement, so the pouch is no longer necessary. Instead a gauze pad is worn over the stoma to provide protection from clothing.

Helping the Client to Care for the Ostomy

The client usually is taught how to care for the ostomy before leaving the hospital. The caregiver may also be shown how to help the client. Even so, there may be times when the home care aide will need to assist the client to care for the ostomy. The care plan will give directions about what needs to be done. Be sure to wear gloves when performing ostomy care to protect yourself. Some of the duties the home care aide may perform include caring for the skin around the stoma, disposing of fecal material, and cleaning the ostomy pouch.

The following information about caring for the ostomy is taught to the client or caregiver. However, the home care aide may need to assist when necessary.

Skin Care   Remove any fecal material on the stoma with toilet paper and discard in plastic trash bag or flush in toilet. Wash the skin around the stoma thoroughly, but gently, with soap and warm water. Pat dry. If you notice any redness or irritation, notify your supervisor, who will give further directions for skin care.

Disposing of Fecal Material From Pouch   If possible, have the client sit on the toilet or commode. He/she holds the pouch and places it between the legs. The bar clamp is removed and the client empties the contents into the toilet. Some clients find it easier to empty the contents into a container first, then into the toilet.

Those with poor eyesight or difficulty handling the bar clamp usually need help with opening and closing it. Wear gloves when assisting the client to empty the pouch.

The pouch should be emptied when one-third to one-half full. If the pouch is allowed to fill completely, the weight of the pouch can cause it to loosen from the skin.

Cleaning the Pouch   Most pouches are odor proof, if cleaned properly. Each time the pouch is emptied, put on gloves and follow these directions:

1. Remove the pouch from the appliance attached to the skin.
2. Fold the end of the pouch back (like a cuff) before emptying to prevent additional fecal material from collecting at the bottom, causing odors.
3. Empty contents into toilet.
4. Rinse inside of pouch with warm water.
5. Wipe the last two inches (10 cm) of pouch with toilet tissue to remove any fecal material.
6. Un-cuff the end of the pouch and put on the clamp.

Providing Emotional Support

Adjusting to the ostomy and its care can be difficult for both the client and the family. It is not unusual for some clients to be sad, withdrawn, or even angry during this time. Your attitude toward caring for the client is very important. When giving care, use a positive approach. Do not give the slightest impression that you are disturbed or disgusted about giving ostomy care. If your client wants to talk about the surgery or has concerns about caring for the ostomy, listen carefully. Record your client's concerns and report them to your supervisor. Remember, clients are usually embarrassed to be eliminating through an opening in the abdomen. Your thoughtful, caring attitude can help the client to adjust to the day-to-day activities of living with an ostomy.

Universal Precautions and Medical Asepsis

Universal precautions and medical asepsis must be followed when handling body fluids, feces, and soiled linens and clothing. Review the rules listed in Box 14-4.

Box 14-4

Universal Precautions and Medical Asepsis Rules When Handling Body Wastes

- Wash hands before and after wearing gloves.
- Wear gloves when:
  - there is risk of contact with urine, feces, sputum, mucous membranes, vomitus, blood, or drainage from wounds
  - assisting clients with toileting who have diarrhea, incontinence of urine and/or feces, or an ostomy
  - measuring client's output
  - handling clothing or bed linens soiled with body fluids.
- Dispose of body wastes carefully; avoid splashing when disposing of contents of bedpan, urinal, or commode; if splashing occurs, clean area immediately.
- Empty bedpans and urinals immediately after use; clean and disinfect properly.

- Follow procedures listed in Chapter 9 for cleaning clothing and bed linens that have been soiled with body wastes.
- Wear goggles if there is danger of splashing body fluids in your eyes.
- Place soiled disposable materials in plastic bags; remove immediately and discard.
- Double bag any soiled linens or clothing; launder as soon as possible

CHAPTER SUMMARY

- Illness, injury, and/or disability may cause clients to have problems with elimination.
- The home care aide can promote normal urinary and bowel elimination.
- Body waste is eliminated as perspiration, carbon dioxide, urine, and bowel movements.
- Many clients are embarrassed when someone who is not a family member helps to meet their needs for elimination.
- Good skin care is essential to prevent skin breakdown in incontinent clients.
- Universal precautions are required when handling body fluids, feces, and contaminated linens and clothing.

STUDY QUESTIONS

1. Describe normal urine and feces.
2. List six ways the home care aide can promote normal urinary and bowel elimination.
3. What is urinary incontinence? What special care is needed by incontinent clients?
4. What is an indwelling catheter? When are indwelling catheters used?
5. List five guidelines to remember when caring for a client with an indwelling catheter.
6. Describe three common bowel problems.
7. Mr. Halpern has a colostomy. Discuss three ways the home care aide may assist him with colostomy care.
8. List five examples of the use of universal precautions when handling body wastes.

15 Collecting Specimens

Objectives

After you read this chapter, you will be able to:

1. Discuss three reasons for collecting specimens.

2. List five general rules for specimen collection.

3. Practice universal precautions and medical asepsis when collecting and handling specimens.

4. Demonstrate procedures for collecting urine, stool, and sputum specimens.

5. Assist clients to perform blood sugar monitoring.

Specimens

Specimens are small amounts of body tissue or fluids that are collected for examination and **analysis** in the medical laboratory. Tests are performed on the specimens to:

- Evaluate the health of organ systems
- Determine the cause of illness
- Identify infecting microorganisms
- Evaluate results of treatment
- Observe client's progress
- Check for presence of abnormal substances, chemicals, drugs, and cells.

When clients are unable to leave home, specimens are obtained and taken to the medical laboratory according to agency policy. A few tests can be done in the home; for example, urine is strained for the presence of stones.

Avoid confusion and mix-up by properly labeling the specimen container with:

- Client's name and address
- Date
- Time of specimen collection

Be sure the specimen container is tightly sealed and placed in a plastic bag for transportation to the laboratory. It is important that specimens are collected properly. Follow the general rules listed in Box 15-1.

Mrs. Grant complained of frequent and painful voiding. The home care aide, Janet, noted that Mrs. Grant's urine was cloudy and had a dark color. The aide reported these observations to her supervisor. The agency nurse visited Mrs. Grant to assess her condition. Janet was told to collect a urine specimen from her client and to be sure that Mrs. Grant drinks eight glasses of fluid a day.

analysis
determining the substances present in a specimen.

Box 15-1

General Rules for Obtaining and Handling Specimens

- Follow agency's directions for collecting specimens from clients.
- Complete all information requested on the label (Fig. 15-1):
  - client's name
  - address
  - date
  - time specimen was collected.
- Be sure all information is spelled correctly and is readable.
- Collect the specimen at the time specified.
- Use a clean container for each specimen.

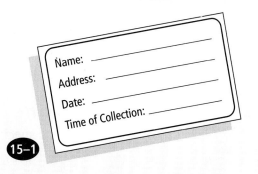

15–1

- Do not touch the inside of the container or the lid.
- Put the lid on the container immediately.
- Follow directions for storing the specimen.
- Store the specimen immediately.
- Inform the client or family member where the specimen is stored.
- Follow the agency's instructions about sending the specimen to the laboratory.

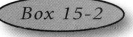

Box 15-2

Universal Precautions and Medical Asepsis Rules for Obtaining and Handling Specimens

- Wash hands before putting on gloves.
- Always wear gloves when obtaining a urine, stool, or sputum specimen.
- Pour urine into container carefully; do not splatter or allow urine to contaminate the outside of the container.
- Wear goggles when there is risk of splashing urine.
- Do not fill the urine specimen container to the top to avoid the chance of spilling over.
- Place stool specimen in container carefully—avoid contaminating the outside of the container.
- Have client cough directly into the sputum specimen container; wear mask, if necessary.
- Remove and discard gloves after placing specimen in container, securing the lid, and cleaning and storing materials.
- Wash hands after removing gloves, goggles, or mask.
- Dispose of used lancets according to agency policy and community regulations.

The usual specimens collected in the home are urine, stool, and sputum. When handling these body substances, all rules of universal precautions and medical asepsis must be followed (Box 15-2). Always wear disposable gloves when collecting and handling specimens.

Urine Specimens

Urine specimens are analyzed to determine the presence of:

- Normal contents
- Abnormal contents, such as blood, bacteria, and protein

Results of laboratory tests help in making the diagnosis and establishing a treatment plan. Repeated or "follow-up" analysis of urine is used to determine the effectiveness of the treatment and to evaluate the client's condition.

When you collect a urine specimen from a client who is on intake and output (I and O), measure the amount of urine in the specimen and record on the I and O form.

Routine Urine Specimen

A routine urine specimen may be collected any time the client voids. The urine may be voided into the bedpan, urinal, commode, or speci-

Procedure 15-1

Collecting a Routine Urine Specimen

Materials Needed

- Bedpan, urinal, commode, or urine collector (hat) for toilet
- Bedpan cover
- Urine specimen container and lid
- Label for specimen container
- Disposable gloves
- Graduate
- Small plastic bag (sandwich bag size)
- Small paper bag (lunch bag size)

Procedure

1. Explain what you are going to do.
2. Wash your hands.
3. Obtain materials listed above.
4. Label container and place in bathroom.
5. Put on gloves.
6. Assist client to bathroom or commode or offer bedpan or urinal (Procedures 14-1 and 14-2).
7. Have client void into commode, bedpan, urinal, or hat.
8. Remind client not to drop toilet paper into specimen. Ask client to discard paper into waste basket.
9. Take bedpan/urinal or commode pail into bathroom.
10. Pour urine into graduate and then into specimen container until ³/₄ full. Discard remaining urine into toilet.
11. Put lid on specimen container.
12. Place container into a plastic bag and then into a paper bag.
13. Clean materials and store in proper location.
14. Remove and discard gloves.
15. Wash your hands.
16. Help client, as needed, back to bed, chair, etc.
17. Store specimen in refrigerator.
18. Record what you have done. Report any abnormal conditions to your supervisor.

men-collecting pan ("hat") placed in the toilet. Tell your client not to discard toilet paper into the voided specimen because it will affect the quality of the specimen. Do not collect a urine specimen from a container that contains a bowel movement. This will also affect the quality of the specimen. Follow Procedure 15-1, Collecting a Voided Urine Specimen for Urinalysis. Assist client as needed.

"Clean Catch" or Midstream Urine Specimen

This specimen is collected to determine the presence of bacteria in the urine. Before voiding, the perineal area is cleansed. The "clean" urine specimen is collected in the middle of the voiding process. First, the client begins to void. Then, the client stops voiding, and the specimen container is positioned to "catch" the urine when voiding is restarted. After the specimen is collected, voiding is stopped again, and the container is removed. The client may then complete the voiding process as usual.

Many clients are unable to perform this procedure without assistance. You will assist by cleaning the perineum and positioning the specimen container properly. Always wear gloves. The agency will provide a special kit that contains all the materials necessary for collecting a clean catch urine specimen. Follow Procedure 15-2.

Collecting a Clean Catch or Midstream Urine Specimen

Materials Needed

- Midstream Urine Specimen Kit—from agency
- Disposable gloves
- Bed pan/urinal or commode
- Small plastic bag (sandwich bag size)
- Small paper bag (lunch bag size)

Procedure

1. Explain what you are going to do.
2. Wash your hands.
3. Obtain materials listed above.
4. Open kit (Fig. 15-2). Remove contents and label container.
5. Assist client to bathroom or commode, or offer bedpan or urinal. (See Procedures 14-1 and 14-2)
6. Tell client how to perform procedure. Be sure client understands what to do and how to do it. Instruct client to call you when finished.
7. If assistance is necessary, put on gloves.

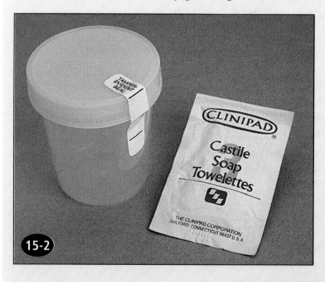

15-2

8. Give perineal care using towelettes in specimen kit.
9. Keep labia separated until specimen has been collected so that urine will not flow over skin surfaces. In uncircumcised males, the foreskin is retracted until the specimen has been collected.
10. Collecting the specimen:
    a. Ask client to begin voiding into urinal, bedpan, commode, or toilet.
    b. Instruct client to stop voiding.
    c. Hold specimen container under urinary meatus, but do not allow it to touch the skin surface. Do not touch the inside of container with your hands.
    d. Ask client to restart voiding.
    e. Catch enough urine to fill the container about half way.
    f. Ask client to stop voiding.
    g. Remove container.
    h. Instruct client to finish voiding.
11. Put lid on specimen container. Be careful not to touch inside in order to keep the specimen clean.
12. Place container into a plastic bag and then into a paper bag.
13. Assist client to complete toileting, if necessary.
14. Clean materials and store in proper location.
15. Remove and discard gloves.
16. Wash your hands.
17. Help client, as needed, back to bed, chair, etc.
18. Store specimen in refrigerator.
19. Record what you have done. Report any abnormal conditions to your supervisor.

24-hour Urine Specimen

Twenty-four-hour specimens are collected to evaluate the body's elimination of certain chemicals and hormones. Your agency will provide a large container for storing the collected urine. This is kept in the refrigerator or stored in a bucket of ice to prevent growth of bacteria in the specimen. Sometimes a preservative may be added to the container for the same purpose. When you begin to collect the specimen, discard the first voided specimen because it was produced by the kidneys during the previous 24-hour period. Then save all other urine for the next

calculi
abnormal stones formed in the body due to accumulation of mineral salts.

24 hours. Place each specimen in the large container and keep cold. The last voided specimen is also added to the container. For example:

- Tuesday, 8 AM, voided 250 ml; DISCARD and begin 24-hour collection
- Wednesday, 8 AM, voided 300 ml; INCLUDE in 24-hour specimen

Always explain the procedure to both client and family. Usually, you will not be in the home for a 24-hour period, and the client and caregiver need to know what to do with the urine. Be sure they understand. If there are any problems, check with your supervisor. Follow Procedure 15-3, Collecting a 24-Hour Urine Specimen.

Straining Urine

Urine is strained to detect the presence of **calculi** that can develop in the urinary tract. They can be very large or as small as grains of sand. Large stones may need to be removed surgically. Very small stones may be passed when the client voids. When the care plan calls for urine to be strained, ALL the urine is poured through a paper filter or a gauze 4" x 4" dressing to remove any calculi. If any stones are found, they are saved for laboratory examination.

Be sure to explain the procedure to the client and family members because they will need to strain the urine when you are not in the home. Show them what to do and ask them to demonstrate the procedure to you. If there are questions or problems, notify your supervisor. For clients on I and O, measure and record the amount of urine in each strained specimen. Also, remind your client not to put toilet tissue into the specimen and to defecate separately from urinating. Follow Procedure 15-4, Straining Urine.

Testing Urine

Occasionally you will be asked to test a client's urine for the presence of abnormal substances. This is done by inserting a chemically treated "dipstick" into the urine. Compare color changes on the chemical to the chart on the dipstick container (Fig. 15-3). Each test has its own set of instructions to follow. Your supervisor will tell you how to do he test. Instructions are also found on the dipstick container. Several rules apply to the use of these products:

1. Check the container for date. Do not use if outdated.
2. Recap dipstick container immediately after use. Store in a dry location.
3. Some chemicals used in testing products may be poisonous. Store out of children's and confused adults' reach.
4. Always use gloves when handling and testing client's urine.

Note the results of the test and record in writing. Report abnormal or unusual findings to your supervisor.

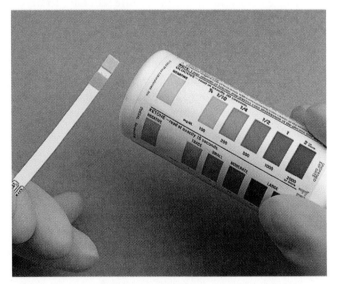

15-3 Compare results on dipstick to chart on container.

Collecting a 24-Hour Urine Specimen

Materials Needed

- 24-hour urine container (with preservative, if needed)
- Container lid and label
- Bucket with ice, if needed
- Disposable gloves
- Graduate or funnel

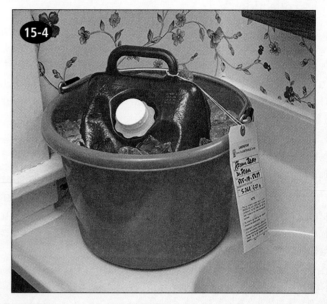

Procedure

1. Explain procedure to client and family.

2. Wash your hands.

3. Obtain materials listed above.

4. Label container.

5. Arrange urine container in bucket of ice in the bathroom (Fig. 15-4). Place preservative in container, if needed.

6. Place a sign saying "Save All Urine" in bathroom near toilet.

7. Put on gloves.

8. Have client void first specimen. Discard. Record time.

9. Remove and discard gloves. (Wear gloves each time you handle another urine specimen. Wash hands after removing gloves. Discard gloves.)

10. Collect all urine for the next 24 hours. Pour into specimen container.

11. Remind client not to have bowel movement when urinating. If feces comes in contact with the urine, the entire procedure will have to be repeated.

12. Record I and O if needed.

13. Add each urine specimen to the container immediately following voiding. Pour into graduate and then into large container to avoid spilling and splashing (Fig. 15-5). A funnel may also be used.

14. Add ice to the bucket as necessary to keep the specimen cold.

15. At the end of 24 hours, have client void as before. Place final specimen in large container.

16. Record what you have done. Report any problems or abnormal conditions to your supervisor.

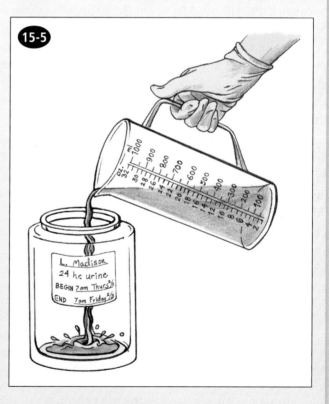

17. Keep specimen on ice until ready for transfer to laboratory.

18. Remove container from ice and dry outside of container. Place in large grocery bag for delivery to lab.

Procedure 15-4

Straining Urine

Materials Needed

- Graduate
- Strainer (disposable paper filter or gauze 4"x 4")
- Specimen container
- Disposable gloves
- Goggles (if needed)

Procedure

1. Explain procedure to client and family.
2. Obtain materials listed above and place in bathroom.
3. Place sign saying "Strain all Urine" near toilet.
4. Wash your hands.
5. Put on gloves and goggles, if needed.
6. Have client void into bedpan/urinal, commode, or urine collector (hat) in toilet.
7. Transfer urine into graduate.
8. Place strainer or gauze over specimen container.
9. Pour urine through strainer and into specimen container (Fig. 15-6).
10. Inspect filter paper or gauze. If stones are present, wrap them in the filter material and place into the specimen container for transport to the laboratory. Label container. Store in refrigerator according to directions in Procedure 15-1.
11. If no stones are found, discard urine. Discard used disposable materials. Clean used reusable materials and prepare for reuse the next time the client voids.

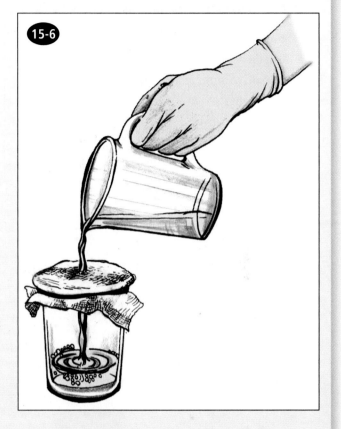

15-6

12. Remove and discard gloves. Remove goggles. Use gloves each time you handle a urine specimen.
13. Wash your hands.
14. Record what you have done. Report any abnormal conditions to your supervisor.

Stool Specimens

Small amounts of stool are collected for laboratory examination for the presence of blood, fats, microorganisms, **parasites,** and other abnormal contents. Only a small amount of stool is needed for examination; about two tablespoons is sufficient. Do not use stool that has come in contact with urine. Sometimes a warm specimen is needed. In that case, the specimen must be transported to the laboratory quickly. Follow your supervisor's instructions regarding delivery of the stool specimen. Follow Procedure 15-5, Collecting a Stool Specimen.

parasites
organisms that live in or on another organism.

Collecting a Stool Specimen

Materials Needed

- Stool specimen container and label
- Tongue depressor
- Bedpan, commode, or toilet "hat"
- Toilet paper
- Disposable gloves

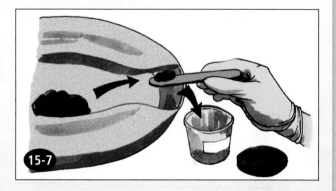

Procedure

1. Explain what you are going to do.
2. Wash your hands.
3. Obtain materials listed above.
4. Label container.
5. Assist client to bathroom or commode or offer bedpan.
6. Ask client not to urinate, if possible, while having the BM.
7. Put on gloves.
8. Transfer stool to specimen container using tongue depressor (Fig. 15-7) and put on lid.
9. Flush remaining feces down toilet and assist client to complete toileting, as necessary.
10. Remove and discard gloves.
11. Wash your hands.
12. Help client, as needed, back to bed, chair, etc.
13. Store specimen according to agency policy or supervisor's directions.
14. Record what you have done. Report any abnormal conditions to your supervisor.

Sputum Specimens

Sputum is thick mucus produced by the respiratory tract when disease or infection is present. Sputum specimens are obtained to check for the presence of blood, bacteria, and abnormal cells. The client coughs up sputum from the trachea and bronchi. Sputum specimens are usually easier to collect in the morning because this material collects in the lungs during sleep. Be sure that you collect sputum, not saliva (the fluid found in the mouth). Rinse client's mouth with plain water to remove saliva. Encourage the client to cough sputum directly into specimen container, close the lid, and then place the container into a plastic bag. If you handle the specimen, wear gloves. Never let a client cough on you. Follow Procedure 15-6, Collecting a Sputum Specimen.

Assisting Clients to Self-Monitor Blood Sugar Levels

Clients with **diabetes** may monitor their blood sugar levels. They use a small electronic monitor called a "glucometer" (Fig. 15-8A). The client collects a sample of his/her own capillary blood on a specially treated dipstick. The sample is inserted into the glucometer, which displays the amount of sugar in the blood. This procedure is the client's responsibil-

diabetes
disease resulting from lack of insulin secreted by special cells of the pancreas; causes blood sugar to be elevated.

lancets
short, pointed blades used to obtain blood from capillaries.

Procedure 15-6

Collecting a Sputum Specimen

Materials Needed

- Sputum specimen container with lid
- Label
- Tissues
- Small plastic bag (sandwich bag size)
- Small paper bag (lunch bag size)
- Disposable gloves
- Disposable mask (if needed)
- Glass of water and emesis basin

Procedure

1. Explain procedure to client.
2. Wash your hands.
3. Obtain materials listed above.
4. Label container.
5. Provide privacy.
6. Put on gloves.
7. Assist client to rinse mouth with plain water.
8. Have client hold sputum specimen container in one hand, tissue in the other.
9. Instruct client to take a deep breath, hold it for a second, and then cough into tissue. Do not let client cough on you. Use disposable mask, if needed. Have client repeat the coughing two or three times to loosen the sputum deep in the respiratory tract.
10. When client has loosened sputum, have client cough sputum directly into the specimen container. Approximately two tablespoons of sputum will be needed.
11. Do not touch the inside of the container. Keep the outside clean and free of any sputum.
12. Put lid on specimen container.
13. Place container into plastic bag, then into a paper bag.
14. Remove and discard gloves.
15. Wash your hands.
16. Record what you have done. Report any abnormal conditions to your supervisor.
17. Specimen is sent to laboratory according to agency policy.

---

ity. If necessary, the agency nurse will teach the client how to perform this test and will evaluate his/her accuracy in performing the test. You may need to take the equipment to the client so he/she can perform the test. Observe the results and assist client to record them in the blood sugar diary. This diary contains a record of blood sugar levels for each day. Clients may monitor their blood sugar several times a day. You may be asked to write the results in the client care record. Report abnormal blood sugar levels as instructed by your supervisor and the care plan. Teach the client to dispose of used **lancets** and dipsticks (Fig. 15-8B) according to agency and local community policies. Do not handle lancets because of the risk of skin puncture. Both lancet and dipstick are contaminated with client's blood. Dispose of any other used materials, such as cotton balls, in the correct manner. Review Chapter 9 for disposing of materials safely. Return glucometer to proper storage area.

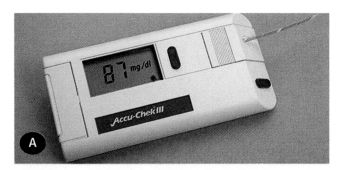

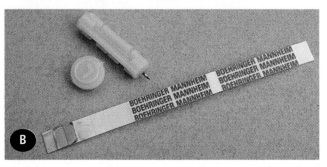

15-8 A, A glucometer with a blood sample in place and a normal reading. *B,* To reduce risk of infection from blood-borne pathogens, be sure lancets and dipsticks are disposed of properly.

CHAPTER SUMMARY

- Specimens are small samples of body tissues and fluids that are examined in the medical laboratory for the presence of normal and abnormal contents.

- The results of laboratory tests are used to determine the cause of illness and to evaluate client's progress.

- Usual specimens collected by home care aides are urine, stool, and sputum.

- Proper labeling of specimen containers includes: client's name, address, and date and time of specimen collection.

- Practice universal precautions and medical asepsis when collecting and handling specimens.

STUDY QUESTIONS

1. What are three reasons for collecting specimens?

2. List five rules to follow when collecting specimens.

3. Give two examples of the use of universal precautions and medical asepsis when collecting the following specimens:
   a. routine urine specimen
   b. clean catch urine specimen
   c. 24-hour urine specimen
   d. stool specimen
   e. sputum specimen

Measuring Vital Signs

16

Objectives

After you read this chapter, you will be able to:

1. Discuss the importance of measuring vital signs.

2. List three factors that may affect vital signs.

3. List normal range of vital signs for adults.

4. Discuss guidelines for taking temperature, pulse, respirations, and blood pressure.

5. Perform the procedures listed in this chapter.

6. Identify three measures the home care aide can use to avoid the spread of infection when taking vital signs.

Temperature, pulse, respirations, and **blood pressure** are called the **vital signs.** They give information about essential body processes: circulation, breathing, and heat regulation. See Box 16-1 for a review of the circulatory and respiratory systems.

Home care aides measure temperature, pulse, and respirations. Some agencies may also require you to measure blood pressure. This will vary according to the agency and state. Vital signs are taken and recorded according to the client's plan of care.

Take the vital signs while the client is at rest. Exercise and activity can cause the vital signs to increase. Other factors that influence vital signs are sleep, age, anxiety, fear, pain, illness, foods and fluids, and medications.

Temperature

Temperature is the amount of heat produced by the body as it uses food for energy. Normally, the amount of heat produced should be the same as the amount of heat lost from the body. Heat leaves the body through urine, feces, exhaling, and skin surfaces. When heat produced by the body is not removed through normal means, it builds up in the body. This increase in body temperature is called a **fever.**

Measuring body temperature is an important way to observe the client's response to illness and treatment. Pulse and respirations are usually measured at the same time the temperature is taken.

Some factors may change the reading of the body temperature for a short time. These include:

- drinking hot or cold liquids
- eating hot or cold foods
- smoking
- taking a hot or cold bath or shower
- exercising

If your client has participated in any of these activities, wait 15 minutes before taking the temperature.

temperature
the amount of heat produced by the body as it uses food for energy.

pulse
throbbing felt over the arteries with each beat of the heart.

respiration(s)
act or process of breathing.

blood pressure
the pressure of blood in the large arteries.

vital signs
essential signs of life: temperature, pulse, respirations, and blood pressure.

fever
an abnormal elevation of body temperature.

thermometer
an instrument for measuring temperature.

Box 16-1

Circulatory/Respiratory/System Review

- The heart is a muscular organ that pumps blood through the arteries to all parts of the body.
- The heart beat has two parts:

    systole—when the heart muscle is contracting.

    diastole—when the heart muscle is resting.
- The act of breathing has two parts:

    inhaling—when oxygen is taken into the body.

    exhaling—when carbon dioxide is expelled from the body.
- The heart and lungs are located in the chest cavity.

There is a vast difference in normal temperature from person to person. Some older adults may have a very low normal temperature. It is important to know what is normal for each person. This is part of the information collected by the nurse during the first visit to the client. See Box 16-2, Vital Signs—Normal Adult Ranges.

Location

Temperature may be taken in several areas of the body:

- oral temperature (mouth)
- axillary temperature (arm pit)
- rectal temperature (rectum)
- tympanic temperature (ear canal)
  NOTE: This type of thermometer is very expensive and is found in very few homes.
- forehead

Follow the care plan's directions for taking your client's temperature. Speak with your supervisor if you are unsure about how your client's temperature should be taken.

Thermometers

A **thermometer** is an instrument used to take the temperature. There are several different kinds of thermometers: oral, rectal, electronic, tympanic, disposable, and forehead. They may be made of glass, plastic, or paper. The client should have his/her own personal thermometer, not one shared with others. If a thermometer is brought from the agency for a single use, a disposable one is best to avoid any risk of transmission of infection.

Reading a Thermometer

Glass Thermometer The glass thermometer has three important parts (Fig. 16-1):

1. Bulb or tip where the mercury is stored
2. Mercury
3. Stem or tube that contains the scale for reading the temperature

The heat of the body causes the mercury to expand and rise in the stem. Long lines on the tube mark 94° to 108° F. Short lines indicate two tenths of a degree. An arrow marks the normal adult oral temperature of 98.6° F.

Read the thermometer in the following manner:

1. Hold the thermometer at eye level, handling only the end of the stem.

Box 16-2

Vital Signs— Normal Adult Ranges

Temperature

Oral	97.6° – 99.6° F	(36.5° – 37.5° C)
Rectal	98.6° – 100.6° F	(37.0° – 38.1° C)
Axillary	96.6° – 98.6° F	(36.0° – 37° C)

Pulse Rate
60–100 beats per minute

Respiratory Rate
12–20 respirations per minute

Blood Pressure

Systolic	100–140
Diastolic	70–90

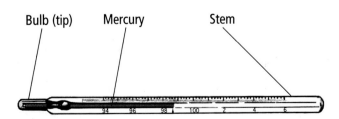

16-1 A glass thermometer—note the bulb (tip), mercury, and stem.

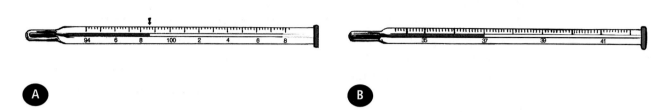

16-2 **A,** A Fahrenheit thermometer. **B,** A Celsius thermometer.

2. Find the column of mercury. Turn the thermometer slowly until you see a silvery line along the scale.
   Fahrenheit Thermometer:
   a. Find the mark to indicate 94° F. Each long line marks one degree of temperature.
   b. Only every other degree is labeled with a number— 94° F, 96° F, 98° F, etc.
   c. Between each long line there are four short lines. Each represents two tenths of one degree ($^2/_{10}$ or 0.2) (Fig. 16-2A)
   Celsius (Centigrade) Thermometer:
   a. Find the mark to indicate 35° C.
      Each long line marks one degree of temperature.
   b. Each degree is marked with a number— 35° C, 36° C, 37° C, etc.
   c. Between each long line there are nine short lines. Each line represents one tenth of one degree ($^1/_{10}$ or 0.1) (Fig. 16-2B).
3. Read the temperature at the point where the mercury ends.

Electronic Thermometer These thermometers give a digital (number) reading of the results. If the battery is working, you will see the results in the readout area. The letter *F* after the reading indicates the Fahrenheit scale of measurement, and the letter *C* indicates Celsius (centigrade) (Fig. 16-3).

16-3 An electronic thermometer —note on and off button.

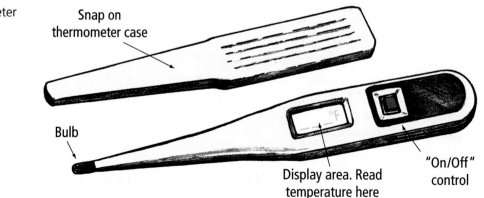

Snap on thermometer case

Bulb

Display area. Read temperature here

"On/Off" control

Disposable (Single Use) Thermometer (Fig. 16–4) The last dot on the thermometer to change color indicates the temperature reading. These thermometers come in Fahrenheit or Celsius scale. Wait 10 seconds after removing the thermometer from the client's mouth before you read it. Other single use thermometers may be applied directly to the skin surface, usually the forehead. They are read in the same manner.

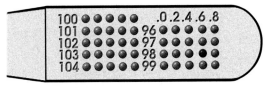

16-4 A disposable Fahrenheit thermometer. This example reads 98.6° F. The last colored dot shows the correct temperature.

Cleaning a Thermometer

Thermometers are cleaned before and after each use. Handle the thermometer by its stem only. For both glass and home use electronic thermometers, follow Procedure 16-1, Cleaning a Thermometer.

Shaking Down a Glass Thermometer

The mercury in a glass thermometer will not go back into the bulb unless you shake it down. In order to get an accurate reading, shake the mercury down to 95° F or 35° C.

- Grasp thermometer firmly by the stem end with thumb and two fingers.
- Stand away from areas where you might hit the thermometer and break it.
- Shake thermometer with a movement that snaps the wrist, as in a vigorous shaking to remove water from the hands.
- Shake over bed or sofa if there is danger of dropping the thermometer.

Procedure 16-1

Cleaning a Thermometer (Glass or Oral Electronic)

Materials Needed:
- Thermometer
- Cotton balls or tissues
- Soap and cold water

Procedure

1. Wash your hands.
2. Obtain materials listed above.
3. Wet cotton ball (or tissue) with soap and water.
4. Hold thermometer by stem over sink or wastebasket.
5. Begin at stem end. Wash from stem to bulb end, twisting cotton ball firmly.
6. Discard used cotton ball.
7. Rinse thermometer with a clean, wet cotton ball using the same twisting, downward movement.
8. Repeat washing and rinsing.
9. Dry with a tissue, wiping in same downward movement.
10. Discard tissue.
11. Take client's temperature or store thermometer properly.

Taking an Oral Temperature

The usual way to take the temperature is by mouth. The glass thermometer is left in the mouth for three minutes. Electronic thermometers signal with a "beep" when the reading is complete. Single use thermometers will give results in 60 seconds.

For certain clients, taking an oral temperature is not recommended. These include:

- Unconscious, restless, or confused clients
- Mouth breathers
- Those receiving oxygen
- Paralyzed clients
- Those with sore mouths
- Infants and young children

Procedure 16-2

Taking an Oral Temperature (with Glass Thermometer)

Materials Needed

- Glass oral thermometer
- Tissues or cotton balls
- Watch with sweep second hand
- Pencil
- Paper

Procedure

1. Explain what you are going to do. (Remind client not to eat, drink, or smoke for 15 minutes.)

2. Have client lie down or rest in a chair.

3. Wash your hands.

4. Obtain materials listed above.

5. Clean thermometer. (See Procedure 16-1)

6. Shake down mercury to 95° F (35° C), if necessary.

7. Place thermometer under client's tongue, as far back as possible, into either heat pocket (Fig. 16-5).

8. Tell client to keep mouth closed and not to talk.

9. Leave thermometer in place for three minutes. (You may take the pulse and respirations at this time.)

10. Remove thermometer.

11. Wipe thermometer with tissue from stem end to bulb end. Discard tissue. Do not touch any part of the thermometer that has been in the client's mouth.

12. Read the thermometer and then place it on a tissue.

13. Write the temperature (pulse and respirations) on the paper.

14. Clean and dry thermometer.

15. Shake down thermometer to 95° F (35° C).

16. Store thermometer in holder in proper location.

17. Wash your hands.

18. Record temperature on client record. Indicate (O) for oral temperature.

19. Report abnormal temperature to your supervisor.

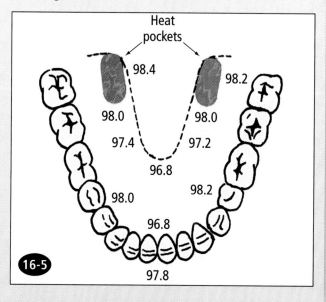

16-5

Remember, if your client has had something hot or cold to eat or drink or has smoked, wait 15 minutes before taking the temperature. Follow Procedures 16-2, 16-3, and 16-4—Taking an Oral Temperature with Glass, Electronic, or Single Use Thermometers.

Taking an Axillary Temperature

Axillary temperatures are taken when the oral method cannot be used. This method may be used for adults, children, and infants. It is the least accurate method of measuring temperature. However, it is preferred over the rectal temperature because it is not damaging to body tissue. Also, since there is no contact with body fluids, there is reduced risk of infection.

The axilla (armpit) is dried before beginning the procedure. Hold the thermometer in contact with the skin surfaces. This will ensure an accurate reading. Have your client sit or lie down during the procedure. The glass thermometer remains in place for 10 minutes; the single use thermometer for three minutes. The electronic thermometer remains in

---

Procedure 16-3

Taking an Oral Temperature (with Electronic Thermometer)

Materials Needed

- Electronic thermometer
- Tissues or cotton balls
- Pencil
- Paper

Procedure

1. Explain what you are going to do. (Remind client not to eat, drink, or smoke for 15 minutes.)
2. Have client lie down or rest in a chair.
3. Wash your hands.
4. Obtain materials listed above.
5. Clean thermometer. (See Procedure 16.1)
6. Turn on thermometer.
7. Wait until it reads "0" or shows "- - -" on the digital display window (Fig. 16-6).

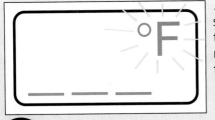

...with the °F sign flashing, the thermometer is ready to take a temperature.

16-6

8. Place thermometer under client's tongue, as far back as possible, into either heat pocket.
9. Tell client to keep mouth closed and not to talk.
10. Leave thermometer in place until you hear it "beep." (You may take pulse and respirations at this time.)
11. Remove thermometer.
12. Wipe thermometer with tissue from stem end to bulb end. Discard tissue. Do not touch any part of the thermometer that has been in the client's mouth.
13. Read the thermometer and then place it on a tissue.
14. Write the temperature (pulse and respirations) on the paper.
15. Clean and dry thermometer.
16. Turn off thermometer.
17. Store thermometer in holder in proper location.
18. Wash your hands.
19. Record temperature on client record. Indicate (O) for oral temperature.
20. Report abnormal temperature to your supervisor.

Taking an Oral Temperature (with a Single Use Thermometer)

Materials Needed

- Single use thermometer
- Watch with sweep second hand
- Tissues
- Pencil
- Paper

Procedure

1. Explain what you are going to do. (Remind client not to eat, drink, or smoke for 15 minutes.)
2. Have client lie down or rest in a chair.
3. Wash your hands.
4. Obtain materials listed above.
5. Remove thermometer from wrapper.
6. Place thermometer under client's tongue, as far back as possible, into either heat pocket.
7. Tell client to keep mouth closed and not to talk.
8. Leave thermometer in place for at least one minute. (You may take pulse and respirations at this time.)
9. Remove thermometer. Wait 10 seconds and read the last colored dot on the thermometer. Place the thermometer on a tissue.
10. Write the temperature on the paper.
11. Discard thermometer.
12. Wash your hands.
13. Record temperature on client record and indicate (O) for oral.
14. Report abnormal temperature to your supervisor.

place until a "beeping" sound is heard, about two to three minutes. See Procedure 16-5, Taking an Axillary Temperature.

Taking a Rectal Temperature

Rectal temperatures are taken when the oral and axillary routes cannot be used. Rectal temperatures are not taken when clients have diarrhea, rectal disease or surgery, and certain types of heart and blood diseases.

A glass rectal thermometer is usually used. NOTE: RECTAL THERMOMETERS ARE USED IN THE RECTUM ONLY. They are NEVER to be used in the mouth. If a single use thermometer is used, its transparent plastic cover is left on while the temperature is taken. Both types should be lubricated for ease in insertion and to prevent damage to rectal tissues. Electronic thermometers are usually not appropriate for taking rectal temperatures. Gently insert the tip of the thermometer into the rectum. Do not push if you have difficulty inserting the thermometer. Always hold the thermometer in place to prevent breakage and its being lost in the rectum. Follow Procedure 16-6, Taking a Rectal Temperature.

Reporting Changes from Normal Temperature

Notify your supervisor if your client's temperature is above the normal range listed in Box 16-2. When a fever is present, a client may have other symptoms: headaches, chills, and sweating. Keep the client warm with extra clothing or blankets. Remove these if the client sweats and complains of feeling hot. Change wet clothing as needed. Make sure the client drinks fluids. Check with your supervisor before increasing the fluid intake.

Taking an Axillary Temperature

Materials Needed

- Thermometer—glass, electronic, or single use
- Watch with sweep second hand
- Dry towel or washcloth
- Tissues
- Pencil
- Paper

Procedure

1. Explain what you are going to do.

2. Have client lie down or sit down.

3. Wash your hands.

4. Obtain materials listed above.

5. Clean thermometer, if glass or electronic. (See Procedure 16-1)

6. Shake down mercury (glass thermometer) to 95° F (35° C). Turn on electronic thermometer. Or, remove single use thermometer from wrapper.

7. Provide privacy.

8. Remove client's arm from sleeve. Expose axilla.

9. Dry axilla with towel or washcloth.

10. Put client's arm across chest to hold thermometer in place (Fig. 16-7). For infant or child, hold arm in place as necessary.

11. Leave thermometer in place:
    glass—10 minutes
    electronic—until "beep" is heard
    single use—3 minutes
    (You may take pulse and respirations at this time.)

12. Remove thermometer.

13. Wipe with tissue from stem end to bulb, if glass or electronic thermometer is used. Then discard tissue.

14. Read the thermometer and then place it on a tissue.

15. Write the temperature on the paper.

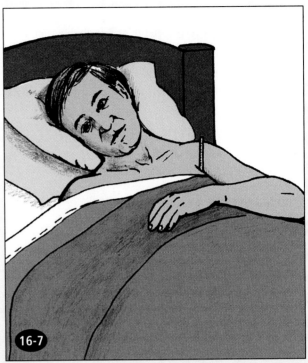

16-7

16. Help client put arm back in sleeve.

17. Turn off electronic thermometer, if used.

18. Clean and dry glass or electronic thermometer. Discard single use thermometer.

19. Shake down glass thermometer, if used.

20. Store thermometer in holder in proper location.

21. Wash your hands.

22. Record temperature on client record. Indicate (A) for axillary temperature.

23. Report abnormal temperature to your supervisor.

Taking a Rectal Temperature

Materials Needed

- Glass rectal thermometer or single use rectal thermometer with wrapper
- Watch with sweep second hand
- Toilet tissue
- Disposable gloves
- Water soluble lubricant
- Pencil
- Paper

Procedure

1. Explain what you are going to do.
2. Put client in bed.
3. Wash your hands.
4. Obtain materials listed above.
5. Clean glass thermometer. (See Procedure 16-1)
6. Shake down mercury in glass thermometer to 95° F (35° C), if necessary.
7. Provide privacy (close door, shut drapes, pull shades).
8. Place client in Sims' position.
9. Put on gloves.
10. Place small amount of lubricant on toilet tissue. Lubricate bulb end of thermometer.
11. Fold back top linens and remove clothing to expose anal area.
12. Raise upper buttock to expose anus (Fig. 16-8).
13. Gently insert thermometer one inch (2.5 cm) into the rectum.
14. Hold in place for three minutes (Fig. 16-9).
15. Remove thermometer.
16. Wipe thermometer with toilet tissue from stem end to bulb end. Place soiled tissue on several folded layers of toilet tissue.
17. Place thermometer on clean toilet tissue.
18. Cleanse excess lubricant and feces from anal area using toilet tissue.
19. Replace clothing and cover client.
20. Discard soiled toilet tissue into toilet.
21. Remove gloves and wash your hands.
22. Read the thermometer and then place it back on tissue.
23. Write the temperature on the paper.
24. Clean and dry glass thermometer. Discard single use thermometer.
25. Shake down glass thermometer to 95° F (35° C).
26. Store thermometer in holder in proper location.
27. Wash your hands.
28. Make sure client is safe and comfortable.
29. Record temperature on client record. Indicate (R) for rectal temperature.
30. Report abnormal temperature to your supervisor.

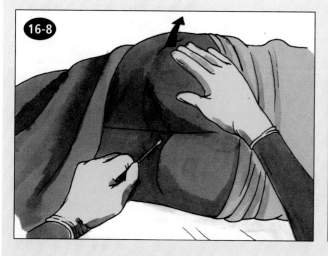

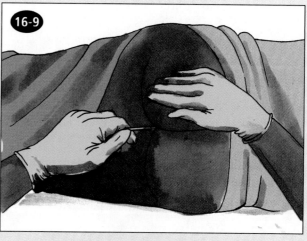

Pulse

The pulse is caused by the beating of the heart. With each beat, the heart forces blood to flow out through the arteries of the body. The pulse rate, then, shows the number of heart beats that are felt in an artery during one minute. The pulse rate can be slower or faster depending on several factors:

- *Exercise*—immediately after climbing stairs, the rate will be higher than when sitting and watching TV
- *Age*—infants have higher pulse rates than older adults
- *Fever*—elevated temperature and pulse usually go together
- *Excitement or fear*—causes the heart to beat faster
- *Pain*—may also cause the heart to beat faster
- *Medications*—some are used to slow down the pulse rate; others are used to raise the pulse rate

Force and Rhythm

When taking the pulse, you will also need to note its force and rhythm. The force shows the strength of each beat. A strong pulse is usually easy to feel. A weak pulse is usually hard to feel. The rhythm, or pattern of beats, should be regular. This means that the time between each beat is the same. An irregular pulse is caused by the heart beating unevenly or skipping beats. It is very important to note the force and rhythm of the pulse rate. Record and report weak and/or irregular pulse rates to your supervisor. See Box 16-3.

Box 16-3

Report to Your Supervisor...

Changes in vital signs

Temperature:

- Increased (Fever):
  Oral—   Above 99.6° F (37.5° C)
  Rectal—   Above 100.6° F (38.1° C)
  Axillary—   Above 98.6° F (37° C)
- Decreased:
  Oral—   Below 97.6° F (36.5° C)
  Rectal—   Below 98.6° F (37° C)
  Axillary—   Below 96.6° F (36° C)
- Major change from what is "normal" for your client

Pulse:

Below 60 beats per minute

Above 100 beats per minute

Change in rhythm or force of beats

Respirations:

Below 12 respirations per minute

Above 20 respirations per minute

Changes in pattern or depth of respirations

Difficulty breathing

Noisy breathing

Blood pressure:

Any blood pressure reading that is not within normal range or is changed from what is "normal" for your client

According to instructions in care plan

Taking a Radial Pulse

Materials Needed

- Watch with sweep second hand
- Pencil
- Paper

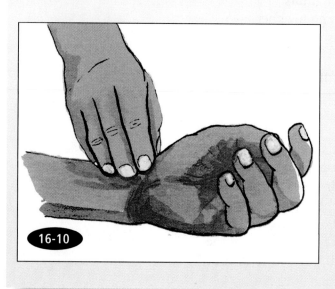

16-10

Procedure

1. Explain what you are going to do.
2. Ask client to sit or lie down.
3. Wash your hands.
4. Obtain materials listed above.
5. Locate radial pulse. Use your middle three fingers to press down on radial artery (Fig. 16-10).
6. Note the following:
   Strong or weak
   Regular or irregular
7. Count the beats for one minute.
8. Write the pulse rate on the paper. Also note the strength and regularity of beats.
9. Assist client, as needed, into desired position.
10. Record pulse on client record.
11. Report any abnormal pulse conditions to your supervisor.

Taking a Radial Pulse

Usually, the pulse is taken on the radial artery. This artery is located on the palm side of the wrist at the base of the thumb. Using your three middle fingers, press against the wrist bone to feel the blood pumping through the radial artery. Do not use your thumb to take the client's pulse. Your thumb has its own artery and you may mistake your pulse for the client's. Take the pulse for one full minute and note the rate, force, and rhythm of the beats. See Procedure 16-7, Taking a Radial Pulse.

Do not take your client's pulse immediately after any physical activity such as climbing stairs or using the bathroom. Wait for 15 minutes before taking the pulse to get an accurate reading.

The normal pulse rate is:

Adults—60–100 beats per minute

Record and report the following abnormal conditions to your supervisor immediately:

Adults	**Rate**	**Force**	**Rhythm**
	above 100	weak	irregular
	below 60	weak	irregular

Respirations

The act of inhaling oxygen and exhaling carbon dioxide is called respiration. During one respiration, the chest usually rises as air enters the lungs (inhalation) and falls as air is pushed out of the nose and mouth (exhalation). The rate of respirations means the number of times the chest rises and falls during a one-minute period of time. You may find that some clients use their abdominal muscles rather than chest muscles to help them breathe. In these cases, the chest may not rise and fall. Rather, the abdomen rises and falls with each breath.

The rate of respirations is one way to tell the health of the respiratory system. Since both the circulatory and respiratory systems work closely together, the pulse and respiratory rates are affected by similar factors. For example, running to the bus stop causes the heart rate to increase (pulse) and breathing (respirations) to increase also. Exercise, age, fever, excitement or fear, and medications influence the respiratory rate.

In healthy persons, the normal respiratory rate is:

Adults   12–20 respirations per minute

Depth, Pattern, and Effort of Respirations

When taking the client's respirations, also note the depth, pattern, and effort of breathing while counting each respiration. In normal respirations, both sides of the chest rise and fall equally. The respirations are regular in pattern and depth; they are quiet and without effort. Use the following guidelines when observing your client's respirations.

Rate
Normal   12–20
Abnormal   under 12 or over 20

Depth
Normal   both sides of chest rise and fall equally
Shallow   breath is short
Deep   breath is long and deep

Pattern
Regular   each inhalation and exhalation is at the same rate
Irregular may have periods where no breath is taken followed
             by rapid or slow, shallow breaths

Noise
Normal   breathing is quiet
Abnormal   raspy, gurgling, wheezy breathing

Effort
Normal   breathing is easy, without effort
Abnormal   breathing is difficult, painful, or takes great effort

Report any changes from normal respirations to your supervisor immediately (see Box 16-3 on page 285).

Taking Respirations

Take the client's respirations when he/she is resting. Wait 15 minutes after exercise or activity to allow the respiratory system time to adjust to normal. Have client sit or lie down so that you can see the chest rise and fall. For abdominal breathers, you may need to rest your hand on the abdomen and notice the rise and fall of your hand.

Respirations can be controlled to some extent by the client, especially if he/she knows you are taking the respirations. This may result in an

Taking Respirations

1. Continue holding client's wrist after taking the pulse.

2. Do not tell the client that you will count the respirations.

3. Count each rise and fall of the chest or abdomen as *one* respiration (Fig. 16-11).

4. Count respirations for one minute.

5. Observe for the following:
   Deep or shallow breathing
   Painful or difficulty breathing
   Noisy breathing

6. Record respirations on paper, noting information listed above.

7. Assist client, as needed, into desired position.

8. Wash your hands.

9. Record respirations on client record.

10. Report any abnormal respirations to your supervisor.

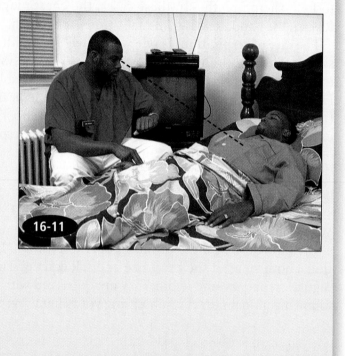

16-11

incorrect count. So, do not tell the client you are taking respirations. After taking the pulse, just keep your fingers on the pulse while watching the rise and fall of the client's chest. In this way the client will think that you are still taking the pulse. Follow Procedure 16-8, Taking Respirations.

Measuring Blood Pressure

Blood pressure is the force of the blood that pushes against the walls of the blood vessels. When taking the client's blood pressure, you are measuring the force of the blood flowing through the arteries. This force is caused by the heart pumping blood into the arteries. It is this force that makes the blood circulate to all parts of the body.

The amount of pressure in the arteries depends on two factors: the client's heart rate, and how easily blood flows through the blood vessels.

Two Readings

When taking your client's blood pressure (BP), you are measuring two pressures:

- **Systolic pressure**—the force of the blood pushing against the walls of large arteries when the heart is contracting. This is the higher reading and is listed first— 120.
- **Diastolic pressure**—the force of the blood pushing against the walls of the arteries when the heart is *resting*. This is the lower reading and listed below the systolic reading— 80.

systolic (blood) pressure
force of blood pushing against walls of the large arteries when the heart is contracting.

diastolic (blood) pressure
force of blood pushing against walls of large arteries when the heart is relaxing.

hypertension
high blood pressure.

hypotension
low blood pressure.

Factors Affecting Blood Pressure

Like the client's temperature, pulse, and respirations, blood pressure also is affected by many factors. For example, pain, anxiety, and fear can cause an increase in blood pressure. Exercise can also cause the blood pressure to rise due to the increased effort of the heart to pump blood to the body. This rise is usually only temporary. Have the client sit and rest for 15 minutes before taking the blood pressure. See Box 16-4, Guidelines for Taking Vital Signs.

Illnesses of the circulatory system may cause the blood pressure to become higher or lower. Clients with disease conditions that affect the heart, blood, or blood vessels will usually have their blood pressure taken regularly. These conditions include:

- **hypertension**—high blood pressure
- **hypotension**—low blood pressure
- certain heart diseases
- kidney diseases
- problems with pregnancy

Your supervisor will explain what to look for when taking your client's blood pressure. It is important to know your client's usual blood pressure. The normal adult blood pressure is considered to be $\frac{120}{80}$. However, the normal range is between $\frac{100}{70}$ and $\frac{140}{90}$. Notify your supervisor when the pressure is higher or lower than the "usual" reading for your client.

Box 16-4

Guidelines for Taking Vital Signs

- Take vital signs when client has been resting for 15 minutes.
- Take vital signs when client is sitting or lying down.
- Wait for 15 minutes before taking the temperature, if your client has been:
  - smoking
  - exercising
  - drinking hot or cold liquids
  - eating hot or cold foods.
- Ask client not to talk while you take the vital signs.
- Take the temperature while taking the pulse and respirations.
- Record vital signs immediately after taking them, using paper and pencil; transfer this information to the client's care record.
- Record the method of taking the temperature: (O) for oral; (R) rectal; or (A) axillary.

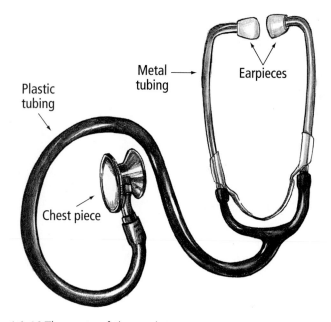

Metal tubing → Earpieces

Plastic tubing

Chest piece

16-12 The parts of the stethoscope.

Equipment Needed

There are two items needed to take a blood pressure reading: the stethoscope, and the blood pressure cuff. Your agency or the client will have these available for you to use.

Using a Stethoscope The stethoscope is an instrument used to listen to sounds produced in the body. Invented in the early 1800s, it is said to be one of the 10 greatest contributions to medical science. By hearing the sounds of the heart, arteries, lungs, abdomen, and other body cavities, health care professionals are able to diagnose illnesses more easily.

Basically, the stethoscope makes body sounds easier to hear. It magnifies sound like a hearing aid. The three parts of the stethoscope are (Fig. 16-12):

1. *Earpieces*—block out outside noises and receive sound from the tubing.
2. *Metal and plastic tubing*—connect earpieces to chest piece (diaphragm) or bell. Sound travels through the tubing to the earpieces.
3. *Chest piece (diaphragm) or bell*—transmits sound to the tubing when placed over a part of the body:
   a. Chest piece (diaphragm)-a round, flat piece
   b. Bell-a bell-shaped piece

The following are tips to follow when using a stethoscope:

- Wipe earpieces and chest piece with antiseptic wipes before and after using to prevent spread of pathogens.
- Shut off radio, TV, and reduce other external noises before using stethoscope.
- Ask client not to talk or move during the procedure.
- Warm the chest piece (diaphragm) or bell with your hands before placing it on the client's body.
- Do not touch the metal or plastic tubing after earpieces are inserted—the noise will be very irritating to you.
- Store stethoscope in the proper location after use.

Using the Blood Pressure Cuff The blood pressure cuff is an instrument placed over an artery to measure the pressure of the blood. There are four parts to this instrument (Fig. 16-13):

1. *Dial*—shows numbers from 20 to 300 and has a pointer. Each line represents 2 millimeters (mm) of mercury. This part can also be called the gauge or scale.
2. *Cuff*—contains a cloth-covered rubber bag that can be inflated. The cuff fits around the client's arm with the rubber bag positioned over the artery.

Measuring Blood Pressure

9. Find the brachial artery by feeling the pulse at the inner side of the elbow (Fig. 16-15).

10. Wrap the cuff around the client's arm, at least one inch above the bend in the arm. Make sure cuff is secure and even. Position rubber bag over the artery (Fig. 16-16).

11. Put stethoscope earpieces in your ears.

12. Place fingers over radial pulse. Inflate the cuff until you cannot feel the radial pulse. Inflate the cuff 30 mm beyond the point at which you last felt the pulse.

13. Place stethoscope chest piece (diaphragm) or bell over the brachial artery (Fig. 16-17).

14. Keep your eyes on dial and begin to deflate the cuff slowly and evenly (two to four millimeters per second) by turning the valve of the bulb counterclockwise.

15. Note the first sound you hear and read the dial at this point. This is the systolic pressure reading.

16. Keep eyes on dial and continue to deflate the cuff. Note the last sound you hear and read the dial at this point. This is the diastolic pressure reading.

17. Deflate the cuff completely. Remove the stethoscope and cuff from the client's arm.

18. Write the blood pressure on the paper.

19. Assist client, as needed, to desired position.

20. Clean earpieces and chest piece (diaphragm) or bell of stethoscope with antiseptic wipes. Discard used wipes.

21. Return all materials to proper storage place.

22. Wash your hands.

23. Record blood pressure results on client record.

24. Report blood pressure readings that are above or below normal to your supervisor.

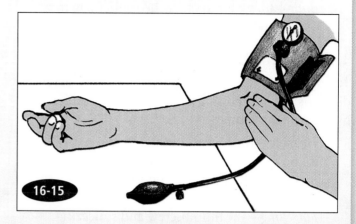

16-15

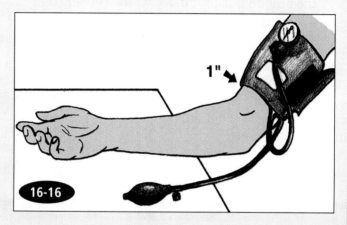

1"

16-16

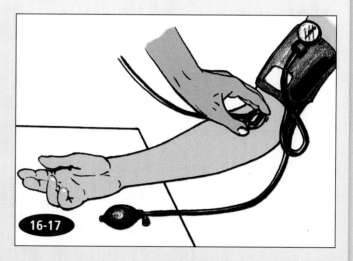

16-17

3. *Valve*—a thumbscrew opens and closes the valve. The valve controls the air that goes in and out of the cuff.

4. *Bulb*—allows air to enter the rubber bag in the cuff when the bulb is squeezed.

Taking the Blood Pressure

Taking an accurate blood pressure requires a great deal of skill. Several skills are involved and all are used at the same time.

Hearing—the sounds of the blood in the artery.

Seeing and Reading—the pointer on the dial.

Handling—the thumbscrew and squeezing the bulb to inflate and deflate the rubber bag in the cuff.

Remembering—the readings so they can be accurately recorded when you finish taking the blood pressure.

See Procedure 16-9, Measuring Blood Pressure, and Box 16-5 for steps and reminders for measuring blood pressure.

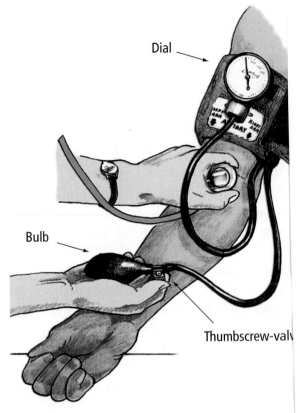

Dial

Bulb

Thumbscrew-valv

Fig. 16-13 The blood pressure cuff.

Procedure 16-9

Measuring Blood Pressure

Materials Needed

- Blood pressure cuff
- Stethoscope
- Antiseptic wipes
- Paper
- Pencil

Procedure

1. Explain what you are going to do.
2. Ask client to sit or lie down.
3. Wash your hands.
4. Obtain materials listed above.
5. Wipe stethoscope earpieces and chest piece (diaphragm) or bell with antiseptic wipes.
6. Place client's arm in position level with the heart, palm up, supported by a pillow(s), table, or arm of chair (Fig. 16-14).

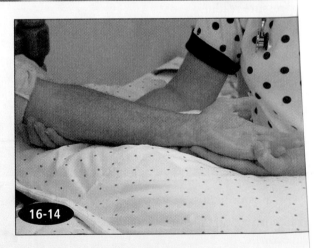

16-14

7. Expose the client's upper arm. Remove clothir so that area is bare.

8. Squeeze the blood pressure cuff to expel any a Close the valve of the bulb.

Continue

Box 16-5

Reminders When Measuring Blood Pressure

- Ask client not to talk during the procedure.
- Shut off radio, TV, and reduce other background noises (if possible).
- Remove clothing from the arm.
- Wrap the cuff snugly around the client's arm; make sure the edge of the cuff is above the bend in the arm and the rubber bag is over the artery.
- Place the dial in the holder attached to the cuff; make sure you have a clear view of the dial.

- Do not take the blood pressure in the client's arm that:

    is injured or paralyzed

    has a cast

    has an IV infusion.

- Write the results on your paper immediately, including the time BP was taken; remember to record information on the client's care record.

Preventing Infection

It is important to prevent the spread of infection when taking the client's vital signs. Infection may be spread by improper cleaning of equipment and by contact with the client's body fluids. Follow the infection control rules listed in Box 16-6 when taking the client's vital signs.

Box 16-6

Infection Control Rules When Taking Client's Vital Signs

- Wash your hands before and after taking vital signs.
- Use client's own personal thermometer, not another family member's.
- Wash glass or electronic thermometer before and after use.
- Clean glass thermometer from stem to bulb.
- Discard cotton balls after cleaning thermometer.
- Use rectal thermometer for rectal temperature only.
- Wipe stethoscope's earpieces and chest piece with antiseptic wipes before and after use.
- Wear gloves when there is risk of coming in contact with the client's body fluids.

CHAPTER SUMMARY

- Vital signs give information about essential body processes—circulation, breathing, and heat regulation.

- Temperature, pulse, respirations, and blood pressure are the vital signs.

- The range of normal vital signs varies from person to person and is influenced by many factors, including: sleep, age, fear, anxiety, food and fluid intake, medications, and activity.

- Home care aides observe, record, and report vital signs according to the care plan.

- Home care aides are expected to know the normal range of vital signs for adults.

- Practice measures to avoid the spread of infection when taking vital signs.

STUDY QUESTIONS

1. Explain the meaning of the term *vital signs.*

2. List four vital signs and three factors that may affect each.

3. List the normal adult range for:
   a. oral temperature
   b. axillary temperature
   c. rectal temperature
   d. pulse
   e. respirations
   f. blood pressure

4. Describe the procedure for taking:
   a. oral temperature
   b. axillary temperature
   c. pulse
   d. respirations
   e. blood pressure

5. Discuss three ways the home care aide prevents the spread of infection when taking vital signs.

Special Procedures

17

Objectives

After you read this chapter, you will be able to:

1. List seven guidelines to follow when performing or assisting with special procedures.

2. Explain the difference between assisting clients to take medications and administering medications.

3. Discuss the role of the home care aide in assisting clients to take medications.

4. List 10 guidelines to follow when assisting clients to take medications.

5. Give two desired effects of hot applications and two desired effects of cold applications.

6. Describe five safety rules to follow when applying heat or cold.

7. Discuss six safety precautions to follow when oxygen is used by the client.

8. Describe four conditions that must be reported to the supervisor when the client is receiving intravenous infusions.

9. Identify three responsibilities of the home care aide for each of the following:
   - client needing clean, dry dressing
   - client wearing elastic stockings
   - client wearing elastic bandages

10. Demonstrate procedures listed in this chapter.

As a home care aide, you perform client care procedures according to the care plan. Most of these will be personal care procedures where you assist clients with grooming, hygiene, elimination, and mobility.

The procedures in this chapter are *not* routine. They are special because they are important in the treatment of a client's condition. Some of the procedures are done by the home care aide. Examples are: applications of heat and cold and changing dressings, according to agency policy. Other procedures, such as administration of medications, will be done by the client. The home care aide assists the client to carry out these procedures according to the care plan. Certain special procedures, such as oxygen administration and intravenous therapy, are done by a health care professional. The home care aide observes the progress of the therapy and reports any problems or client complaints.

Guidelines for Special Procedures

The following guidelines apply to all special procedures:

1. Follow the care plan.
2. Know your limits—do only what you have been taught.
3. Notify your supervisor if you are not sure that you are permitted to perform a certain procedure.
4. Observe the immediate effects of the procedure on the client.
5. Observe any changes in the client's condition as a result of a special procedure.
6. Record on the care plan what you have done and observed.
7. Report any unusual symptoms to your supervisor.

Medications

Medications (drugs) are substances used in the treatment of disease or illness. They are very powerful and cause many effects. For example, a medication taken for pain relieves the pain. However, that medication may also cause drowsiness, nausea, and constipation. These symptoms are known as side effects or adverse effects. Many of these side effects are predictable, and the care plan or medication sheet will include which side effects to expect and which to report. Some side effects are so serious that the medication must be stopped until the physician is notified.

Medications come in many different forms, both solid and liquid. They are available as tablets, capsules, ointments, drops, lotions, suppositories, and other forms. See Table 17-1.

Clients may take:

* *Over-the-counter (OTC) drugs,* which can be bought without a prescription; for example, aspirin or Tylenol
* *Prescription (Rx) drugs,* which are available through a pharmacist according to the doctor's order.

However, there MUST be a written order from the physician for each medication the client takes. This includes both prescription and OTC drugs.

medications
substances used in the treatment of diseases or illness; drugs.

Table 17-1

Types of Medication

SOLIDS

Capsules   Small gelatin containers that hold medication.

Lozenges   Flat discs containing medication in a flavored base. Lozenges are held in the mouth where they dissolve and slowly release medication.

Tablets   Dry, powdered drugs that have been formed into small discs.

Ointments   Semi-solid material containing medication. These are applied externally.

Suppositories   Solid form of medication for insertion into a body cavity, usually the rectum or vagina. Body temperature causes the suppository to melt and medication is released.

Transdermal Discs or Patches   Medication is located on a small disc or strip that is applied to unbroken skin. Drug is absorbed through the skin over a 24-hour period.

LIQUIDS

Elixirs   Drug is dissolved in liquid containing alcohol or water and flavorings.

Suspensions   Drug is suspended in a liquid and may be labeled "shake before using."

Syrups   Medication is dissolved in a concentrated sugar solution.

Drops   Liquid form of medication in a special container that allows one drop at a time to be administered. Usual types are eyedrops, ear drops, or nose drops.

OTHER

Metered Dose Inhalers (MDI)   Small cylinders (used with a special delivery system) containing a drug that is inhaled through the mouth in specifically measured (metered) doses.

Assisting with Medications

Most clients are able to take medications by themselves. Some may need assistance from the home care aide because they are unable to reach the medicines or get them out of the container. Assist means *to help;* administer means *to give.* Home care aides NEVER administer medications of any type—prescription or OTC. They assist clients to take their own medications. You are legally responsible for your own actions. As a home care aide, you are not licensed or certified to administer medication of any type. Only registered nurses (RNs) and licensed practical/vocational nurses (LPNs, LVNs) are permitted to administer medications according to the regulations of the state nurse practice act. Never assume this responsibility. Always follow your agency's policies and state laws to protect yourself and your employer.

When assisting clients to take medications, you may:

- bring medication containers to the client
- loosen and remove container lids
- supervise client as he/she pours the medication into hand, spoon, or cup
- steady client's hand while pouring medications; direct hand as needed for eyedrops, nose drops, etc.
- bring prepoured medications and prefilled syringes to client according to care plan and medication sheet (Fig. 17-1).
- record what medications the client has taken
- watch for desired effect of medication
- watch for and report side effects according to care plan and medication sheet.

The nurse will teach the client about the medications he/she is taking. Clients should be able to follow the medication sheet and take drugs accurately. They should know the drug's desired effect, when and how to take the drug, any side effects to watch for, and foods or other medications to avoid or omit. If your client does not know this information, notify your supervisor.

Medications may be prepoured by the nurse, client, or family member and stored in a "reminder" device (Fig. 17-2). These containers help clients to remember what they have taken and what medications remain to be taken each day. If the client is unable to prepour, a nurse or family member may do so. This is *not* the responsibility of the home care aide.

Six "Rights" of Assisting with Medications

In order to assist clients to take medications accurately and safely, the home care aide follows the Six "Rights" of Assisting with Medications (Box 17-1).

1. Right drug
2. Right client
3. Right dose
4. Right route
5. Right time
6. Right documentation

MEDICATION RECORD

Name	Delbert Sullivan							
Day		SUN	MON	TUE	WED	THUR	FRI	SAT
Date		7/11	7/12	7/13	7/14	7/15	7/16	7/17
Drug Name	Lasix (water pill)							
Dose	1 tablet							
Action	Increases urination							
Time	One (1) daily	8 a.m.	8 a.m.	8 a.m.	8 a.m.	8 a.m.	8 a.m.	8 a.m.

Special Instructions	Daily weight at 8 a.m.
	Drink plenty of fluids.
	Watch for and report any weight gain or swelling.
	Do not omit or increase dosage.
	Call doctor if unable to take medication.

Immediately Report

Day		SUN	MON	TUE	WED	THUR	FRI	SAT
Date		7/11	7/12	7/13	7/14	7/15	7/16	7/17
Drug Name	Ferrous Sulfate (iron pill)							
Dose	1 tablet							
Action	Replaces iron in blood.							
Time	Three (3) times daily	9 a.m.	9 a.m.	9 a.m.	9 a.m.	9 a.m.	9 a.m.	9 a.m.
		1 p.m.	1 p.m.	1 p.m.	1 p.m.	1 p.m.	1 p.m.	1 p.m.
		5 p.m.	5 p.m.	5 p.m.	5 p.m.	5 p.m.	5 p.m.	5 p.m.

Special Instructions	Take between meals.
	Take with full glass of water.
	Do not take with milk or antacids.
	Will change color of stool to black.
	Do not crush tablet.
	May cause constipation.
Immediately Report	Nausea, vomiting, and diarrhea
	Abdominal pain

17-2 Medication reminder boxes can help clients keep track of their daily medications.

17-1 A sample medication sheet.

Box 17-1

The Six "Rights" of Assisting with Medications

When assisting clients to take medications, remember the six "rights":

1. **Right Drug** — Read container label. Check against medication list.

2. **Right Client** — Check label of container; be sure the drug is for the client. In some homes, two people may have the same name.

3. **Right Dose** — Be sure you understand how much medication your client should be taking.

4. **Right Route** — Be sure you know the correct route and form of the drug.

5. **Right Time** — Bring drug to client at correct time or remind client about taking medications.

6. **Right Documentation** — Observe as client records what was taken. If client is not able, you record. Record what you observed.

If you have any questions or problems with the six "rights," notify your supervisor.

Right Drug The name of the drug will be listed on the medication sheet and on the medication container. Read the label and compare with the medication sheet. Be sure you are assisting the client to take the right drug.

Right Client Check the label on the medication container; be sure the drug is for your client (Fig. 17-3). The label should have your client's first and last name on it. In some homes, two people may have the same name. Be certain you are assisting your client to take medications that are for his/her use only.

Right Dose The dose is listed on the medication sheet and on each prescription container. For example: "Take one tablet daily," or "Apply ointment to left elbow twice a day." The correct amount of medication must be taken. For example, if Mrs. Jones takes two tablets from the container but should take only one tablet, you must remind her that she is to take only one tablet.

When the medication is in a liquid form, the dose may be in teaspoons or tablespoons. Be sure to bring the client the correct standard measuring spoon to use when pouring the medicine.

Right Route The method in which the medication is taken is called the route. This includes:

1. *Oral medications*—solids or liquids taken by mouth. Examples are tablets and cough syrup.
2. *Sublingual medications*—placed under the tongue where they dissolve.
3. *Topical medications*—applied to skin and mucous membranes. For example, ointments and eyedrops.

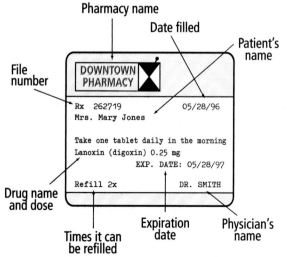

17-3 Read the label before client takes any medications.

4. *Transdermal discs, patches*—forms of topical medications applied to the skin.
5. *Metered dose inhaler*—medication is sprayed into throat and inhaled into the lungs.
6. *Injections* (sometimes called parenteral medications) may be:
    subcutaneous—under the skin
    intramuscular—into the muscle
    intravenous—into the vein.

Right Time Medications must be taken at the correct time in order to work properly. Some are given only once a day; others may be given two, three, or four times a day. The directions on the prescription will give instructions on the time the medication is to be taken. For example, a client may have medication that must be taken every six hours—this means four times during a 24-hour period. Your client's medication schedule should be in the care plan or medication sheet. Some drugs have to be taken at times when the stomach is empty—that is, one hour before or two hours after eating. Other medications need to be taken at mealtime to reduce stomach upset and help with absorption. These prescriptions usually have labels that say "take on empty stomach" or "take with food or milk."

A client may also need to avoid certain foods or beverages when taking some medications. The prescription container may carry such special instructions, as "avoid alcoholic beverages." If they are not avoided, internal bleeding or kidney damage could occur. Also, mixing certain drugs with alcohol and tobacco can cause serious harm, such as depressed respirations, unconsciousness, or even death. For these reasons, clients must *never* take any drugs without the doctor's knowledge, including over-the-counter medications.

Sometimes clients are confused about when to take their medications. For example, a client may say, "I can never remember. Do I take two tablets at 3 o'clock, or three tablets at 2 o'clock?" Alert your supervisor if this happens. Your client may need a "refresher" course on taking medications properly. Assist your client to take all medications at the right time.

Right Documentation Ideally, clients should keep their own medication records. The nurse is the one who teaches the client how to do this. However, some clients may be unable to write on the medication sheet because of physical disability or vision problems. In these cases, the home care aide will record the information for the client. Always follow your agency policies regarding documentation (recording), and ask your supervisor for help, if needed.

Guidelines for Assisting with Medications

When assisting clients with medications, the following guidelines should be observed:

1. Always follow agency policy.
2. Carefully review care plan with your supervisor before assisting client with medications. Follow the Six "Rights" of Assisting with Medications (see Box 17-1).

3. Make sure you bring the correct medication containers to the client. Read the labels carefully. There may be more than one person in the home with the same name. Compare container labels with the medication sheet list to be sure you have the correct medication.

4. Know the correct dose of each medication. Check the care plan.

5. Give a glass of water (or other liquid) with oral medications as ordered.

6. Store medications:
   - separately from those of other family members, in a special location, just for client's medications
   - in a dry, cool place (not in the bathroom medicine cabinet)
   - out of reach of children and confused persons
   - in original containers
   - with lids tightly closed
   - according to any special storage directions; for example, "store in refrigerator"

7. Do not leave medications at the bedside and assume that the client will take them correctly. Remain with the client until he/she has finished taking the medications.

8. Do not remove labels from medication containers.

9. Never use any medication container that is not labeled or take medication from a container where the label cannot be read.

10. Do not use discolored or deteriorated drugs. Notify your supervisor.

11. Be sure prescriptions are refilled before medications are completely used. Remind client/family to reorder medication when only a few days' supply remains.

12. Listen to your client. If he/she questions something about a medication, STOP—do not assist with administration. Call your supervisor immediately.

13. Report to your supervisor if your client:
   - does not use medication sheet and/or does not take drugs correctly
   - does not know why the drug is being taken, the dosage, the time schedule
   - refuses to take the medication, forgets, or omits a dose; the client should not take a double dose if one is omitted
   - shows any side effects (e.g., vomiting, rash, breathing difficulty, itching, diarrhea)
   - takes any medications that are not listed on the medication sheet, particularly OTC drugs.

14. Discard any unused medication. Check with your supervisor for instructions.

15. Record what you have done on the care plan. Client should record on the medication sheet. Assist as necessary.

16. Record if a medication is not taken or omitted, and why. Follow Procedures 17-1 through 17-5 for assisting clients with medications.

Procedure 17-1

Assisting With Oral Medications

Materials Needed

- Oral medications
- Teaspoon or tablespoon, if needed (use standard measuring spoon)
- Glass of water
- Straw, optional

Procedure

1. Explain what you are going to do.
2. Check care plan and medication sheet.
3. Wash your hands.
4. Obtain materials listed above.
5. Help client to wash hands.
6. Check label on each prescription (see Fig. 17-3) or on each prepoured medication for:

    Right Drug   Right Dose   Right Time
    Right Client   Right Route

7. Loosen lid(s) on container(s) if client is unable to do so. Tell client name of each medication (read from label).
8. Place containers where client can reach them or hand container to client. Let client read name of medication to you. Be sure client is wearing eyeglasses if client needs them to read.
9. Assist client with oral medications:
    - Give sip of water to moisten mouth.
    - Support hand as necessary to pour medication.
    - Give a full glass of water or other cool liquid after client puts medication in mouth.
    - Remind client to lower chin while swallowing.
10. Close containers.
11. Have client record medications taken. Home care aide may record for client, if necessary.
12. Store materials in proper location.
13. Wash your hands.
14. Record what you have done. Report any abnormal conditions to your supervisor.

Procedure 17-2

Assisting With Rectal Suppositories

Materials Needed

- Suppository
- Water soluble lubricant
- Disposable glove
- Toilet tissue
- Hand-washing supplies

Procedure

1. Explain what you are going to do.
2. Check care plan and medication sheet.
3. Wash your hands.
4. Obtain materials listed above.
5. Provide privacy. (Close door, shut drapes, pull shades.)
6. Assist client into bed and Sims' position.
7. Remove clothing to expose anal area.
8. Check label on the suppository for:

    Right Drug   Right Dose   Right Time
    Right Client   Right Route

9. Unwrap suppository.
10. Apply water soluble lubricant to suppository. Do not use petroleum jelly because it is not water soluble.
11. Give glove to client to put on.
12. Hand suppository to client to insert into rectum. Guide client's hand, if necessary.
13. Observe as client inserts medication and wipes anus with toilet tissue.
14. Have client remove and discard glove into waste container.
15. Assist client to wash hands.
16. Discard used materials in waste container.
17. Have client record medication taken. Home care aide may record for client, if necessary.
18. Remind client to remain on side for 15–20 minutes to allow suppository to melt and medication to be absorbed.
19. Wash your hands.
20. Record what you have done. Report any abnormal conditions to your supervisor.

Assisting With Eye Medications or Ointment

Materials Needed
- Eye medication or ointment
- Tissues or cotton balls
- Small hand mirror
- Disposable gloves (if necessary)

Procedure

1. Explain what you are going to do.
2. Check care plan and medication sheet.
3. Wash your hands.
4. Obtain materials listed above.
5. Help client to wash hands.
6. Check label on prescription container for:
   Right Drug—be certain the preparation is for use in the eyes only
   Right Client
   Right Dose—be certain the strength of the solution/ointment in the container is correct
   Right Route—which eye, or both eyes
   Right Time
7. Loosen lid on container, if client is unable to do so.
8. Place container within client's reach or hand to him/her as necessary. Be sure client is wearing eye glasses, if client needs them to read.
9. Hold mirror so client can see to administer eye medication.
10. Remove client's eyeglasses, if worn.
11. Assist client with:
    Eye medications
    - Guide client's hand to grasp lower lid.
    - Observe that client looks up and releases drops into lower lid.
    - Observe that client closes eye to distribute medication.
    - Make sure that dropper does not touch client's eye.

    Ointment:
    - Guide client's hand to grasp lower lid.
    - Observe that client looks up and squeezes a small ribbon of ointment into the lower lid from inner corner of eye to outer corner of eye.
    - Observe that client closes eye to allow medication to melt and be distributed.
    - Make sure that tip of tube does not touch eye surface.
12. Reseal container.
13. Have client record medications taken. Home care aide may record for client, if necessary.
14. Store materials in proper location.
15. Wash your hands.
16. Record what you have done. Report any abnormal conditions to your supervisor.

Applications of Heat and Cold

Heat and cold are applied to parts of the body to treat many types of problems, such as pain, swelling, and soreness. Applying heat or cold to the body is only done when the doctor orders such treatment. The care plan indicates the type of treatment and the number of times each day the treatment is to be given. In some states, the home care aide is not permitted to apply heat or cold. Be sure you know what your state (and agency) allows you to do.

There are two types of hot or cold applications—dry and moist.

1. *Dry*—the heat or cold does not come in direct contact with the client's skin. For example, hot water bag or ice bag. Dry heat or cold does not produce its effects as deeply or as quickly as moist heat or cold. But, there is still risk of skin damage.
2. *Moist*—the heat or cold comes in direct contact with the client's skin. For example, hot water soaks and cold **compresses.** Moist heat or cold produce the desired effects more quickly and more effectively. However, because heat or cold comes in direct contact with the skin, risk of skin damage is greater.

compress (compresses) gauze, washcloths, or small towels applied to a body area; may be moistened with hot or cold solution.

Procedure 17-4

Assisting With Transdermal Discs

Materials Needed
- Medicated transdermal disc
- Disposable gloves (if necessary)

Procedure

1. Explain what you are going to do.
2. Check care plan and medication sheet.
3. Wash your hands.
4. Obtain materials listed above.
5. Provide privacy. (Close door, shut drapes, pull shades.)
6. Help client to wash hands.
7. Check label on disc container for:

   Right Drug   Right Dose   Right Time
   Right Client   Right Route

8. Have client remove and discard old disc into waste container. Wash skin that had been covered by old disc.
9. Ask client to select new site for new disc (any area without hair) usually the chest or upper arm.
10. Observe as client applies new disc to skin surface. Be sure that the medicated surface of the disc is not touched with ungloved fingers. (Your skin may absorb some of the drug.)
11. Discard disc wrapper and other used materials.
12. Have client record medications taken. Home care aide may record for client, if necessary.
13. Store materials in proper location.
14. Wash your hands.
15. Record what you have done. Report any abnormal conditions to your supervisor.

Procedure 17-5

Assisting With Metered Dose Inhalers

Materials Needed
- Metered dose inhaler container of prescription drugs
- Disposable gloves (if necessary)

Procedure

1. Explain what you are going to do.
2. Check care plan and medication sheet.
3. Wash your hands.
4. Obtain materials listed above.
5. Provide privacy.
6. Help client wash hands.
7. Check label on prescription container for:
   Right Drug   Right Dose   Right Time
   Right Client   Right Route
8. Hand metered dose inhaler (MDI) to client, who then uses it to inhale the medication (Fig. 17-4).
9. Have client record medication taken. Home care aide may record for client, if necessary.

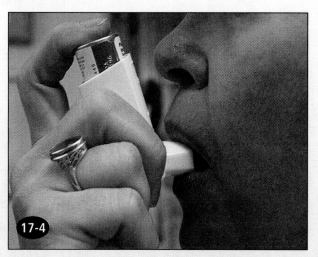

17-4

10. Clean inhaler according to manufacturer's instructions and store in proper location.
11. Wash your hands.
12. Record what you have done. Report any abnormal conditions to your supervisor.

Effects of Heat

Applying heat to a part of the body causes blood vessels in the area to **dilate.** These enlarged blood vessels help bring more blood, containing oxygen and nutrients, to the surrounding tissues. Heat applications are used to:

- Provide warmth and comfort
- Help to relax sore muscles
- Relieve soreness in joints
- Increase blood circulation to the area

Effects of Cold

Applying cold to a part of the body causes blood vessels in the area to **constrict.** As the blood vessels become smaller, circulation to the area is reduced. The sensation of pain is usually reduced because nerve endings in the skin become less sensitive. Cold applications are used to:

- stop bleeding
- reduce pain
- reduce swelling
- reduce heat in the tissues

Safety

Whenever heat or cold is applied to the body, there is risk of skin damage. Clients at greatest risk include:

- *fair-skinned—*
  skin is delicate, thin, and fragile and is injured more easily
- *infants, young children, and confused adults—*
  cannot tell you when the application is too hot or too cold
- *older adults—*
  skin is thin and reaction to heat or cold may be delayed
- *unconscious or paralyzed—*
  cannot feel the effects of heat or cold
- *diabetics—*
  nerve endings are not as sensitive to changes in temperature

Check your client's skin frequently after applying heat or cold. If the client complains of pain or numbness in the area, remove the application immediately and notify your supervisor. Record the client's reaction, appearance of skin, and time the treatment was stopped. See Box 17-2, Signs of Skin Damage When Applying Heat and Cold.

The following general safety rules should be used when applying heat or cold:

- Use a cooking thermometer, if available, to check the temperature of the water.
- Follow manufacturer's directions for operating equipment safely; contact your supervisor when in doubt.
- Follow your agency's guidelines for temperature ranges for hot and cold applications.
- Cover hot water bag, hot or cold pack, or ice bag with towel or other covering before placing it on client's skin.

dilate
expand or open wider.

constrict
to narrow.

Box 17-2

Signs of Skin Damage
When Applying Heat and Cold

Heat Applications

- Client complains of burning sensation or pain in area
- Skin is:
  red
  blistering

Cold Applications

- Client complains of burning sensation, numbness, or pain in area
- Skin is:
  red
  pale
  bluish

- Check client's skin every 10 minutes; for those at risk of skin damage, check more frequently.
- Remove the application immediately if there are signs of skin damage (see Box 17-2).

Applying Dry Heat

The most common ways of applying dry heat are by hot water bag, heating pad, or hot pack. The care plan will indicate how long dry heat should be applied and how frequently. Sometimes, the client may ask you to apply dry heat even though it is not listed in the care plan. "I feel so cold—please get the heating pad and put it on my shoulders." This may sound like a reasonable request. But remember, as a home care aide, you may only apply heat when ordered by the doctor and approved by your agency. In this case, helping the client to put on an extra sweater or placing a blanket over the shoulders may be a good substitute. Explain why you are not able to apply the heating pad.

Before applying dry heat by heating pad or hot pack, read the manufacturer's directions and be sure you understand how to use the appliance. Do not allow the client to lie on top of the heating pad or pack because this position increases the risk for burns.

Your client may use commercially made hot packs (pads, pillows, cushions, or wraps) (Fig. 17-5). These items have gel in the center of the pack. They are prepared by heating in the microwave. The gel becomes hot and radiates warmth to the rest of the pack. Read the manufacturer's directions about heating, applying, and reheating this type of hot pack. Heat the pack for the lowest time recommended by the manufacturer. Cover the pack with a towel or cover provided by the manufacturer before applying it to the client's skin. Hot wraps

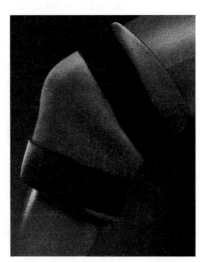

17-5 Commercially made hot packs. *(Courtesy Southwest Technologies, Inc., Kansas City, MO.)*

may have Velcro closures that can be easily wrapped around the ankle, elbow, or wrist.

See Procedures 17-6 for Applying A Hot Water Bag and 17-7 for Applying Hot/Cold Pack.

Applying Moist Heat

Moist heat is used when there is a need to provide warmth deeper in the tissues. The most common forms of moist heat are hot soaks, compresses, and sitz baths. It is very important to check the temperature of the water before the client's skin comes in contact with the water. Burns can occur immediately if the water is too hot. When the client's skin is prone to burns, Vaseline or other protective substance may be used around the outer part of the skin to protect it from the heat of the hot compress. Contact your supervisor for instructions.

While the client is receiving moist heat, check the skin every 10 minutes for signs of burns. Also, add water as needed to maintain the proper water temperature. See Procedures 17-8 and 17-9 for Applying Hot Compresses and Hot Soaks.

Sitz Bath The sitz bath is a method of applying moist heat to the client's perineum and pelvic area. The purpose of the sitz bath is to increase the circulation of blood to the area. It also helps to promote healing, clean a wound of the rectal or perineal area, or ease discomfort after surgery or childbirth.

Equipment needed includes a plastic sitz bath that fits on the rim of the toilet bowl and a water bag with tubing and a clamp (Fig. 17-6). Warm water is placed in the plastic sitz bath. The client sits in the warm water. The water bag holds additional warmer water. When the water in the sitz bath begins to cool, the tubing is unclamped and warmer water enters the sitz bath. The client may be taught how to control the flow of water. For clients who are unable to handle the clamp, the home care aide will perform this task.

Warm water increases the circulation to the perineal area. When this happens, there is less blood flow to other parts of the body. As a result, the client may become pale, weak, or feel light-headed or dizzy. It is important to check the client every five minutes for these signs. Also, the shoulders and legs may become cold. To avoid chilling during the procedure, cover the shoulders and knees.

Do not use a regular bathtub to give a sitz bath. Keeping the legs under hot water causes blood vessels in the legs to dilate and decreases circulation to the perineal area. See Procedure 17-10, Giving a Sitz Bath.

Applying Dry Cold

Ice bags and cold packs or wraps are commonly used to apply dry cold to a part of the body. Similar to hot packs, cold packs or wraps contain gel in the center of the appliance. They are prepared by placing them in the freezer section of the refrigerator until the gel is frozen. Be sure to follow the manufacturer's directions about freezing, applying, and refreezing these packs or wraps.

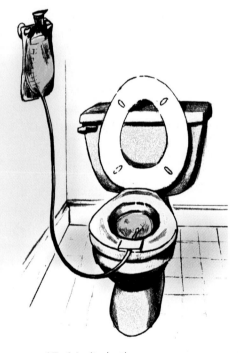

17-6 A sitz bath.

Procedure 17-6

Applying a Hot Water Bag

Materials Needed

- Hot water bag
- Soft cloth or towel
- Cooking thermometer (if available)
- Pencil
- Paper

Procedure

1. Explain what you are going to do.
2. Wash your hands.
3. Obtain materials listed above.
4. Provide privacy.
5. Fill hot water bag with water. Secure with stopper. Turn bag upside down to check for leaks.
6. Remove stopper and empty bag.
7. Run more hot water and test with cooking thermometer; adjust water temperature to 115°–130° F or 45°–54.4° C.
8. Fill bag ⅓ to ½ full.
9. Lay bag flat to remove air. Place stopper in bag while it is still flat.
10. Cover bag with soft cloth or towel and apply to client's affected area.
11. Write on paper the time the bag was applied.
12. Refill bag when it becomes cool.
13. Check client's skin every 10 minutes for danger signs (see Box 17-2).
14. Remove bag according to time required. Write time of removal on paper.
15. Remove stopper, empty bag, and hang bag upside down to dry. Place cloth or towel in laundry container to be washed.
16. Wash your hands.
17. Record what you have done. Report any unusual conditions to your supervisor.
18. When bag is dry, blow air into it and replace stopper to prevent insides of bag from sticking together. Store in proper location.

Procedure 17-7

Applying Hot/Cold Pack

Materials Needed

- Hot or cold pack
- Soft cloth, towel, or cover
- Pencil
- Paper

Procedure

1. Explain what you are going to do.
2. Wash your hands.
3. Obtain materials listed above.
4. Provide privacy.
5. Place hot pack in microwave and heat according to manufacturer's directions. Or, remove cold pack from freezer.
6. Cover pack with soft cloth, towel, or cover and apply to client's affected area.
7. Write on paper the time the pack was applied.
8. Check client's skin every 10 minutes for danger signs (see Box 17-2).
9. Remove pack according to time required. Write time of removal on paper.
10. Store pack according to manufacturer's directions. Place cloth, towel, or cover in laundry container to be washed.
11. Wash your hands.
12. Record what you have done. Report any unusual conditions to your supervisor.

Applying Hot Compresses

Materials Needed

- Basin or container
- Hot water
- Cooking thermometer (if available)
- Compresses (small towel, washcloth, or gauze squares)
- Bath towel
- Waterproof protector pad
- Disposable gloves
- Plastic wrap
- Tape
- Pencil
- Paper

Procedure

1. Explain what you are going to do.

2. Wash your hands.

3. Obtain materials listed above.

4. Provide privacy.

5. Place waterproof protector pad under the body part where compress is to be applied.

6. Fill basin or container ½ to ⅔ full of water at 105°–115° F (40.5°–46.1° C). (Check temperature with cooking thermometer.)

7. Put on gloves.

8. Place compress in the water.

9. Wring out compress and apply to area (Fig. 17-7). Note time applied.

10. Cover compress quickly with plastic wrap. Secure edges of plastic wrap with tape. Cover with bath towel.

11. Write on paper the time compress was applied.

12. Apply, according to directions, a hot water bag or rubber-protected heating pad over the plastic wrap to keep compress hot.

13. Check client's skin every 10 minutes for danger signs (see Box 17-2).

14. Change compress, if cooling occurs.

15. Remove compress according to time required.

16. Write time of removal on paper.

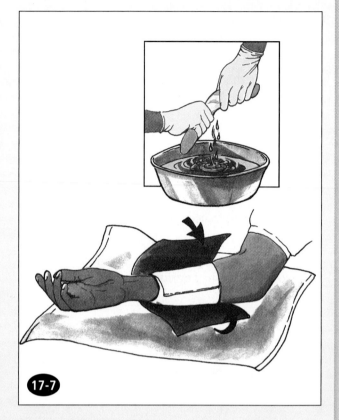

17-7

17. Pat area dry with towel. Discard used gauze or compress. Place used cloths or towels in laundry container to be washed.

18. Remove and discard gloves.

19. Wash your hands.

20. Clean and store materials in proper location.

21. Record what you have done. Report any unusual conditions to your supervisor.

Procedure 17-9

Applying Hot Soaks

Materials Needed

- Basin or other container
- Hot water
- Cooking thermometer (if available)
- Waterproof protector pad
- Towel

Procedure

1. Explain what you are going to do.
2. Wash your hands.
3. Obtain materials listed above.
4. Provide privacy.
5. Assist client to comfortable position.
6. Place waterproof protector pad under the area to be soaked.
7. Fill basin or container $1/2$ full of water 105°–110° F (40.5°–43.3° C). (Check temperature with cooking thermometer.)
8. Expose only the part to be soaked.
9. Place area to be soaked into the water.
10. Check water temperature and skin of area being soaked every 10 minutes. Remove from water if danger signs are noticed (see Box 17-2).
11. Remove body part from water according to time required.
12. Write time of removal on paper.
13. Pat body part dry. Assist client to replace clothing and to get comfortable.
14. Clean and store materials in proper location.
15. Put used towel in laundry container to be washed.
16. Wash your hands.
17. Record what you have done. Report any unusual conditions to your supervisor.

Inexpensive substitutes for an ice bag are: a freezer bag or heavy duty plastic bag filled with crushed ice, or a bag of frozen peas or corn. When the treatment is finished, the bag of peas or corn can be refrozen for later use. Be sure to mark the bag so that it is not used as food.

Change the cover of the ice bag, cold pack, or wrap when you feel moisture. You may need to refill the ice bag or get another bag of frozen peas when the contents begin to melt. Sometimes the client may feel chilly while receiving applications of cold. This is not unusual. A sweater or blanket may help to relieve the feeling. See Procedure 17-11, Applying an Ice Bag.

Applying Moist Cold

Cold compresses are the usual way to apply moist cold. Just as moist heat is more penetrating than dry heat, moist cold is more effective than dry cold. Covering the cold compress with plastic wrap or a piece of plastic helps to retain the cold. Cold compresses become warm quickly because of the body's heat. Change the compress as soon as it becomes warm. Cold compresses are often used for areas such as the eyes. Be careful to avoid pressing on the area that is usually sensitive to the touch. See Procedure 17-12, Applying Cold Compresses.

Giving a Sitz Bath

Materials Needed

- Portable plastic sitz bowl
- Hot water
- Water bag and tubing
- Pitcher
- Blanket or large towel
- Cooking thermometer (if available)
- Clean dressing or sanitary pad (if needed)
- Disposable gloves (2 pairs, if needed)
- Paper bag

Procedure

1. Explain what you are going to do.
2. Wash your hands.
3. Obtain materials listed above.
4. Assist client to bathroom or commode.
5. Provide privacy.
6. Put on gloves.
7. Help client to remove clothing from below waist.
8. Ask client to remove and discard dressing or pad, if worn. Assist, if needed. Observe amount and color of drainage.
9. Ask client to void before beginning the procedure.
10. Raise toilet seat. Place sitz bowl so that drainage holes are at the back of the toilet. Fill half of plastic sitz bowl with warm water, 94°–98° F (34°–37° C). (Check temperature with cooking thermometer.)
11. Close side clamp of bag tubing. Fill water bag with warm water, 120° F (49° C). Hang bag so that it is higher than the toilet (on towel bar, top of toilet tank, or vanity).
12. Assist client to sit in sitz bowl. If client feels cold, cover shoulders and knees with blanket or towel.
13. Place tube end of water bag in outlet at front of the bowl.
14. Instruct client to open clamp of water bag to let warmer water into the bowl when water begins to cool. Assist as needed.
15. Instruct client to call for assistance, if needed. Explain that the procedure will take 15–20 minutes.
16. Remove and discard gloves.
17. Wash your hands.
18. Check client's condition every seven minutes or more frequently, if needed.
19. When time is up, clamp tubing and remove from sitz bath.
20. Put on second pair of gloves.
21. Assist client to slowly assume standing position.
22. Inspect perineal area; note any drainage in water. Dry area and reapply dressing or pad, if needed.
23. Assist client to dress, as needed, and to return to chair or bed.
24. Empty and disinfect plastic bowl. Flush tubing with water and clean end of tubing. Return equipment to proper location.
25. Remove and discard gloves.
26. Wash your hands.
27. Straighten bathroom.
28. Record on care record, noting color and amount of drainage on dressing or pad. Report any unusual conditions to your supervisor.

Procedure 17-11

Applying an Ice Bag

Materials Needed

- Ice bag
- Crushed ice
- Paper
- Soft cloth or towel
- Pencil

Procedure

1. Explain what you are going to do.
2. Wash your hands.
3. Obtain materials listed above.
4. Provide privacy.
5. Fill ice bag with water. Secure with stopper. Turn bag upside down to check for leaks.
6. Remove stopper and empty bag.
7. Crush the ice and fill bag ($1/2$ to $2/3$ full).
8. Lay bag flat to remove air. Place stopper in bag while it is still flat.
9. Cover bag with soft cloth or towel and apply to client's affected area.
10. Write on paper the time bag was applied.
11. Add ice as bag warms. Change towel if it becomes moist.
12. Check client's skin every 10 minutes for danger signs (see Box 17-2).
13. Remove bag according to time required. Write time of removal on paper.
14. Remove stopper, empty bag, and place bag upside down to dry. Place cloth or towel in laundry container to be washed.
15. Wash your hands.
16. Record what you have done. Report any unusual conditions to your supervisor.
17. When bag is dry, blow air into it and replace stopper to prevent insides of bag from sticking together. Store in proper location.

Procedure 17-12

Applying Cold Compresses

Materials Needed

- Basin or container
- Bath towel
- Plastic wrap
- Pencil
- Compresses (small towel, washcloth, or gauze squares)
- Ice water
- Disposable gloves
- Tape
- Paper
- Waterproof protector pad

Procedure

1. Explain what you are going to do.
2. Wash your hands.
3. Obtain materials listed above.
4. Provide privacy.
5. Place waterproof protector pad under the body part where compress is to be applied.
6. Fill basin or container $1/2$ to $2/3$ full with ice water.
7. Put on gloves.
8. Place compress in water.
9. Wring out compress and apply to area.
10. Cover compress quickly with plastic wrap. Secure edges of plastic wrap with tape. Cover with bath towel.
11. Write on paper the time compress was applied.
12. Check client's skin every 10 minutes for danger signs (see Box 17-2).
13. Change compress if warming occurs.
14. Remove compress according to time required.
15. Write time of removal on paper.
16. Pat area dry with towel. Discard used gauze square or compresses. Place used cloths and towels in laundry container to be washed.
17. Remove and discard gloves.
18. Wash your hands.
19. Clean and store materials in proper location.
20. Record what you have done. Report any unusual conditions to your supervisor.

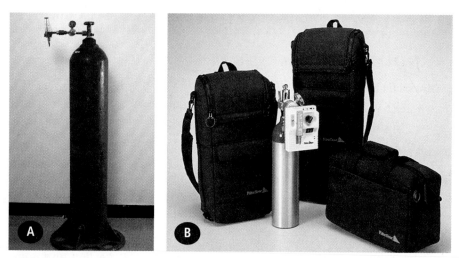

17-8 Oxygen tanks. *A,* A standing tank. *B,* A portable tank with carrying case. *(Courtesy DeVilbiss Health Care, Inc., Somerset, PA.)*

Oxygen Therapy

Clients who have difficulty breathing and are not receiving enough oxygen through the air may need additional amounts of oxygen. The doctor orders the amount and the method to be given—usually by nasal tube or mask. Oxygen is a drug and is part of the client's treatment or therapy.

Oxygen is supplied to homes by companies that specialize in delivering and providing breathing equipment. The respiratory therapist or company representative explains the correct use of the equipment to the client and family caregiver. Care of equipment, including ways of disinfecting parts and proper maintenance, is also explained. If your client is receiving oxygen therapy, the name, address, and phone number of the oxygen supplier should be available in case of an emergency.

Types of Equipment

There are two basic types of oxygen systems used to deliver oxygen in the home:

1. *Gas cylinders*—oxygen is stored under pressure in metal cylinders (Fig. 17-8A & B). They may be *stationary*—usually at the side of the bed for clients who are immobile—or *portable*—wheeled in a cart or worn by the client in a shoulder bag to permit easy movement.
2. *Oxygen concentrators*—this equipment separates oxygen from the other gasses in the air and stores it in a tank (Fig. 17-9). The concentrator runs on a continuous supply of electricity. Backup power sources or an oxygen cylinder must be available in case of an electrical failure.

Oxygen Safety

One of the three requirements needed to produce a fire is oxygen. Therefore, the danger of fire and explosion in the home is always present when oxygen is being used. It is very important that everyone in the home—you, the client, family members, and visitors—follow the rules of oxygen safety.

17-9 An oxygen concentrator. *(Courtesy DeVilbiss Health Care, Inc. Somerset, PA.)*

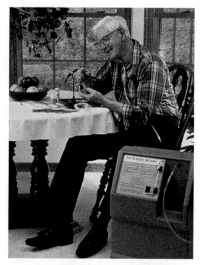

nasal cannula
a two-pronged device that delivers oxygen; short prongs are inserted into client's nostrils.

The home care aide should make sure that:

- *"No Smoking"* and *"Oxygen in Use"* signs are placed on the front door of the client's home, apartment, or room and in the client's room where oxygen is being used
- Fire hazards are removed (see Chapter 6)
- Client uses oxygen in areas free from the danger of fire
- Client stays out of areas where open flames (pilot lights) and electrical equipment may cause sparks (kitchen, basement, garage)
- Cigarettes, cigars, lighters, and matches are removed from client's area
- Client does not use alcohol and other flammable liquids (nail polish, perfume, aftershave lotion) when receiving oxygen
- A working, fully charged fire extinguisher is available for use in case of an emergency
- Name and phone number of oxygen supplier is available
- Oxygen tanks are properly secured in the floor stand provided by the supplier and should be at least six inches from walls, drapes, and heating units
- Oxygen tanks are stored away from sun and other heat sources

Caring for the Client Receiving Oxygen

Nasal Cannula In the home, the most common method of administering oxygen is by **nasal cannula.** It is easy to use, and the client can talk and eat while the cannula is in place (Fig. 17-10). There are two prongs that project from the plastic tubing. They are inserted about $1/2$ inch into the nostrils. The respiratory therapist adjusts the length of the prongs to make them comfortable for the client. A strap above the ears and around the back of the head keeps the cannula in place. The tubing is attached to the source of oxygen.

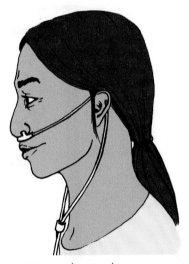

17-10 A nasal cannula.

When caring for a client with a nasal cannula:

- Note any skin irritation around the nostrils and ears.
- Place padding (cotton balls, gauze) between the straps and the ears, if needed.
- Wash and dry the area around the nostrils and ears carefully.
- Apply water soluble lubricant around nostrils, if irritation is present.
- Do not use petroleum jelly (Vaseline) as a lubricant because it can act as a fuel to produce fire.
- Notify your supervisor of any skin irritation (redness, broken skin) and its location immediately.

Face Mask When oxygen is needed on an occasional basis, a face mask may be used (Fig. 17-11). Talking is difficult when wearing a mask, and it must be removed before eating. The mask fits snugly over the client's nose and mouth. Straps are adjusted around the head and over the ears. Some masks have small holes on both sides that allow carbon dioxide to escape during exhaling. These holes also allow air from the room to enter during inhaling.

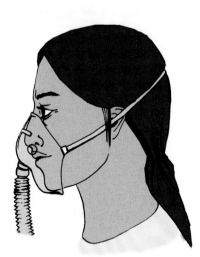

17-11 A face mask.

humidifier
equipment used to increase the amount of moisture in an oxygen delivery system.

distilled water
water that goes through a special process to remove minerals and other substances.

When caring for a client with a face mask:

- note any irritation on the nose or face where the mask touches the skin
- place padding (cotton balls, gauze) between the strap and the ears, if needed
- wash and dry the face carefully
- report signs of irritation (redness, breaks in skin) and location to your supervisor immediately

Oxygen dries the membranes of the mouth and respiratory system. An oxygen **humidifier** may be used to add moisture to the oxygen. This special container for **distilled water** is attached to the oxygen delivery system. When the oxygen is turned on, it will bubble through the distilled water.

Humidifiers must be cleaned and refilled on a regular basis. Your supervisor will explain how to check the water level in the humidifier and how to add more. Store the distilled water supply in the refrigerator; write the date it was opened on the container and discard if not used within two weeks. Clean the humidifier as instructed by your supervisor or the respiratory therapist.

Clients receiving oxygen therapy need frequent mouth care. Check with your supervisor about the frequency of giving mouth care. Encourage the client to drink water and other fluids to provide added moisture to the mouth's mucous membranes.

Intravenous Infusions

Intravenous (IV) infusions are used to administer medications and to supply needed fluids. IV equipment includes (Fig. 17-12):

- Fluid container—plastic bag with fluid
- Pole—holds fluid container
- Tubing—plastic tubing carries fluid from the bag to the client
- Needle or catheter—inserted into a vein in the client's arm or hand and secured with tape
- Meter—controls the flow of fluid (number of drops per minute)

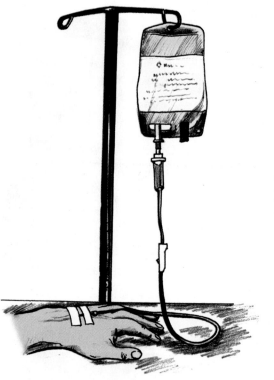

17-12 Intravenous equipment.

Caring for the Client Receiving IV Therapy

The home care aide has limited responsibilities regarding the use of IV therapy in the home. Most of the responsibilities are those of the nurse. The nurse is the person who adjusts the rate of flow of the medications and performs all procedures regarding the use and disposal of IV equipment. Your responsibility is to observe and report any problems with the equipment and to observe and report any changes in the client as follows:

Equipment
- Rate of fluid is too slow or too fast
- Fluid is leaking around the needle
- Meter is "beeping"
- Fluid bag is low and needs to be changed

Client
- Has swelling (edema) where needle is inserted
- Complains of pain or burning sensation around needle
- Feels itchy, nauseous (vomits)
- Has sudden chills, headache, skin rash, or difficulty breathing
- Becomes restless and may be injured by needle or equipment
- Tries to pull needle out

After you have talked with your supervisor, be sure to record on the care record the time you called, what your supervisor told you to do, and what you did.

Dry Dressings

Dressings are gauze squares that are used to cover wounds or surgical openings. They protect the area from clothing and microorganisms in the air and help to absorb any drainage from the wound. There are two types of dressings: sterile and unsterile. The home care aide does not apply or remove sterile dressings or apply dressings with ointments or other types of medication. These tasks are the responsibility of the nurse.

Applying and Removing Dry Dressings

You may be required to apply and remove unsterile dry dressings or to reinforce a dressing already in place. Dressings are reinforced when drainage is leaking from the dressing or when the dressing becomes loosened. Use universal precautions when applying and removing dressings because of the risk of blood-borne pathogens. Observe the area carefully. Note the size of the area and color of the skin around the area; also note the color, amount, and odor of drainage, if any. Record this information on the care record. Any changes in the appearance of the area should be reported to your supervisor.

Tape is used to secure the dressing to the skin. Make sure the edges of the dressing are taped to prevent movement of the dressing (Fig. 17-13). When removing tape, pull tape toward the dressing, not away from the dressing. Injury can occur if pressure is applied when pulling tape away from the bandaged area. Inspect the skin under the tape. If reddened or broken, notify your supervisor. Do not reapply tape over irritated skin.

The dressing may stick to the skin if drainage from the wound or opening dries. If this happens, do not pull off the dressing, as this may break the skin or damage the wound. Apply water to the dressing, and wait for it to soak through and soften the drainage. Then, gently remove it. Notify your supervisor if there is bleeding or drainage as a result of removing the dressing. Follow Procedure 17-13, Removing a Soiled Dressing and Applying a Clean, Dry Dressing.

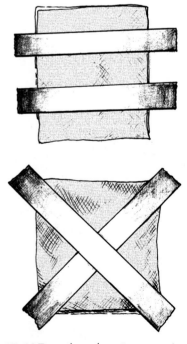

17-13 Tape the edges to prevent movement of the dressing.

Removing a Soiled Dressing and Applying a Clean, Dry Dressing

Materials Needed

- Gauze dressing pad
- Tape
- Scissors
- Waterproof protector pad (if needed)
- Tongs or spring clip clothespin (if available)
- Paper or plastic bag
- Disposable gloves (if needed)

Procedure

1. Explain what you are going to do.
2. Wash your hands.
3. Obtain materials listed above.
4. Provide privacy.
5. Cut length of tapes needed and hang them on edge of table for use later.
6. Put on gloves, if needed.

Removing soiled dressing

7. Expose area where dressing is to be removed.
8. Place paper or plastic bag nearby.
9. Remove all tape from skin by pulling tape toward the dressing/wound.
10. Gently remove soiled dressing using tongs or clothespin to grasp the edges. If tongs or clothespin is not available, grasp the cleanest part of the dressing and remove. Inspect dressing and skin. Note color, amount of drainage, and odor. Discard into paper bag.

Applying clean, dry dressing

11. Remove clean, dry dressing from cover, touching the edge of dressing only.
12. Apply dressing to area.
13. Take strips of precut tape and apply to secure dressing.
14. Place dressing cover in paper bag and discard.
15. Remove and discard gloves in paper or plastic bag.
16. Wash your hands.
17. Record what you have done. Report any unusual conditions to your supervisor.

Promoting Circulation

Many factors affect clients' circulation, including:

- inactivity and immobilization
- paralysis
- disease conditions of the heart, blood, and blood vessels
- surgery
- **trauma**
- pregnancy

Clients with these conditions may have slow or sluggish circulation. In some cases, an abnormal blood clot, or **thrombus,** may form. If a thrombus, or some part of it, travels through the circulatory system, it may damage vital organs—heart, lungs, brain. A moving blood clot is called an **embolus.**

Moving, exercising, coughing, and deep breathing can improve circulation. Encouraging clients to do as much as possible for themselves is one method of improving circulation. Blood collects in the lower extremities, and leg exercises help the blood to return to the heart. Walking is the best exercise, but, if this is not possible, leg exercises may be ordered. The nurse or therapist will teach the leg exercises. Follow

trauma
injury caused by external force or violence.

thrombus
blood clot.

embolus
a blood clot that travels through the circulatory system until it lodges in a distant blood vessel.

antiembolism stockings
elastic stockings worn to prevent the formation of blood clots in the legs.

the care plan and assist your client to perform the exercises as scheduled. Follow Procedure 13-15 (see page 239) for range of motion leg exercises. Never massage a client's legs. You may dislodge a thrombus causing it to travel to a vital organ.

Elastic Stockings

Elastic stockings, called TEDs or **antiembolism stockings** are used to improve circulation of the legs and feet and prevent the formation of blood clots. They create pressure on the leg veins, increasing the return of blood to the heart. These stockings come in many sizes and in both knee-high and thigh-high lengths. The client's legs are measured by the nurse to determine the proper size stockings. Ideally, clients will apply their own stockings. You may or may not be permitted to apply elastic stockings; it depends on your agency policies.

Stockings are removed three times a day to check for color and warmth of feet and toes. Improper application can block circulation and damage tissues. See Box 17-3 for hints on checking client's circulation when elastic stockings or bandages are worn. Change stockings daily after bathing the legs. Stockings are washed regularly. Hand wash and air dry according to manufacturer's instruction. See Procedure 17-14, Applying Elastic Stockings.

Box 17-3

Caring for the Client Who Wears Elastic Stockings or Bandages

- Check toes (or fingers) for
  - coldness
  - bluish skin
- Check with client to see if he/she has any complaints of
  - numbness
  - pain
  - tingling
- Remove elastic stocking (bandage) and observe skin condition.
- Report abnormal observations to your supervisor.
- Record what you have done.

Elastic Bandages

Elastic bandages, sometimes called ACE bandages, are used for the same purpose as elastic stockings. In addition, elastic bandages are used to provide support and reduce swelling after musculoskeletal injuries. These may be applied to arms and/or legs. Ideally, clients will apply their own elastic bandages. If they require assistance, follow the care plan. Not all agencies permit home care aides to apply elastic bandages; follow agency policy.

When applying elastic bandages, follow these guidelines:

- Use bandages of proper length and width.
- Leave furthest part of limb (fingers, toes) exposed in order to check for proper circulation.
- Keep limb elevated while applying bandage.
- Wrap evenly with no wrinkles or folds.
- Do not wrap too tightly.

Wash and dry bandages according to manufacturer's instruction. Avoid heat, as it will destroy the elastic. Overstretched elastic bandages should be replaced with new ones. Follow Procedure 17-15, Applying Elastic Bandages.

Applying Elastic Stockings

Materials Needed

- Clean elastic stockings

Procedure

1. Explain what you are going to do.

2. Wash your hands.

3. Obtain elastic stockings.

4. Provide privacy.

5. Put client in supine position.

6. Expose legs. Check to see that legs are clean and dry.

7. Turn stockings inside out, down to heel (Fig. 17-14A).

8. Place foot of stocking over client's toes, foot, and heel. Fit client's foot into heel and toe portion of stocking (Fig. 17-14B).

9. Pull leg of stocking up over foot and up the leg. The stocking will turn right side out as you pull it up (Fig. 17-14C).

10. Adjust stockings to fit smoothly without folds or wrinkles.

11. Make sure client is safe and comfortable.

12. Wash your hands.

13. Record what you have done. Report any unusual conditions to your supervisor.

14. Check circulation regularly according to care plan.

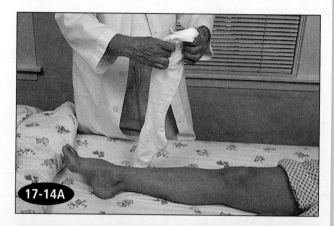

17-14A

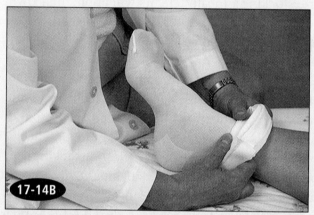

17-14B

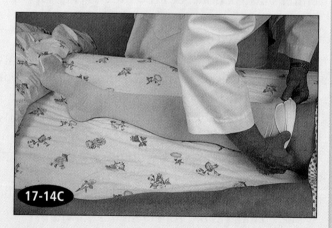

17-14C

Protecting Yourself

It is very important to use universal precautions when in contact with the client's body fluids and waste materials. To prevent the spread of possible infection, also practice medical asepsis techniques discussed in Chapter 9. Box 17-4 reviews important rules of universal precautions and medical asepsis when performing procedures discussed in this chapter.

Procedure 17-15

Applying Elastic Bandages

Materials Needed

- Elastic bandages
- Fasteners (clips, safety pins, tape)

Procedure

1. Explain what you are going to do.
2. Wash your hands.
3. Obtain materials listed above.
4. Provide privacy.
5. Assist client to comfortable position—supine for legs and feet; other positions according to care plan and part to be bandaged.
6. Expose part. Check to see that it is clean and dry.
7. Hold the bandage with roll up (Fig. 17-15).
8. Apply one end of bandage to the smallest part (e.g., wrist, ankle).
9. Wrap two turns to anchor bandage.
10. Continue wrapping in spiral turns upward (overlap previous turn by $^2/_3$). Apply firmly but NOT TOO TIGHTLY.

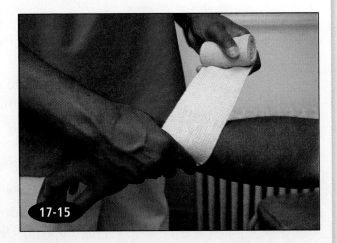

17-15

11. Fasten end with clip, pin, or tape.
12. Wash your hands.
13. Record what you have done. Report any unusual conditions to your supervisor.
14. Check for proper circulation regularly according to care plan.

Box 17-4

Protecting Yourself When Performing Special Procedures

- Wash your hands before and after wearing gloves.
- Wear gloves when:
  - there is risk of contact with body fluids, including drainage from wounds
  - disposing of soiled dressings and perineal pads
  - cleaning oxygen equipment
- Dispose of soiled dressings, pads, and gloves in paper or plastic bag, then in trash bag; discard in trash immediately.

CHAPTER SUMMARY

- Special procedures are important in the treatment of the client's condition.
- Special procedures are listed in the care plan. Some procedures are done by the home care aide, some by the client, and other procedures are the responsibility of other members of the home care team.

- Home care aides assist clients to take their own medications; home care aides never administer medications of any type.

- Applications of heat and cold are used for their helpful effects. Improper use of heat and/or cold may cause a client to have a severe injury. Home care aides must follow all safety rules about applications of heat and/or cold.

- Oxygen is used for clients who have difficulty breathing and cannot get enough oxygen through the air. There is great risk of fire when oxygen is being used in the home. Home care aides must know and follow safety rules pertaining to oxygen use.

- Home care aides observe and report problems with intravenous equipment or any client complaints during IV therapy.

- Home care aides may be responsible for other treatments, including: applying clean, dry dressings and assisting clients to apply elastic stockings or bandages.

- Three important responsibilities of the home care aide in every special procedure are: observing, recording, and reporting to the supervisor.

- Use universal precautions and medical asepsis rules when performing the special procedures discussed in this chapter.

STUDY QUESTIONS

1. List seven guidelines for special procedures.

2. What is the difference between administering medications and assisting with medications?

3. List 10 guidelines to follow when assisting clients to take medications.

4. What are two desired effects of hot applications? Cold applications?

5. Describe two safety rules to follow for each procedure listed below:
   a. Application of hot water bottle   b. Hot compresses
   c. Sitz bath   d. Ice bag
   e. Hot soak

6. List six rules of safety to follow when the client is receiving oxygen.

7. Your client is receiving an intravenous infusion. List four observations you would report to your supervisor.

8. How does the home care aide practice infection control and universal precautions when removing a soiled dressing and applying a clean, dry dressing?

9. Identify three responsibilities of the home care aide when caring for clients with elastic stockings.

10. When checking a client's extremities for proper circulation, what will you look for?

Understanding The Older Adult

Objectives

After you read this chapter, you will be able to:

1. Define the terms aging, young old, middle old, and oldest old.

2. Identify three common myths about older adults and the realities about those myths.

3. Discuss four adjustments older adults need to make for meaningful aging to occur.

4. Identify eight common physical changes experienced by older adults and eight ways the home care aide can assist the client to cope with them.

5. Discuss three safety factors to consider when caring for older adults.

6. Define and describe three signs of possible physical abuse, emotional abuse, and material or financial abuse.

7. Discuss five guidelines to follow when caring for older adults.

8. Discuss the problem of alcoholism in older adults.

9. Identify two warning signals of suicide in older adults.

Narina is a home care aide in a large city. She has noticed that most of her clients are older adults. In the past few weeks, she has cared for several people in their late 80s and one woman who was 99 years old. Narina thinks to herself, "There must be a lot of old people around here.

How Old is Old?

Aging is the process of growing old that begins at birth and continues until death. Aging is inevitable. The rate at which aging takes place differs with each person, but it increases and becomes more noticeable during the later years.

The term *old* has a very personal meaning for each of us. If you are 22 years old, then age 35 may seem very "old" to you. At age 75, a person may consider "old" to be anyone five years older than himself. And a 95 year old may consider herself to be "old."

No one really knows what causes aging to occur. Much research is being done in this area, and **gerontologists** have many theories. These include:

- cells wear out
- each person has a personal "time clock" that controls aging
- the genes determine the rate of aging

This is the first time there have been so many older adults. Because of this, we are able to learn more and more about the aging process. For example, certain conditions, such as Alzheimer's disease, have been recognized as disease processes—not a part of the normal aging process. As research continues, the secrets to the aging process may be uncovered.

While 65 is the usual age for retirement and social security benefits, gerontologists classify the older adult population according to the following groups:

- *Young old age*   70 to 80 years
- *Middle old age*   80 to 90 years
- *Oldest old age*   90 to 100+ years

Facts About Older Adults

Narina's observation that there are "a lot of old people" is correct. More than 13% of the total United States population is over the age of 65. Elders aged 85 and over are the fastest growing group.

At the beginning of the twentieth century, one out of every 25 people was 65 or older, about 4% of the population. At the beginning of the twenty-first century, the year 2000, more than 35 million people will be over the age of 65. This elderly population will increase greatly as the population group known as the "**baby boomers**" begins to turn 65. It is expected that older adults will account for 21% of the United States' population by the year 2030. Of this group, approximately three million people will be 85 or older.

gerontologists
specialists in the study of aging.

baby boomers
those born between 1946 and 1964.

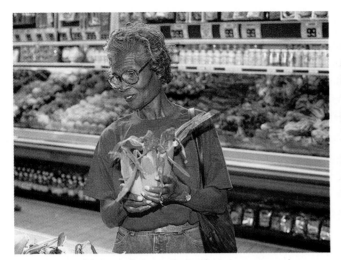

18-1 Most older adults remain in their homes and continue with daily routines, such as shopping.

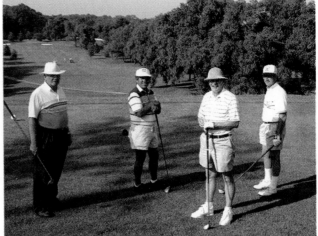

18-2 Many older adults enjoy the popular sport of golf.

Box 18-1

Facts About Older Adults

- There are 32 million adults aged 65 and older living in the United States; This represents 13% of the population.

- There are more older women than men; for every two men older than 65, there are three women; for every two men 85 and older, there are five older women.

- Women living alone make up one of three elderly households.

- About 12% of older adults live below the poverty level; women make up 72% of the elderly poor.

- About 13% of the white population is above 65; other groups include:
  - African Americans 8%
  - Asian Pacific Islanders 6%
  - Hispanics 5%
  - Native Americans 5%

- About 30% of older adults live alone.

- A 65-year-old man can expect to live to 80; a 65-year-old woman can expect to live to 84; the upper limit of life expectancy rises with changes in health care and education.

- About 5% of the elderly are institutionalized.

- About 10% of the elderly have a child over the age of 65.

Most older adults are well and continue to live at home. They continue with daily routines, like shopping, and persue recreational activities (Fig. 18-1 and Fig. 18-2). Only 5% are in institutions, and these are usually the oldest old. See Box 18-1 for more facts about the older population.

Myths and Realities

In the United States the focus is on youth. TV commercials sell creams and lotions to reduce wrinkles; give smooth, young skin; and erase the effects of aging. We get the idea that to be young is "ok" and to be old is dull, boring, not "cool." Older adults are portrayed as grouchy, forgetful, rigid, helpless, worthless, useless, unproductive, stupid, and slow. Society has created an unfair and untruthful **stereotype** of the older population.

There is no typical older adult. Each is a unique individual who will age at his/her own rate and in his/her own way. For example, if Mr. Felder was a happy, pleasant person in his younger years, chances are that he will have the same personality as he becomes an older adult. Grouchy, complaining Mr. Green will be even better at complaining when he gets older. After all, he has years of practice. Grandma Bennett likes to sit in the rocker on her porch and watch the flowers grow, but her 76-year-old sister runs in the marathon each year and says she doesn't have time to waste "watching the roses bloom."

As people age from young old to oldest old, they usually become more frail and have more chronic illnesses. They experience an increasing loss of strength and mobility. There is a big difference between the 70 year old and the 90 year old. The oldest old require more help with performing activities of daily living and caring for and maintaining their homes.

Many older adults enjoy reminiscing about the "old days" and the "old times." Listen to them; it is a wonderful opportunity to learn about their history and culture (Fig. 18-3). Sometimes, you may hear the same story over and over and over again. Be patient; those older adults who have memory problems will forget what they have told you and repeat it frequently. This can be trying for the listener; but smile, be patient, and listen again. Table 18-1 lists some myths and realities about older adults.

stereotype
a generalization about a form of behavior in an individual or a group.

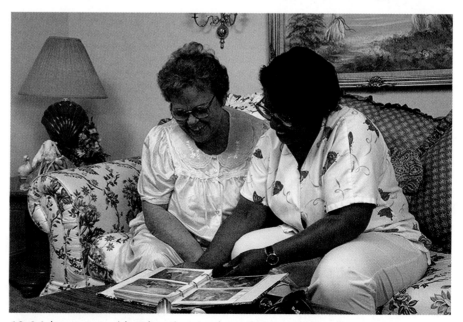

18-3 A home care aide takes time to share the past with a client.

Table 18-1

Myths and Realities of Aging

The Myth	The Reality
Other adults can't learn new things or adjust to changes.	It may take longer, but older adults can learn new routines and new skills. They can adjust to changes with help and support from others.
Incontinence is a sign of aging.	Incontinence is a sign of an abnormal condition that requires medical treatment.
Most older adults are sick and are in nursing homes.	Only about 5% of older adults are in nursing homes and other institutions.
Mental confusion is a normal part of growing old.	Mental confusion is an abnormal condition that must be reported to your supervisor.
Older adults are no longer concerned about looking attractive.	The need to look attractive does not change as the aging process continues.
Forgetfulness is a sure sign of illness.	Forgetfulness is not necessarily a sign of illness or disease.

Ageism

Ageism is a form of discrimination practiced against older adults. Younger generations may "look down" on older adults and treat them as mindless, stupid, and worthless beings. Ageism puts older adults into categories such as senile, rigid in thought and behavior, and old fashioned in morality and skills. It allows younger persons to see older people as different from themselves. They no longer identify older people as human beings. Ageism may take many forms, including:

- being denied a job because of age
- discrimination in housing
- "rip-offs" in home repairs and maintenance
- treating older adults as if they are not able to think or make decisions for themselves.

Our cultural background and personal experiences with older persons influence our views of aging. In some cultures, older adults are revered and respected. They are always cared for at home and would never be sent to a nursing home. In other cases, older adults live far away from children and grandchildren, and younger persons have little or no experience with their elders. This may lead to a stereotyped view of older adults. Also, ageism protects younger persons from thinking about the future—and the issues of their own illness, aging, and death.

Adjusting to Growing Older

As a person grows older, there are many changes that occur. These changes are not only physical, but social and emotional, too. The older person must face these changes and learn how to adjust to them in order for meaningful aging to occur (see Box 18-2).

Box 18-2

Adjusting to Growing Older

- Adjusting to retirement and reduced income
- Finding meaning in life
- Maintaining satisfactory living arrangements
- Finding satisfaction within the family
- Facing the reality of death
- Accepting oneself as an aging person
- Adjusting to decreasing health and physical strength

Retirement and Reduced Income

The usual age for retirement is age 65. With downsizing and restructuring of government and industry, some people retire at an earlier age, some as early as 50. The change from working outside of the home to not going to work requires a lot of adjustment. Many people associate employment with a feeling of worth and not working with a feeling of uselessness. Some view retirement as a permanent vacation and are delighted to do nothing. Others can't sit still and are easily bored. Whatever the case, the income may be reduced or, at best, remains the same. Budgeting, wise use of credit and credit cards, and careful shopping are now a necessary way of life. Social Security checks are not enough to live on, and some pensions are barely enough. Health care costs are so high, especially medications, that the older adult may be forced to choose between food or medicine.

If one is wealthy, there is no problem with finances. But for most people, the money they do have now has to last for a lifetime. As a result, most older adults are cautious and very careful about their money. Notify your supervisor if your client is having financial problems. There are community agencies to help older adults with everything from financial counseling to food stamps.

Meaningful Life

Older adults find meaning in life in many ways. Most will continue to do what they have always done: participate in the same clubs, church activities, social groups, and volunteer activities and enjoy their children and grandchildren. Others need to fill the gap created by retirement. This is done by finding part-time or full-time employment (Fig. 18-4), beginning a new career, developing new hobbies or interests, participating in volunteer activities (Fig. 18-5), continuing one's education, and joining senior citizens' clubs.

Loneliness is a common experience for older adults. Advancing age and the inability to drive or use public transportation isolates them

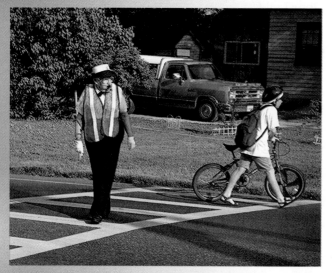

18-4 Part-time employment fills social and financial needs.

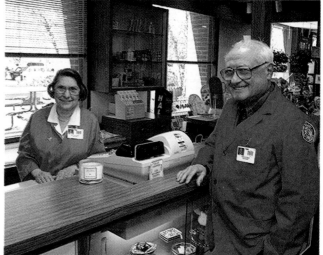

18-5 Volunteer service provides meaningful activity and the chance for socializing.

from the community. They are lonely because they have outlived many of their own generation, and they continue to experience what seems to them an ongoing, never-ending series of losses. They feel these losses very deeply. After a lifetime of human contact, they may now be alone without the loving touch of another human being. They need the nonverbal communication of hand-holding, a gentle touch or hug. Sometimes, the home care aide is the only person visiting the client, providing personal care, and meeting the need for human contact. Remember to give older clients a smile, a comforting touch (Fig. 18-6), and a hug (if appropriate to their culture).

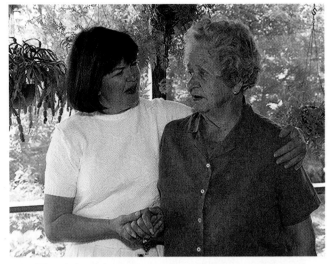

18-6 Touch is an important means of communicating.

Pets provide companionship and love, especially for the person who is alone. Animals enjoy hugs and kisses; humans enjoy giving this love to their pets. These animals may become the older adult's "family." Be kind to your client's animals. If you are afraid of the pet, or allergic to its hair, or dislike dogs or cats, ask the client to secure the animal where you will not have contact with it. Tell your client that you can't be around animals because of health reasons. If you are very allergic to animals, you should tell your supervisor.

Satisfactory Living Arrangements

Most older adults stay in the home where they have always lived. Others may live with one of their children. Some older adults live in assisted living facilities, senior citizen apartments, retirement communities, group homes, single-room occupancy hotels, or adult foster homes. Still others may live in a Continuing Care Retirement Community (CCRC). They "buy into" the community, live in an apartment, then move to the community nursing home when necessary and remain a resident of the CCRC until death. Clients in all of these living facilities will use the services of a home care aide.

Satisfaction Within the Family

With retirement, married couples spend a great deal of time together. Some partners may not have had so much togetherness since their honeymoon. It is a time of adjustments and getting to know one another again.

Older adults have the opportunity to build adult relationships with their grown children and resolve any problems of the past. For most elders, grandchildren are a special delight. Some older adults provide child care for their grandchildren while the children's parents work. Some grandparents raise their grandchildren because the children's parents are sick, deceased, unemployed, divorced, or in prison. In other cases, older adults have no families; may be abandoned or ignored by family members; or outlive relatives. There may be no opportunity for satisfaction within the family.

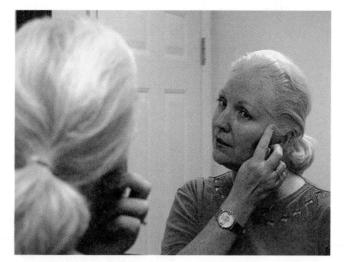

18-7 Accepting the physical changes of aging is a task of older adults.

Reality of Death

Older adulthood is the final stage of life, the next step is death. Older adults are very aware of the reality of death. They have lost friends, relatives, perhaps a spouse. Preparing a will, purchasing a burial site, preplanning with a funeral director, and making advance decisions about care and treatment all remind the older adult of what is to come.

The death of a partner causes deep sadness and grief. **Mourning** has many physical, social, and emotional effects. It may take the survivor several years to recover from the death. Even then, life is changed forever, and many adjustments must be made to living on one's own.

Self Acceptance

We all need to accept ourselves just as we are (Fig. 18-7). Some older adults have difficulty facing the fact that they are "older adults." They do not like the changes caused by the aging process. They long for their youth and the "good old days." But most older adults adjust to the changes in their lives and learn to accept things as they are.

Exercise, proper diet, and rest are important factors in feeling good and staying healthy. Grooming, hygiene, and cleanliness are important factors in looking good. An interest in life, getting out, reading, and being a part of the community help to promote a positive attitude and emotional well-being. All these things help a person with self-image and self-acceptance.

Decreasing Health and Physical Strength

Some older adults may ignore problems with seeing, hearing, and walking—saying that they are "just a part of old age." These difficulties can interfere with daily living. They can also lead to medical problems and increasing dependence. For example, a person who cannot see to read the medication labels may take the wrong drug at the wrong time. As a result, he/she may become confused, may fall, or need to be hospitalized.

As aging progresses, most people do not have the strength they formerly had. It takes longer to do the tasks they used to do, and these jobs are very tiring. Many of the oldest old are unable to perform household duties or activities of daily living because chronic illness interferes with mobility. These older adults require assistance with home maintenance and personal care, such as bathing and grooming. It is hard for the independent-minded older adult to accept help with such personal activities. They may become frustrated and angry with their slowness and dependency. Be patient; give them time and assistance as needed.

Older adults cherish their independence and will do almost anything to remain living "at home." They have a basic need to make their own decisions and choices about their care and future.

mourning
a reaction to a great personal loss.

Physical Signs of Aging

While the aging process begins at birth, the physical signs of this process do not become noticeable until later in life. Aging affects all the body systems but at different rates of speed. Physical changes begin gradually and may not be obvious right away. For example, hair begins to lose its color very gradually—a few hairs at a time—until there are many gray hairs. The ability to perform strenuous physical activity without rest periods also decreases gradually as we age. But there are always exceptions: the 80-year-old woman who does not have one gray hair, or the 85-year-old man who runs in the marathon race.

The changes that occur are influenced by many factors: heredity, health practices and lifestyle (rest, sleep, exercise, eating habits, smoking, alcohol use, illegal drug use, etc.), stresses of life, and one's occupation.

The following are a few of the signs of aging:

- *wrinkling of the skin—*
  due to loss of fatty tissue and elastic quality of the skin
- *thinning and graying of hair—*
  due to glandular changes and loss of color of the hair
- *decrease in physical strength and endurance—*
  due to changes in the skeletomuscular, circulatory, and respiratory systems
- *difficulty in adjusting to shadows, glare, or dim lights—*
  due to changes in the eye
- *increase in time needed to react to emergency situations—*
  due to changes in the nervous system

The material that follows explains: (1) the basic changes in each body system, (2) common situations experienced by the client, and (3) ways that the home care aide can assist the client to cope with these normal changes.

Changes in the Skeletomuscular System

"I used to be 5′4″—now I'm only 5 feet tall! And I just don't seem to have as much energy as I had when I was younger."

Perhaps the change that is most noticeable in this body system is that older adults are just not as tall as they used to be. As aging occurs, there is a shortening of the spinal column. This is a very gradual process. In some people, the upper spine becomes curved and the head bends forward. Bones lose calcium, causing them to become weak and brittle. So, older adults are more prone to fractures. When fractures occur, healing takes longer, too.

Changes also occur in the joints and muscles. Generally, there is a decrease in the strength and flexibility of the muscles. Joints stiffen, especially after a period of sleep or rest. Lack of exercise, including walking, contributes to further muscle weakness and joint stiffness.

Common Situations	Suggestions for Helping Client
Stiffness in joints and muscles	Assist client to put joints through range of motion during ADL. Help client to change position at least every two hours.
Difficulty removing and recapping jars, toothpaste tubes, medication containers, or opening cereal boxes	Remove caps or lids on containers, or open boxes, as needed.
Difficulty handling heavy cups, mugs, and glassware	When possible, use lightweight plasticware with handles. Fill cups $^{1}/_{2}$ full to reduce weight and prevent spills.
Takes more time to perform activities	Assist client when needed but do not perform activity for the client. Allow extra time for activities— do not rush the client.
Tires easily	Allow for rest periods between activities to avoid exhaustion. Schedule hygiene activities at a time when energy levels are highest, if possible.

Changes in the Integumentary System

"My skin used to be very oily. Now, it's so dry and flaky."

Most of the changes that occur in this system do not produce major physical problems. Rather, they are outward signs of the aging process. There is a redistribution of fatty tissue under the skin. These fatty deposits are gradually lost from the face, arms, and legs; they may seem to "reappear" in the abdomen and hips. Glands do not produce as much oil to lubricate the skin naturally. So, the skin becomes dry and flaky. The elbows, hip bones, and shoulder blades become more visible because of the lack of fatty tissue covering the bones. Also, the skin loses its elastic quality, and blood vessels near the surface of the skin are more visible, especially in the hands and arms.

The fingernails become ridged and brittle, while the toenails tend to become hard and thick. They can be very difficult to cut.

Prolonged exposure to the sun's damaging rays hastens the aging of the skin, especially of the face. Wrinkles and crow's feet around the eyes are the results of repeated use of facial muscles over a long period of time.

Common Situations	Suggestions for Helping Client
Dry, flaky skin	Use soap sparingly. Do not give daily tub bath or shower unless care plan indicates. Apply moisturizing creams or lotions to skin <u>after</u> bathing. Do not put oils in bathtub due to risk of falls. Avoid alcohol-based products, as they tend to dry skin.
Brittle fingernails	File, as needed. Apply lotion to soften nails.
Thick, hard toenails	Do not cut or file toenails. Notify supervisor; a podiatrist may need to be contacted.

Changes in the Circulatory and Respiratory Systems

"I'm so cold all the time. Even when it's warm outside, I wear an extra sweater."

Generally, these two body systems become less effective as the body ages. The muscles of the heart and blood vessels gradually begin to lose their strength and efficiency in transporting blood to all parts of the body. The process of returning blood through the veins to the heart also becomes less efficient. The openings of the blood vessels narrow due to the deposits of calcium, cholesterol, and other fatty substances.

The number of alveoli decreases, and each one becomes less elastic, so the exchange of oxygen and carbon dioxide is less efficient. Secretions of the mucous membrane that lines the entire respiratory tract tend to thicken. They can be difficult to expel. See Box 18-3 for normal vital signs of clients 85 years and over.

The body's resistance to infection and disease is lowered because the immune system does not function as efficiently as before. Therefore, older adults are at great risk for infection. It is very important for the home care aide to observe, record, and report beginning signs of infection immediately so that treatment can begin promptly.

Box 18-3

Normal Range of Vital Signs for Clients 85 Years and Over

Temperature

Oral	95°–97°F (35°–36.1°C)
Rectal	95.2°–98.6°F (35.1°–37°C)
Axillary	94°–96°F (34.4°–35.5°C)

Pulse   70–76

Respirations   20–22 (more shallow than younger adult)

Blood Pressure $\frac{120}{80} - \frac{140}{90}$

Common Situations	Suggestions for Helping Client
Complains of being cold, especially in hands and feet	Assist client to put on sweater, socks, gloves; use an extra blanket in bed. Dress by layering. Place thermostat on higher setting. Caution client not to use hot water bottles or heating pads to keep warm. Encourage client to avoid crossing legs when sitting. Avoid use of constricting clothing—tight socks and waistbands, knee-high stockings, round garters.
Rapid heart beat when stressed; takes longer to return to "normal" heart rate	Pace activities to avoid rushing. Allow plenty of time to perform care procedures. Try to reduce stressful situations.
Shortness of breath with increased activity	Provide frequent rest periods when assisting client with ADL.

Changes in the Digestive System

"Food just doesn't taste the same anymore."

Many older clients' concerns result from changes in this aging digestive system. The number of taste buds in the tongue are reduced, especially those that affect the sweet and salty tastes. The sense of thirst is decreased. Lack of teeth or poorly fitting dentures prevent many older clients from eating the foods they once enjoyed. Salivary glands secrete less saliva. Gastric juices produced by the stomach are reduced, and food remains in the stomach longer. As a result, clients complain of bloating and indigestion. Muscles of the large intestine do not work as well, and peristalsis is decreased. The nerve sensation that signals the need to defecate may also be dulled. These factors, coupled with a decreased fluid intake and a diet low in fiber, make constipation a real problem for many older adults.

Common Situations	Suggestions for Helping Client
Dry mouth	Encourage client to drink fluids: 1½–2 quarts (1500–2000 ml) daily. Offer small amounts of fluids frequently. Offer fluids before assisting client to take oral medication to moisten the mouth. Offer frequent mouth care.

Loss of teeth	Provide soft foods (pureed, chopped meat, fruits, and vegetables) according to care plan (See Chapter 8).
Gas, bloating, indigestion, heartburn	Report and record on care record if these complaints are new to the client. Encourage client to eat slowly and to chew food thoroughly. Have client maintain a sitting position for $1/2$ hour after eating. Avoid serving gas-forming, fatty, and highly seasoned foods (see Chapter 8). Offer six to eight small meals daily.
Constipation	Encourage client to eat foods high in fiber (see Chapter 8). Offer fluids frequently— see above. Allow plenty of time in bathroom for bowel movement—do not rush.

Changes in the Nervous System and Senses

"I can remember exactly what I did on my 10th birthday. But, what did I do yesterday?"

Perhaps the best way to describe the normal aging nervous system is that it is slower—slower to receive and send messages to other parts of the body. This slowness is due to loss of nerve cells, which begin to decline around the age of 25. Memory loss for recent events is a common concern for many older adults. Forgetting the home care aide's name or where their eyeglasses are can be embarrassing or frustrating for the older adult. But they are <u>not</u> necessarily signs of illness. One's intelligence does not lessen as aging continues. The ability to learn continues. It may just take longer to learn and remember new information. Adjusting to stress and change in one's life becomes more difficult and takes longer for the older adult.

The sensory organs also become slower in receiving and sending impulses to the brain. The most common of all complaints involving the senses is the decreased ability to hear. This is a very gradual process, hardly noticed, until sounds used in normal conversation become more difficult to hear. Normal changes in the eye result in a decreased amount of tears, decreased side vision, and decreased ability to see certain colors (blues and greens are more difficult to see than reds and yellows).

Other sensory changes include: reduced sense of smell; reduced taste buds; and reduced sense of touch in the fingers and toes.

Many older adults say that their patterns of sleep have changed. Before, they could sleep all night without waking. Now, sleep is disrupted by frequent trips to the bathroom or wakefulness. Lack of physical activity, anxiety, and long naps during the day can cause nighttime insomnia.

Common Situations	*Suggestions for Helping Client*
Forgetfulness	Encourage client to jot down reminders on pad.
Short-term memory loss, such as names of persons who visited yesterday	Provide clues to client to refresh memory.
Difficulty adjusting to depths (going up and down steps and stairs)	Encourage client to use hand rails, if available; provide support as needed. Do not rush—allow plenty of time.
Trouble getting to sleep	Avoid caffeine after evening meal (coffee, tea, chocolate). Avoid alcohol at night. Give back rub. Give warm milk before bedtime, if allowed. Encourage physical activity during the day.
Unsteady balance when changing position suddenly	Encourage client to change position slowly, such as turning around. Count to 10 after client rises from a sitting position, then proceed to assist the client to walk. Provide support when walking. Do not rush client.
Difficulty adjusting to sudden changes in light or darkness	Encourage client to wait a few minutes until the eyes can adjust to the darkness or light. Use a night light.
Changes in ability to see and hear	See Chapter 2 for communicating with the visually and hearing impaired client.

Changes in Urinary and Reproductive Systems

"When I have the urge to go to the bathroom, I have to go fast! I can't hold my water very well."

This comment is usually due to the weakness of the bladder muscles. Some older adults can only hold half as much urine at one time as they could when they were younger. As a result, frequent trips to the bathroom are common. Other older adults retain large quantities of urine because the bladder muscles become stretched and have difficulty contracting. In these situations, the client may complain of leaking. This usually means that the bladder is overfilled.

Urinary incontinence is <u>not</u> part of the normal aging process. There can be many causes for urinary incontinence. It is an abnormal condition that should be reported to your supervisor immediately. See Chapter 14.

As the male reproductive system ages, the prostate gland usually increases in size. This is not a problem unless the gland causes the urethra to constrict and interferes with the normal flow of urine from the bladder. The testes continue to manufacture sperm for much of the older man's life.

In the female, fatty tissue in the breasts and external genitals is reduced. Mucous secretions of the vagina also are reduced. These are due to ovarian hormone changes that occurred during menopause.

Older adults do not lose their interest as sexual beings. The need to continue satisfying sexual relationships is a normal part of aging. Sexual activity may need to be modified because of physical changes. Frail older adults, for example, may find that cuddling, kissing, hugging, and hand-holding can be satisfying types of sexual expression and pleasure. For others, the use of vaginal lubricants to replace the lack of mucous secretions may need to be used; or it may take longer to achieve an erection. But, these changes do not reduce the amount of sexual pleasure. Respect the client's need for privacy.

Common Situations	Suggestions for Helping Client
Urgent need to void; difficulty holding urine	Clothing should be easy to remove—elastic waistband on slacks (no buttons, zippers). <u>DO NOT</u> reduce fluids during the day. May need to help client to bathroom every 2 hours or less.
Interrupted sleep due to nighttime voiding	Avoid drinks with caffeine after evening meal (coffee, tea, colas). Avoid salty and spicy foods for last meal of day. Avoid alcohol, particularly beer, in the evening. Place commode in bedroom. Put on night light. Make sure passage to bathroom is uncluttered, if commode is not used.
Dryness of genital area	Avoid hot tub baths.

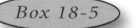

Box 18-4

Older Clients at Greater Risk for Accidents

Clients who are:
- women
- 85 years and older
- living alone

Clients who have:
- poor eyesight
- unsteady gait
- problems with balance

Clients who use:
- canes or walkers incorrectly
- prescription medications, especially blood pressure medications and sedatives
- OTC medications
- alcohol or abuse alcohol

Box 18-5

Safety and the Older Adult

- See Chapter 6 to review home safety practices.
- Confine pets at night or if client may fall over animals.
- Close cabinet and closet doors and drawers after use.
- Keep client areas well lighted; use red-colored night-lights.
- Encourage clients to increase lightbulb wattage, especially in bathrooms, stairways, and other areas frequently used.

Safety and the Older Adult

Because of the physical changes that take place, older adults are at great risk for injury due to accidents. Nursing research indicates that some older adults are at even greater risk because of advanced age, drug use, and severe disability (see Box 18-4). Each year, about one million older adults are treated in hospital emergency rooms for injuries associated with products that they live with and use every day. A recent study of persons aged 75 and over showed that almost 80% of falls occurred at home. Half of the falls were caused by tripping over something. One quarter of those who fell were seriously injured and required hospitalization.

The home care aide must be alert to potential safety hazards and remove them, if possible. When they cannot be removed, inform a family member, if available; record and report the hazard to your supervisor. See Box 18-5 for making the home safer for older adults.

Illness in the Later Years

While older adults make up 13% of the total population, they occupy more than 50% of the acute care hospital beds. More than 70% of available health care services (including home care) are used by older adults. Each year, the average older adult has 11 prescriptions filled. People over 65 take twice as many medications as other age groups. They also have five times more adverse reactions to medicine than younger persons.

Illness can occur very quickly in the older adult because of the many physical changes due to aging (Box 18-6). Beginning signs of illness may be ignored or not reported to the doctor. There are several reasons for not reporting symptoms, these include:

- communication barriers (language, deafness, culture)
- fear of hospital or nursing home admission
- cost of treatment
- fear of outcome

Most commonly, however, the older adult fails to recognize that minor symptoms can quickly develop into a serious medical condition. Prompt treatment can often prevent serious illness and hospitalization.

Important symptoms to recognize and report are:
- sudden confusion and agitation
- urinary incontinence
- eating changes, particularly anorexia
- energy and activity changes
- frequent and recurrent falls

If these symptoms are new, not a part of the client's history, they must be reported to your supervisor immediately. Do not assume that these symptoms are "just a part of getting old." They may be symptoms of drug reaction, infection, or other serious medical problem that requires treatment.

Caring for the older adult can be rewarding and challenging. Some general principles for caring for older adults are listed in Box 18-7.

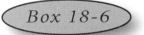

Box 18-6

Watch for Sudden or Gradual CHANGES

C Communicating with others

H Hydration

A Activities of daily living (ability to function); Appearance

N Nutrition, nervous system (memory loss, muscle weakness)

G Gait, gastrointestinal problems

E Environment, emotions

S Sensory problems (seeing, hearing, tasting, balance, smelling, feeling) and vital signs

Box 18-7

Caring for Older Clients—General Principles

- Allow plenty of time for self-care activities of daily living.
- Encourage client to assume as much responsibility for care as possible.
- Help client only when needed—avoid "doing for" clients when they can "do" for themselves.
- Pace activities to avoid rushing the client—rushing can result in frustration for both client and home care aide.
- Offer fluids frequently, even though the client says he/she is not thirsty.
- Encourage physical activity according to the care plan.

- Be aware of possible safety hazards in the client's environment; eliminate them, if possible.
- Respect client's routine—make changes only when necessary.
- Be alert for gradual or sudden changes in the client's physical, mental, or emotional condition; record and report them to your supervisor.
- Watch for signs of infection including: elevation of temperature, pulse, and respirations; cold and flu-like symptoms; record and report them to your supervisor immediately.
- Practice universal precautions because of the great risk for infection.

Who Are the Caregivers

According to national statistics, three fourths of all care given to the frail elderly is provided by **informal caregivers.** About seven million family members give care to older adults 24 hours a day, 7 days a week. While there is no typical caregiver, research indicates that 80% of the caregivers are women: wives or adult daughters. The usual female caregiver is:

- age 57, usually an adult daughter
- working outside of the home
- caring for her own family
- coping with her own health problems
- spends 17 years caring for her own children and 18 years caring for aging parents

About 70% of older adults in the community live with a caregiver. Sometimes an older adult becomes the caregiver. Your client may be cared for by an elderly partner. Or, a 90 year old may be the caregiver for a 70-year-old "child." Adult children, in-laws, or grandchildren may also be caregivers. Sometimes it is elderly siblings, younger nieces or nephews, neighbors, or friends who provide the care.

Home care aides are assigned to give client care, but they also provide assistance to caregivers in the following ways:

- offering emotional support by listening to concerns, problems, and questions
- assuming some of the responsibility for physical care of the client (according to care plan)
- enabling them to get out of the house for a few hours
- encouraging use of agency resources to deal with problem situations

Very often, the care given by the home care aide (if only for a few hours a week) helps the caregiver to feel restored and able to continue with his/her responsibilities.

Elder Neglect and Abuse

Television and radio programs, magazines, and newspapers have brought cases of abuse and neglect of older adults to the public's attention. While only about one in 14 cases of neglect or abuse is likely to be reported, it is estimated by the National Aging Resource Center on Elder Abuse that more than two million older adults are victims each year.

Some Definitions

Neglect is the inability or failure to provide needed care. For example, the older adult, living alone, is unable to care for himself/herself, and no one is assuming responsibility for the care. Or, the caregiver fails to provide adequate food or clothing; leaves the client alone for long periods of time; or withholds needed medications or other necessary items.

Abuse—Mistreating or causing harm. There are three types:

1. *Physical*—Producing physical injury and pain by hitting, kicking, punching, or by other means, including sexual abuse. Confining a person against his/her will is also considered physical abuse.

informal caregivers
unpaid persons who care for clients on a voluntary basis.

neglect
inability or failure to provide needed care.

abuse
mistreating or causing harm.

2. *Emotional*—Threatening or insulting language that produces fear in the person being abused. The types of behavior considered to be emotional abuse vary according to state laws.
3. *Financial or Material*—Stealing money, Social Security checks or other checks, valuables or possessions, or misusing the client's money or possessions.

The Abused

Research shows that those who are at the greatest risk of being abused are older adults who have physical or mental conditions. They may live with another person or may live alone. Isolation and loneliness are key factors in one type of abuse—financial or material—because the older adult, who seeks friendship and companionship from a stranger, trusts the person who later becomes the abuser.

The Abusers

Much of the abuse of the older adult is usually committed by a member of the family—the spouse, adult daughter, or other family member or friend who is assuming responsibility as caregiver. However, employed caregivers also account for about 13% of elder abuse. It is difficult to understand why this happens. The following are some possible reasons:

- The caregiver takes out the frustration and stress of caregiving on the "victim"—the person needing care
- There is history of violence in the family as a way of handling problems
- Alcohol or drug abuse by family members may cause physical or mental conditions leading to abuse
- The abuser is "paying back" the older adult for being abused in the past

Signs of Neglect and Abuse

The following are signs of possible neglect or abuse:

Neglect
- dirty hair, body, and clothing
- urine or feces in the bed, on clothing, or in the client's area
- weight loss

Physical Abuse
- Bruises, cuts, sores, or burns on the skin
- Bruises, cuts, or burns in the genital area
- Unusual vaginal discharge
- Frequent "falls"

Emotional Abuse
- Changes in client's behavior—withdrawn, cries a lot
- Behaves in a fearful manner, especially when abuser is present
- Does not want to be left alone with caregiver or family members
- Yelling at client; using threatening language
- Humiliating or belittling client

Material or Financial Abuse

- Client mentions that money, checks, or valuables are being stolen
- Client tells of being forced to sign over property or other financial documents
- Client tells of being forced to sign checks or pay outrageous prices for services or products

What the Home Care Aide Can Do

Your agency has rules to follow if you suspect that your client is being neglected or abused. It is very important to record your observations and report this information to your supervisor immediately. Record exactly what your client has told you. Do not assume. For example, record the following: "The client said, 'My granddaughter calls me nasty names—I just feel terrible when she does it. She tells me that if I don't turn over my Social Security check to her, she won't give me anything to eat.'" Do not record that the client's granddaughter is abusing the client emotionally and financially. This may or may not be correct. State the facts as clearly as possible so that your agency can investigate the situation further and take the most appropriate steps to protect your client. Elder abuse or neglect is a very serious matter. Many states have laws that require that signs of abuse or neglect be reported to the appropriate authorities. This will be done by your agency as necessary.

Alcoholism

Alcoholism is a serious and often unrecognized problem in older adults. It is estimated that more than 2.5 million older Americans have some drinking problem. Widowers age 75 and older have the highest rate of alcoholism in the country. As a person ages, problems with alcohol may develop. The body's tolerance for alcohol decreases with age, so what was considered moderate drinking in middle age may be problem drinking in old age. Also, the effects of alcohol may be increased by the many medications usually taken by older adults.

Many use alcohol as a sleeping aid or a pain reliever—or as a way to fill up long, lonely, boring days and nights. Alcohol is also used as an escape from the many losses of aging and may hide the symptoms of depression.

Many problems occur as a result of alcohol abuse. These include:

- reduced self-control
- anger, hostility, nastiness, and aggression
- verbal, physical, and/or emotional abuse of family, friends, caregivers
- avoiding others
- social isolation
- falls
- confusion, loss of memory, blackouts
- malnutrition and weight loss

Alcoholism may be suspected when the above problems occur. However, there are often other causes for these symptoms, too. Evidence of a drinking problem may be found in the home. Many empty alcohol containers and a large stock of alcoholic beverages may indicate a drinking problem. If you suspect that your client has a problem with alcohol, notify your supervisor. It is not your job to diagnose or treat alcoholism. You cannot make someone stop drinking. Specialized medical treatment is needed.

If your client or family member asks you what to do about problem drinking, refer them to your supervisor. Home care agencies know of many community resources for assistance with this problem.

Suicide

Older adults have the highest suicide rate of any age group in the United States. Each year as many as 10,000 older adults will die from suicide. There are many theories about the reasons for suicide. These include: changes in brain chemistry; emotional illness, particularly depression; and physical problems, such as heart disease, chronic pain, and loss of a body part or function. Other factors associated with suicide in older adults are:

- a pattern of successive losses with little time in between for grieving and recovery
- alcohol and/or drug dependence
- retirement
- social isolation and lack of a support system

Unlike younger persons, older adults do not make suicide attempts or gestures. Elders who attempt suicide are almost always successful on the first attempt. Methods range from guns to drugs and other poisonous substances. Some people just quietly refuse to eat or drink or take their medications.

Home care aides should be alert for warning signs of suicide (Box 18-8). Pay attention to these signs, take them seriously, and report them to your supervisor immediately. There are many things that can be done to improve the quality of life for older adults. Depression can usually be treated with good results.

Box 18-8

Warning Signs of Suicide in Older Adults

- **Statements such as:**

    "I'm going to kill myself."

    "I just want to end it all."

    "My family would be better off without me."

    "There's no point in going on."

- **Putting life in order, such as:**

    giving valuables away

    making or changing a will

    finalizing funeral or burial plans

- **Self neglect, such as:**

    not eating

    not drinking

    refusing to take medications or taking too much medicine

    overeating, not sticking to prescribed diet

CHAPTER SUMMARY

- Aging begins at birth and becomes more noticeable in the later years.

- Each person ages at his/her own rate and in his/her own way.

- Only 5% of older adults live in institutions.

- Ageism is a form of discrimination practiced against older adults.

- The normal aging process causes many social, emotional, and physical changes. There are many adjustments to be made during this period, including:

  - adjusting to retirement and reduced income

  - finding meaning in life

  - finding satisfaction within the family

  - facing reality of death

  - accepting oneself as an aging person

  - adjusting to decreasing health and physical strength

- Aging causes many changes in the body systems. Home care aides help clients to cope with these changes.

- Older adults are at great risk for injuries from falls and other accidents. Safety is an important factor to remember when caring for older adults.

- Older adults may not report beginning signs of illness because they are not aware of possible serious medical problems that may develop.

- Most older adults are cared for at home by an informal caregiver.

- Elder abuse and neglect are serious problems that must be reported to your supervisor.

- Alcoholism is often unrecognized in older adults.

- Older adults have the highest rate of suicide in the United States.

STUDY QUESTIONS

1. Define: aging, young old, middle old, and oldest old.

2. List three myths about older adults and the reality about each myth.

3. Discuss four adjustments older adults need to make for meaningful aging to occur.

4. List eight common physical changes experienced by older adults. Discuss what the home care aide can do to assist the client to cope with each change.

5. Define: physical abuse, emotional abuse, financial abuse, and neglect. Give an example of each.

6. Why are older adults at risk for accidents? Describe three safety factors to be considered when caring for older adults.

7. List five guidelines to follow when caring for older adults.

8. Why is alcoholism often unrecognized in the older adult?

9. Describe two warning signals of suicide in the older adult.

19

Caring for Mothers, Infants, and Children

Objectives

After you read this chapter, you will be able to:

1. Describe four normal changes that occur in the mother following the birth of the infant.

2. Discuss the responsibilities of the home care aide in caring for mothers of newborns.

3. Identify seven abnormal conditions of the mother that must be reported to the supervisor.

4. Discuss safety factors to be considered when caring for infants.

5. Identify five signs of infant illness that must be reported to the supervisor.

6. List four signs of stress in children.

7. Discuss the difference between discipline and punishment.

8. Identify five ways the home care aide can form positive relationships with children.

9. Recognize five common signs of child abuse.

10. Perform the procedures listed in this chapter.

Caring for mothers, their infants, and children is both demanding and satisfying for the home care aide because of the variety of clients being served. Many are well, for example, the mother and her newborn infant. Other clients, such as children or teenagers, may be recovering from illnesses. Some clients, while not ill, have disabilities that require special care, such as cerebral palsy. The age of the client may range from a two-day-old newborn to a mother who may be past the age of forty. A review of normal growth and development patterns (Chapter 3) will help you to understand each client's needs.

Being *flexible* and *patient* are two important abilities that will be frequently used during visits to these clients. Mothers are usually returning home with their newborns to an established household. This household may include the partner, other children, and relatives. Routines and patterns of behavior may be well-established. Caring for your client means taking into consideration the family's existing routines; being flexible, when possible, so that you can reinforce these routines; and practicing patience when the schedule does not go as planned.

Caring for Mothers

Many years ago, the pregnant woman was admitted to the hospital to have her baby and returned home a week later. Seven or more days in the hospital was not unusual following a normal delivery. Gradually, the length of stay has been shortened. Today, healthy mothers and newborns return home from medical centers or birthing centers within one or two days. As a result, home care services are in great demand to provide care for mothers and their newborns during this important period following childbirth. The home care aide's responsibilities may include assisting the mother in her own physical care and helping her to care for the newborn. Other duties may include supervising an older child or children and performing housekeeping tasks, according to the care plan. Providing emotional support, encouragement, and practicing positive listening skills are also important aspects of client care.

The Postpartum Period

The first six weeks following the birth of the baby is called the **postpartum period.** This is a time when the reproductive organs gradually return to their non-pregnant state. Just as hormones influenced the physical condition and emotions during pregnancy and childbirth, they continue to influence the changes that take place during the postpartum period. Important changes include:

- *Uterus*—Immediately following childbirth, the uterus (about seven inches long and two pounds in weight) contracts. This prevents excessive bleeding from taking place. The uterine muscles continue to contract, causing the uterus to become smaller as muscles tighten. By the end of the postpartum period, the uterus has reached a size similar to its nonpregnant state (about three inches long and two ounces in weight).

postpartum period
the first six weeks following the birth of the baby.

lochia
the discharge from the vagina after childbirth.

hemorrhoids
varicose veins in the rectum or anus.

cesarean birth
surgical procedure where the baby is delivered through an incision in the abdomen.

- *Lochia*—Vaginal drainage following childbirth is dark red and may contain some clots of blood for two to three days. It has a fleshy odor. Gradually, the lochia changes in color as follows:

  Pinkish-brownish—day 4–10
  Creamy—day 11–24

  The amount of lochia gradually decreases until no drainage is present and total healing has taken place.

- *Perineum*—During vaginal childbirth, a surgical incision may have been made in the perineum to increase the size of the birth canal and allow for easier delivery of the baby. Sometimes, the perineum is torn during the birth process. These surgical incisions or tears are repaired by the doctor and are commonly called "stitches." **Hemorrhoids** may be visible in the anal area. These may have been present during pregnancy or appear following delivery because of the pressure experienced during labor and delivery.

- *Breasts*—At the third day following childbirth, the breasts become swollen and tender because of milk "coming in." Hormones are responsible for stimulating the glands in the breast to produce milk. Milk ducts transport the milk to openings in the nipple. Each nipple contains 15 to 20 openings (Fig. 19-1). As the infant sucks the nipple, milk flow is stimulated. Usually, milk will continue to be produced as long as the infant sucks at the breast.

- *Weight Loss*—Losing the weight gained during pregnancy is usually an important goal that the mother wants to accomplish. About 18 to 20 pounds are lost during the first 10 days after giving birth. Getting rid of the remaining weight takes a longer time. Eating a normal, nutritious diet, along with exercise, helps to take weight off slowly. Under normal conditions, it takes six to eight weeks for the mother to return to her pre-pregnancy weight (provided there has been a weight gain of 20 to 30 pounds).

19-1 Milk ducts transport milk to the nipples. *(Courtesy Carnation Company, Los Angeles, CA.)*

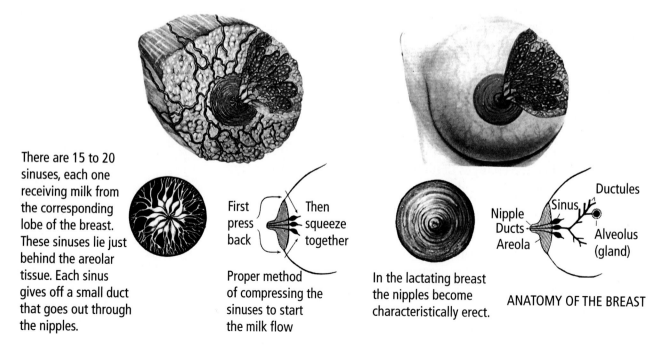

There are 15 to 20 sinuses, each one receiving milk from the corresponding lobe of the breast. These sinuses lie just behind the areolar tissue. Each sinus gives off a small duct that goes out through the nipples.

First press back
Then squeeze together

Proper method of compressing the sinuses to start the milk flow

In the lactating breast the nipples become characteristically erect.

Ductules
Sinus
Nipple
Ducts
Areola
Alveolus (gland)

ANATOMY OF THE BREAST

- *Other Changes*—Some mothers have had a **cesarean birth.** This means that an abdominal incision has been made, and the baby has been delivered through the abdomen rather than through the vagina. In addition to the changes listed above, these mothers also have abdominal sutures and a dressing covering the incision. Healing of the incision takes place gradually.

Caring for the Physical Needs of the Mother

The mother will be instructed about caring for herself before she leaves the hospital, medical center, or birthing center. She is taught to: notice signs that she should report immediately to the doctor; perform perineal care; observe the color of lochia; attend to daily hygiene needs; and care for her breasts. If the mother has had a Cesarean birth, care of the incision and other precautions are also included. The amount of exercise, rest, and sleep should be discussed. Your role, as the home care aide, is to help the mother perform these activities according to the care plan.

Care of the mother includes the following six areas as discussed over the next few pages.

Promote Rest/Sleep

The process of delivering an infant takes lots of energy. Following the delivery, the mother is usually exhausted. Many changes have taken place, both physically and emotionally. The first-time mother needs to learn how to care for her infant and herself. The mother who has other children needs to learn how to schedule time for rest periods between caring for herself and the other children. Encourage the mother to rest or sleep when the infant is sleeping. If another child or children are at home, your role may be to supervise and care for them while the mother takes a much needed rest.

Friends and relatives of the family are usually eager to see the newborn and mother. But, their visits should not interfere with the mother's need for rest and sleep. Be careful that these visits do not tire the mother.

Observe Lochia

The color and amount of lochia are indications of the healing process within the uterus. Therefore, it is very important to observe and record this information on the care record. Check the pad each time it is changed. Always put on gloves before handling the pad. Observe the color (red, pinkish-brownish, creamy). Is it normal for the number of days following delivery? If not, report this to your supervisor. Notify your supervisor immediately if these conditions are present:

- Bright red discharge appears after pinkish-brownish or creamy lochia has been present before
- Lochia has a foul odor
- Large number of blood clots
- More than one pad per hour is saturated for two to three hours in a row or two or more pads used within one hour
- Discharge makes client itch

Box 19-1

Signs to be Reported to Your Supervisor

- Change in color, odor, and amount of lochia
- Bright red bleeding
- Large number of clots
- Two or more pads saturated within one hour
- More than one pad per hour for two to three hours
- Fever of more than 101° F (38.4° C), chills, elevated pulse rate, poor appetite
- Swelling, redness, unusual odor in perineum
- Scant urination, painful urination
- Redness, swelling, unusual odor around abdominal incision (Cesarean birth)
- Changes in behavior (withdrawn, uninterested in surroundings, suspicious)
- Pain, tenderness, or swelling in calf muscle of leg

The soiled pad should be removed by the mother and placed in a plastic or paper bag. It is your responsibility to put it in the trash.

Assist With Personal Hygiene

The mother gives herself perineal care after changing pads, after urinating, and after a bowel movement. If you are responsible for this procedure, follow the instructions given in Procedure 13-8 in Chapter 13. Observe the condition of the perineum for any signs of infection, such as: swelling, redness, or unusual odor or drainage. Also, observe any change in the condition of hemorrhoids, if present. Box 19-1 lists additional information to be reported to your supervisor.

Remove and apply perineal pads from front to back so that any organisms from the anal area do not come in contact with the perineum or vagina. Clients with perineal sutures may find that a sitz bath helps to relieve the discomfort. It is ordered by the doctor. If the care plan indicates the need for this treatment, follow Procedure 17-10 in Chapter 17.

Assist your client to shower or take a sponge bath. Tub baths are usually not allowed until lochia is no longer present and the perineum is healed.

Observe Bladder and Bowel Elimination

It is important that the urinary and digestive systems are working properly following childbirth. Make sure that the mother drinks plenty of fluids. This is particularly important if she is breast-feeding. Constipation may be a problem, especially for mothers who have hemorrhoids. A diet high in fiber and fluids with plenty of fruits and vegetables provides the bulk and fluid needed to soften the stool or for easy elimination. Commercial stool softeners may be recommended by the doctor.

Encourage Proper Diet

The period following the birth of the infant is a time when the mother is regaining energy and repairing body tissues. Therefore, eating well-balanced meals is very important. A diet that includes all the requirements of the Food Guide Pyramid is essential. Some mothers, who are very anxious to lose the weight gained during pregnancy, may go on a "crash diet." This is not the time to diet because the mother's body needs to repair itself following childbirth. Notify your supervisor if your client's eating habits show signs that there is not a proper intake of foods.

Nutrition for Breast-Feeding Mothers The nutritional needs of breast-feeding mothers do not change very much from the needs during pregnancy. However, the need for fluids increases in order to produce enough milk for the baby. Mothers should be encouraged to drink fluids each time they nurse their babies. The doctor orders the type of diet needed and the amount of fluids. For teenage mothers, an additional serving from the milk, yogurt, and cheese group is usually needed (see Chapter 8, Figure 8-3).

The kinds of food and other substances that the mother takes into her body are secreted into her milk. This includes alcohol, any medication, caffeine, chocolate, garlic, and other seasonings. Nicotine, from cigarette smoke, is also transmitted in breast milk. Recent studies have shown that the positive effects of breast milk in providing infants with protection from disease are decreased when the mother smokes. Mothers who are breast-feeding should avoid the use of alcohol and caffeine; stop smoking; and check with the doctor about using prescription and OTC drugs.

If the mother notices a connection between a certain food she has eaten and the infant's reaction (fussiness, diarrhea, gas), she may consider avoiding that food. At a later time, the mother may want to try the food again because the food may not have been the real problem.

Assist With Breast Care

Before leaving the hospital, all mothers are taught how to care for their breasts. This care is very important for those who breast feed and bottle feed. Proper care of the breasts helps to prevent infection.

Clear water is used to clean the breasts, usually once a day. Soap is not used because it has a drying effect on the nipples. Breasts should be supported by wearing a well-fitting bra. It is important that the nipples and breasts are free of any signs of infection or injury (Box 19-2).

For breast-feeding mothers, absorbent breast pads help to keep the breasts dry between feedings, once the milk is flowing. To prevent growth of organisms that produce infection, the pads need to be changed frequently. Following each feeding, the nipples should be exposed to the air to dry thoroughly. Frequent washing of the nipples tends to remove the natural protective body oils. Therefore, washing the breasts and nipples once a day is usually sufficient.

The "Baby Blues"

The body's hormones not only cause physical changes following childbirth, but they influence the mother's emotions as well. It is not unusual for the mother to have periods of feeling sad, or bouts of crying, for no real reason. This is called the "baby blues." Coping with all the body changes and the new responsibilities of parenthood may cause these feelings. It is important to reassure the mother that the "blues" is not a sign of serious emotional problems but a normal reaction to the many changes in her life. Listen to what she has to say and provide positive feedback. As the mother's body returns to the pre-pregnancy state and the family learns new skills in caring for the newborn, the periods of feeling blue decrease.

Box 19-2

Signs of Breast or Nipple Infection

- Painful breasts—red, hard, or hot to the touch
- Cracked skin around the nipples
- Open sores around the nipples
- Cracked nipples
- Bruised nipples
- Bleeding nipples
- Elevated temperature— 101° F (38.4° C) or higher

REPORT ANY OF THESE SIGNS TO YOUR SUPERVISOR IMMEDIATELY

Other Situations

Most babies are born healthy and at **full term.** Bringing baby home is a joyful time for the family. However, these two statements may not apply to all your clients. You may experience the following situations.

The mother returns home without the newborn because:

- the baby was born earlier than expected and remains in the hospital for expert care
- the baby died (before, during, or following birth)
- the baby is being placed for adoption
- the newborn has severe physical or mental disorders
- the mother or father (or both) did not want this pregnancy, and the newborn may not be welcomed
- the mother or father (or both) wanted one baby but, instead, had twins, triplets, or more

The situations listed above may be ones where the usual joys of child-birth are replaced with sorrow, sadness, frustration, or even anger. Your supervisor will advise you about handling these difficult situations. Providing emotional support to the mother and other family members is an important part of the plan of care. Listen to what your client is saying. Use the principles of active listening discussed in Chapter 2.

Caring for Infants

It is true that newborn infants require a lot of care and attention. They are completely helpless and dependent on adults for their care. Even though they may sleep most of the time, it seems that their need for care is almost endless. Consider that the normal newborn's daily needs include:

- changing diapers 6 to 12 times
- feeding every one to four hours
- burping
- bathing
- changing clothing after feeding and at bedtime
- snuggling and loving
- protecting from harm and injury

A newborn infant changes the whole family's routines. Mother is often exhausted after having the baby and needs short-term assistance with infant care. This help may be provided by the home care aide. Duties and responsibilities are listed on the care plan. Mother and aide establish a daily routine that can be followed when the aide is no longer in the home.

The Normal Infant

Appearance

Length and Weight The weight of the average newborn infant is about 7 1/2 pounds (3400 grams). During the first few days of life, 10% of this weight may be lost, but it is quickly regained. At birth, babies are about 18–21 inches (46.4–54.4 cm) long.

Head—The head appears large, and it may be bruised or swollen from the trip through the birth canal. The neck is very weak and must be supported when the baby is lifted or carried (see Box 19-3, Holding an

full term
the completion of the full nine months of pregnancy.

fontanel(s)
space covered by tough membranes between bones of the infant's skull (soft spot[s]).

Infant). There are two soft spots, known as **fontanels,** in the infant's skull. The large anterior fontanel, toward the front of the skull, is closed (becomes hard) by the end of the second year of life. The posterior fontanel, at the back of the skull, is closed after two months. These areas

Box 19-3

Holding an Infant

There are several methods for holding infants:

1. Lift baby by placing one hand under the head and neck for support (Fig. 19-2A). Place the other hand under infant's body. Raise infant's head up to your shoulder. Continue to support head and neck (Fig. 19-2B).

2. Lift up baby, supporting head and neck in bend of your elbow. Trunk rests on forearm. This is called the "football hold." Infant may be held facing up (Fig. 19-3A) or facing down (Fig. 19-3B).

3. Lay baby on his/her tummy across your lap with head turned toward the side (Fig. 19-4).

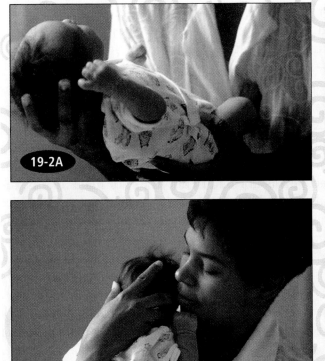

19-2A

19-2B

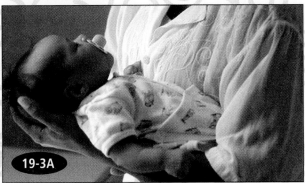

19-3A

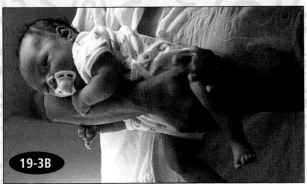

19-3B

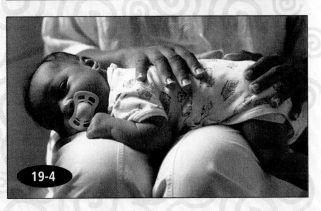

19-4

of soft bone allow for molding of the head during delivery and for brain growth after birth.

The baby may have lots of thick hair, no hair, or just a fuzzy growth on the scalp. There is no average when it comes to infant's hair. Newborns usually have cloudy blue eyes and may have a whitish discharge from the eye for a few days. True eye color appears around six weeks of age.

Skin The newborn's skin may appear reddish. Newborns chill quickly, and their hands and feet become bluish and cold. This is normal. Keep the baby dressed and wrapped as appropriate to the climate and the culture. Infants with black skin tend to be very pale at birth, but the skin darkens as they get older. Fingernails and toenails grow quickly. They may be cut by the parent while the infant sleeps or with help when the child is awake.

Umbilical Cord The stump of the umbilical cord remains in place for about two weeks before it dries up and falls off. It may be cleaned with an alcohol wipe according to the care plan. Keep the cord dry. It should not come in contact with stool, feces, or soiled diapers. Fold diaper down so it does not touch the cord. Likewise, fold the shirt up so it will not touch the cord. Until the cord falls off, babies are given sponge baths. See Procedures 19-1, Bathing an Infant—Sponge Bath, 19-2, Bathing an Infant—Tub Bath, and 19-3, Dressing an Infant.

Genitalia Female genitalia appear large and there may be some mucus or blood-tinged drainage from the vagina. This is normal and comes from exposure to the mother's hormones before birth.

When the male infant's scrotum becomes cold, the testes may move up in the sac in an effort to be warm. Sometimes one testicle appears to be higher than another. This is normal. In about 3% of male infants, the testicles may be undescended. They may descend during the first three months of life. If not, the physician will recommend treatment at the proper age. If the infant has been circumcised, follow instructions for care of the area.

Output

Stools For the first three or four days, the bowel movements are dark and tarry. These are called meconium stools. As the baby takes breast milk, the stools become pasty and mustard colored. Formula-fed infants have stools that are somewhat solid and brownish-yellow in color.

Voiding Infants seem to urinate constantly. They have small bladders and void about every two hours. In fact, infants seem to eliminate at the same time they feed. Diaper changing is a constant responsibility when caring for a newborn. Soiled and wet diapers can cause skin breakdown and infection. See Procedure 19-4, Changing a Diaper, and Box 19-4 for laundering diapers and other garments.

Activity

Sleeping Most infants spend most of their day sleeping. They wake up to be fed and changed. They are not yet able to turn over and to change positions. Pediatricians recommend that babies be placed on their sides or backs when lying down, not on the abdomen. Do not use soft, fluffy

Procedure 19-1

Bathing an Infant—Sponge Bath

Materials Needed

- Basin, bowl, or bathinette with water comfortably warm to the elbow
- Washcloth
- Towels (2)
- Hooded bath towel (optional) or receiving blanket
- Sterile cotton balls
- Rubbing alcohol or alcohol wipes for cleaning umbilical cord stump
- Vaseline or other dressing, if needed for circumcision (according to care plan)
- Mild soap
- Disposable gloves (for diaper change)
- Waste basket
- Clean clothing
- Toilet paper or tissues

Procedure

1. Wash your hands.
2. Obtain materials listed above.
3. Place all materials in easy reach. Spread hooded towel or receiving blanket on flat surface (kitchen table, crib, changing table, etc.) near where you will bathe baby.
4. Place baby on receiving blanket or hooded towel next to basin of warm water. Always keep one hand on baby. Never leave baby unattended. If you have forgotten something, take baby with you to get it.

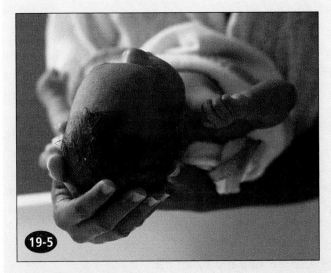

19-5

5. Begin with the head:
   a. Wet a cotton ball with plain water and gently clean eye by wiping from inner corner to outer corner. Discard cotton ball. Use a new one to clean other eye.
   b. Wet washcloth and sponge face, ears, and folds in neck. Pat dry. Do not use cotton swabs to clean nostrils or ears. You may damage delicate tissues.
   c. Pick up baby, holding in the football hold, facing upright. Hold head over basin. With free hand, wet washcloth and wring out over baby's scalp. Put a small amount of soap on the palm of your hand. Rub gently on to the infant's scalp (Fig. 19-5). Rinse by wringing wet washcloth over head. Dry gently. Cover head with hooded towel or receiving blanket.
6. Remove shirt. Wash chest, upper abdomen, arms and hands. Pat dry. Turn baby, wash and dry back.
7. Put on clean shirt.
8. Clean umbilical cord with alcohol (according to care plan).
9. Remove lower clothing. Wash legs and feet. Dry.
10. Put on gloves.
11. Remove diaper. Wipe any feces away with tissue and clean perineal area. Discard diaper or set aside for laundry. Wash perineum:
    a. Girls—wash from front to back. Rinse thoroughly. Gently pat dry.
    b. Boys—wash entire scrotum. Care for circumcision according to care plan.
12. Put on dry diaper.
13. Remove and discard gloves.
14. Finish dressing baby. Wrap in receiving blanket.
15. Place baby in a safe and comfortable position.
16. Clean materials and return to proper location.
17. Record what you have done. Report any unusual observations to your supervisor.

Procedure 19-2

Bathing an Infant—Tub Bath

Materials Needed

- Baby bathtub or Bathinette with water comfortably warm to the elbow
- Washcloth
- Towel
- Hooded towel or receiving blanket
- Mild soap
- Clean clothing
- Toilet paper or tissues
- Disposable gloves (for diaper change)
- Waste basket

Procedure

1. Wash your hands.

2. Obtain materials listed above.

3. Place all materials in easy reach. Spread hooded towel or receiving blanket on flat surface (kitchen table, crib, changing table, etc.) near where you will bathe baby.

4. Place baby on receiving blanket or hooded towel next to basin of warm water. Always keep one hand on baby. Never leave baby unattended. If you have forgotten something, take baby with you to get it.

5. Begin with the head:

   a. Wet a cotton ball with plain water and gently clean eye by wiping from inner corner to outer corner. Discard cotton ball. Use a new one to clean other eye.

   b. Wet washcloth and sponge face, ears, and folds in neck. Pat dry. Do not use cotton swabs to clean nostrils or ears. You may damage delicate tissues.

   c. Pick up baby, holding in the football hold, facing upright. Hold head over basin. With free hand, wet washcloth and wring out over baby's scalp. Put a small amount of soap on the palm of your hand. Rub gently onto the infant's scalp. Rinse by wringing wet washcloth over head (see Fig. 19-5). Dry gently. Cover head with hooded towel or receiving blanket.

6. Lay baby back on flat surface.

7. Remove shirt.

8. Put on gloves.

9. Remove diaper. Wipe any feces away with tissue and clean perineal area. Discard diaper or set aside for laundry.

10. Remove and discard gloves.

11. Hold infant:

    a. Place left hand under baby's shoulders. Your thumb should be over the baby's left shoulder. Your hand is holding the upper left arm.

    b. Use your right hand to support the baby's buttocks. Slide your hand under the thigh. Hold left thigh with your right hand (Fig. 19-6).

12. Lower baby into water, feet first.

covers, pillows, and blankets, as they can block the child's nose and mouth causing suffocation. Not every baby will have a crib to sleep in. Some may sleep in a play pen, bureau drawer, laundry basket, etc. Some safety rules for infants are in Box 19-5.

Crying Infants cry because they are hungry, soiled, or uncomfortable. *Crying is the only way that an infant can communicate its needs. Don't worry about spoiling a newborn baby. Crying means that the child needs attention.* Never let an infant cry for a prolonged period of time. Change, feed, burp, gently rock, sing to the child—whatever is appropriate. Prompt and loving attention helps the infant **bond** with the primary caregiver. An occasional smile may be observed, but real social smiling occurs during the second month of life.

When a baby's cries cannot be quieted by feeding, burping, changing,

bond
emotional attachment between infant and parents, especially the mother.

Procedure 19-2—cont'd

Bathing an Infant—Tub Bath

13. Wash front of infant's body, using your right hand.

14. Change your hold:
    a. Use right hand to support baby in a sitting forward position.
    b. Support and hold fingers around baby's upper arm and your hand under the infant's neck, as in lap position for burping (Fig. 19-7).

15. Wash baby's back.

16. Return to previous position.

17. Wash genital area.

18. Lift baby out of water and onto towel.

19. Wrap in towel, covering head.

20. Pat baby dry.

21. Put on dry diaper.

22. Finish dressing baby. Wrap in receiving blanket.

23. Place baby in safe and comfortable position.

24. Clean materials and return to proper location.

25. Record what you have done. Report any unusual observations to your supervisor.

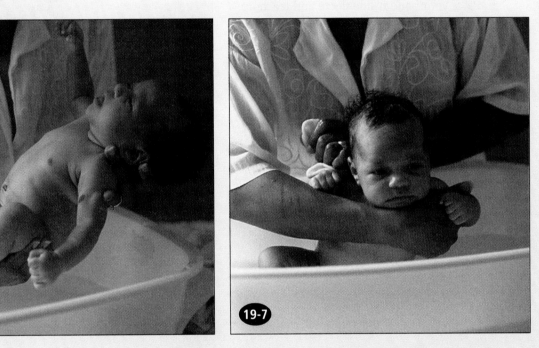

loving, rocking, singing, or other usual means, there may be a problem. The baby may be ill. Notify your supervisor about a baby that cries constantly and cannot be comforted. Other signs of infant illness are listed in Box 19-6, on page 361.

Eating Newborn infants eat every two to four hours. They may be breast-fed or bottle-fed. Breast-feeding is started almost immediately after birth. The first milk is called "colostrum." It is a clear fluid that contains special substances to protect the baby from infection. True milk "comes in" about three days after delivery. Infants who get enough milk will gain weight; appear satisfied after feeding; and produce at least six wet diapers and several fairly liquid, mustard-colored stools each day. For information on assisting a mother with breast-feeding, see Procedure 19-5.

Procedure 19-3

Dressing an Infant

Materials Needed
- Shirt
- Sleeper
- Booties (optional)
- Receiving blanket
- Other garments according to climate

Procedure

1. Apply shirt:
   a. Stretch neck of shirt and pull over baby's head (Fig. 19-8).
   b. Place your hand inside sleeve and reach up through sleeve to grasp baby's hand and pull through (Fig. 19-9).
   c. Repeat on other side.
   d. Pull shirt down over chest. If umbilical stump is still present, fold bottom of shirt up to avoid rubbing.

2. One piece sleeper:
   a. Unfasten all snaps on sleeper.
   b. Lay garment on flat surface.
   c. Place baby on garment.
   d. Insert feet into lower portion of sleeper.
   e. Reach through sleeves (as for shirts) to put on upper portion of sleeper.
   f. Snap up garment.

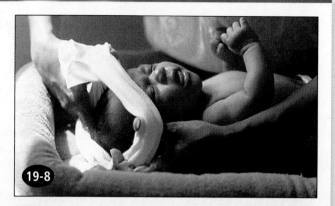

19-8

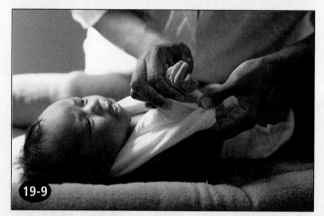

19-9

3. Booties:
   a. Roll bootie over your hand, inside out.
   b. Grasp infant's toes and turn bootie up and over foot with other hand.

Box 19-4

Baby Laundry

Diapers

Keep diapers separate from all other home laundry. Wash diapers daily or every other day.

1. Rinse dirty cloth diaper in cold water after changing baby.
2. Soak in hot water with one-half cup bleach (4 oz, 120 ml) to one gallon (4 L) of water while waiting to be washed.
3. Wash in hot water using detergent and bleach according to label directions. Fabric softener is not recommended. It may irritate the infant's skin.
4. Rinse in cold water. Dry.

Other Baby Clothing

1. If stained with formula or breast milk, rinse in cool water and pre-treat with non-chlorine bleach or detergent according to label instructions.
2. Wash in warm water in a separate load.
3. Rinse in warm water. Dry.

Changing a Diaper

Materials Needed
- Clean diaper—cloth or disposable
- Diaper pail or waste basket
- Diaper pins (for cloth diapers)
- Protective plastic pants (for use with cloth diapers)
- Baby wipes (optional)
- Washcloth (used for diaper changing only)
- Basin of warm water
- Soap
- Disposable gloves

Procedure

1. Wash your hands.
2. Obtain materials listed above.
3. Put on gloves.
4. Place baby on changing surface near materials. Be sure to protect baby from rolling off surface.
5. Open soiled diaper.
6. Wipe genital area with front of diaper (if dry). Wipe from front to back.
7. Roll diaper so that urine and feces are inside. Set aside for later disposal.
8. Wash the perineal area with soap and water or use baby wipes. Rinse and dry thoroughly.
9. Give cord/circumcision care according to care plan.
10. Raise baby's legs. Place clean diaper in place. Cloth diapers may be folded to better fit baby.
    a. Girls—extra fold in back.
    b. Boys—extra fold in front.
11. Pin or fasten diaper in place. Keep diaper below umbilical stump. Be careful not to stick baby with diaper pin. Have your finger under the diaper when you insert pin.
12. Apply plastic pants (if cloth diaper is used).
13. Place baby in a safe and comfortable position.
14. Rinse (or dump) feces from diaper into toilet. Flush. Rinse cloth diaper with cool water and place in diaper pail for laundering (see Box 19-4). Discard disposable diaper in garbage.
15. Remove and discard gloves.
16. Wash your hands.
17. Record what you have done. Report any unusual observations to your supervisor.

Box 19-5

Infant Safety

1. Do not place infants on
   - water beds
   - soft, stuffed bedding, such as fluffy quilts
   - pillows of any type
2. Do not place infants on abdomen in crib or playpen. Position infants on their
   - sides
   - backs
3. Keep sides on cribs raised at all times.
4. Hold baby on changing table. If changing table has belt, use it to secure baby. A good rule to follow when changing or bathing an infant is: **"One hand on the baby at all times."**
5. Do not leave infants unattended on any surface (bed, sofa, table) where they could roll off.
6. Do not place anything in the infant's immediate surroundings that could cause choking or suffocation, such as stuffed toys, pillows, clothing, propped bottle, or plastic bags of any type.
7. Do not bathe infants in kitchen or bathroom sinks. Burns may be caused by hot water dripping on the baby. Older infants may touch hot faucets and be burned.
8. Do not bathe infants in the bathroom tub until they are able to sit up alone. Because of danger of drowning, <u>never EVER</u> leave an infant alone in bath water.
9. Do not place anything around the infant's neck (necklace, cord, pacifier, or string).

Assisting Mother to Breast-feed

1. Wash your hands.

2. Have mother wash hands. Nipples are washed with plain water (if called for in care plan) in a circular motion from nipple outward (Fig. 19-10).

3. Help the mother to a comfortable position
   - in a chair with feet up on a stool
   - in bed with pillows behind back and head for support; adjust pillows until mother is comfortable

4. Change baby's diaper, if needed.

5. Bring baby to mother.

6. Have mother touch infant's cheek on side nearest the breast. This stimulates the **rooting reflex** and causes the newborn to turn toward the nipple.

7. Mother holds back breast tissue so the baby can "latch on" to the entire nipple and most of the **areola.** The infant's lips should cover this area. Baby's tongue should be under the nipple (Fig. 19-11).

8. Baby should nurse for about 10 minutes on each breast. Sucking will be more vigorous on the first breast, and baby will empty that one faster. If baby falls asleep during feeding, mother can remove him/her from the breast. Awaken baby by washing face, changing diaper, or tapping feet. Put baby back to breast.

9. Remind mother how to remove baby from the breast: by inserting her finger into the corner of the baby's mouth to break the suction.

10. Mother burps the baby before moving baby to the other breast.

11. When feeding is over, change diaper.

12. Place baby in a safe and comfortable position.

13. Mother may massage a little milk/colostrum on nipples after feeding. Breasts may be air dried. Nipples should be kept dry. Breast pads may be used as needed and changed when wet.

14. Assist mother with dressing, if necessary. A nursing bra may be worn.

15. Record what you have done and report any abnormal findings.

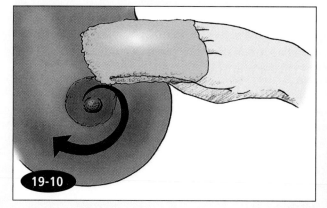
19-10

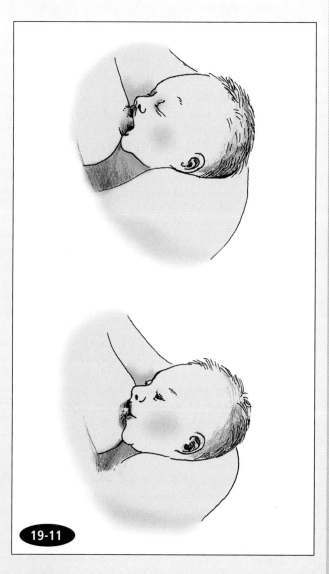
19-11

Box 19-6

Signs of Infant Illness

Notify supervisor if the newborn infant:

- has a axillary temperature over 100°F (37.7°C)
- becomes unusually quiet or limp
- develops skin rash or diaper rash
- vomits (not the usual baby "spit-up") or loses appetite
- develops diarrhea
- may have fallen, been dropped, or bumped
- shows sign of possible injury, such as swelling or bruising
- develops a yellow coloring of the skin or whites of the eyes
- cries constantly and is not comforted by any of the usual methods

Call Emergency Medical Service or 9-1-1 if baby has any trouble breathing or if baby stops breathing.

rooting reflex
normal reaction infants have that makes them begin to suck when their cheeks are stroked.

areola
colored, circular area surrounding the nipple.

The bottle-fed baby will drink a formula suggested by the pediatrician. Formula comes in a variety of forms: as a powder, which is added to sterile water; as a liquid, which is diluted with sterile water; and in disposable, single-feeding containers. Formula preparation is discussed in Procedures 19-6, 19-7, 19-8, and 19-9. Formula is given at room

Procedure 19-6

Sterilizing Bottles

Materials Needed
- Bottles
    - eight—8 oz (240 ml) bottles (glass or plastic)
    - four—4 oz (120 ml) bottles (glass or plastic)
- Nipples
- Bottle brush
- Nipple brush
- Tongs
- Large pot with lid
- Jar with openings in lid for nipples
- Dishwashing liquid
- Clean dish towel

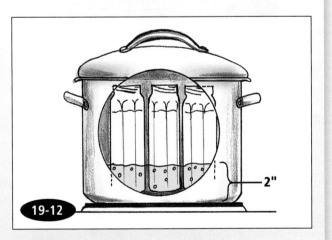
19-12

Procedure

1. Wash your hands.
2. Obtain materials listed above.
3. Wash all bottles and nipples in dish-washing liquid and hot water. Rinse thoroughly.
4. Place bottles and jar of nipples in large pot. Put two inches (five cm) of water in the pot. Place lid on pot and boil for five minutes. Do not lift lid during this process (Fig. 19-12).
5. Let pot cool. Remove contents with tongs.
6. Stand bottles on a clean dish towel to dry.

Preparing Formula from Powder

Materials Needed

- Sterilized bottles and nipples
- Powdered formula and scoop
- Funnel or measuring cup
- Long-handled spoon
- Water

Procedure

1. Wash your hands.

2. Obtain materials listed above.

3. Boil water and allow to cool.

4. Pour cooled water into bottle.

5. Add powdered formula using scoop, according to label instructions (Fig. 19-13).

6. Shake well to mix.

7. Cap, seal, and store bottles in the refrigerator until needed.

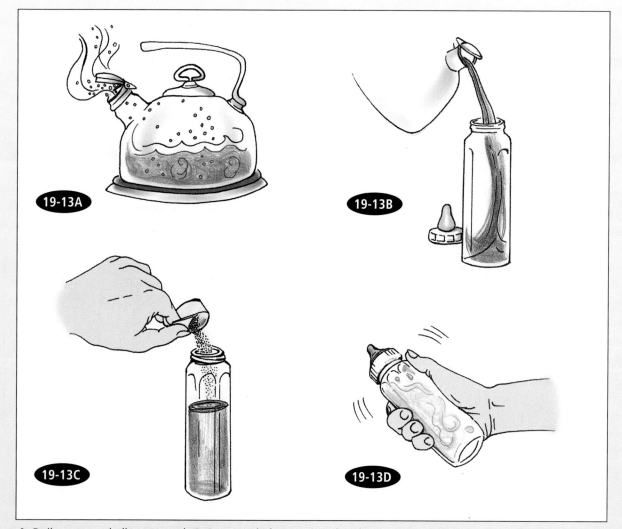

A, Boil water and allow to cool. *B,* Pour cooled water into bottles. *C,* Add proper amount of powder to bottles. *D,* Put lids on bottles and shake well to mix.

Preparing Formula Using Concentrated Formula

Materials Needed

- Sterilized bottles and nipples
- Canned concentrated formula
- Water Funnel or measuring cup

Procedure

1. Wash your hands.
2. Obtain materials listed above.
3. Boil water.
4. Wash can lid with hot soapy water. Rinse. Open can.
5. Pour appropriate amount of formula through funnel into bottle. Add appropriate amount of water (Fig. 19-14).
6. Prepare enough bottles to use all formula concentrate.
7. Cap, seal, and store bottles in the refrigerator until needed.

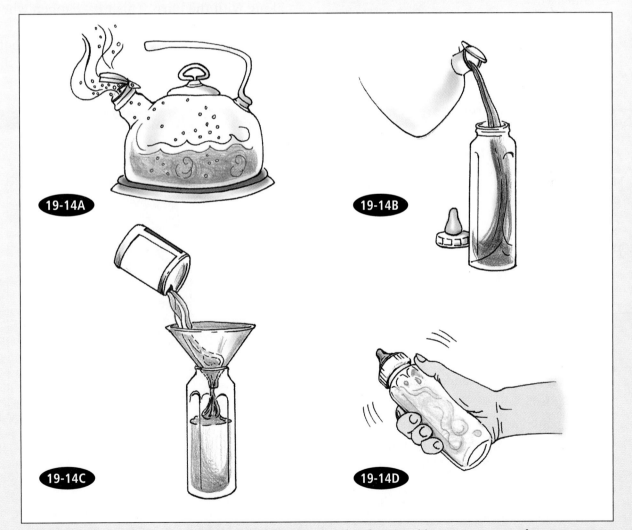

19-14A

19-14B

19-14C

19-14D

A, Boil water and allow to cool. *B,* Pour cooled water into bottles. *C,* Add proper amount of concentrate to bottles. *D,* Put lids on bottles and shake well to mix.

Procedure 19-9

Preparing Formula from Ready-to-Use Supply

Materials Needed
- Sterilized bottles and nipples
- Funnel or measuring cup

Procedure

1. Wash your hands.

2. Obtain materials listed above.

3. Wash off can lid with hot soapy water. Rinse. Open can.

4. Pour formula into bottle using funnel.

5. Cap, seal, and store formula until needed.

temperature. Cold formula may be warmed by placing the bottle in a container of warm water. **NEVER WARM A BOTTLE OF INFANT'S FORMULA IN A MICROWAVE.** The newborn will take about two to three ounces (60–90 ml) at each feeding. With growth, the infant will drink more formula at a feeding and will need to eat less often. Do not prop a bottle in a baby's mouth because the baby may suffocate. See Procedure 19-10, Assisting the Mother to Bottle-Feed.

Infants swallow a lot of air when they are feeding. Babies need to be burped to help get rid of this air, or gas. Some babies are very "gassy," others are not. For ways to burp a baby, see Box 19-7. Be sure to use a cloth or diaper to protect your clothing when burping a baby. Some infants will "spit up" some of the feeding along with the burp. This may happen when the baby has eaten too fast or too much.

Some pediatricians will add one or two bottles of sterile water to the feeding routine if the baby seems thirsty.

Procedure 19-10

Assisting Mother to Bottle-Feed

Materials Needed
- Bottle of formula
- "Spit-up" cloth

Procedure

1. Wash your hands.

2. Obtain materials listed above.

3. Warm bottle (if cold) by placing in a pan of warm water until it is about room temperature.

4. Have mother wash her hands.

5. Help the mother to a comfortable position.

6. Change baby's diaper, if necessary.

7. Bring bottle and baby to mother.

8. Bottle should be tilted so that neck and nipple are always covered with formula (Fig. 19-15). Never prop the bottle.

9. Have mother burp the baby halfway during the feeding and at the end.

10. Feeding is discontinued when baby is no longer eating.

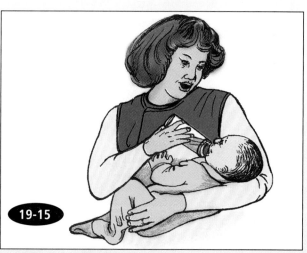

19-15

11. Change diaper.

12. Place baby in a safe and comfortable position.

13. Wash your hands.

14. Record what you have done and the amount of formula taken. Report any unusual observations to your supervisor.

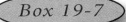

Box 19-7

Burping an Infant

There are several methods for burping an infant:

1. Place diaper or "spit-up" pad over your shoulder. Hold the baby up to your shoulder. Remember to support head and neck. Gently pat or rub infant's back until burp is heard (Fig. 19-16A).

2. Sit infant in your lap. Support with hand under infant's chin. Hold "spit-up" pad in this hand. Rub or pat back until burp is heard (Fig. 19-16B).

3. Lay baby across your lap with head a little higher than rest of body. Place "spit-up" pad under infant's head. Rub or pat back until burp is heard (Fig. 19-16C).

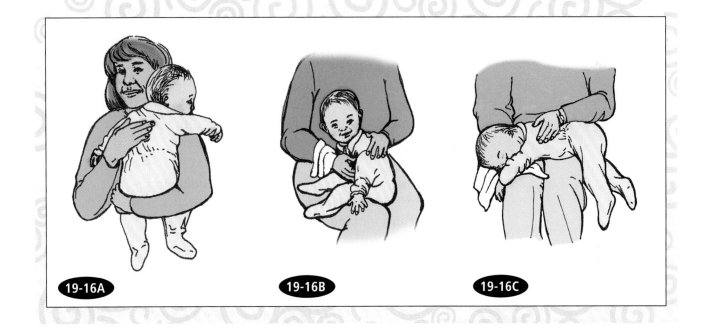

19-16A   19-16B   19-16C

The Premature Infant

The premature infant is any baby born before 37 weeks' **gestation.** They have a low birth weight and their organs are not fully developed. There is great variety in the condition and **prognosis** for each infant. With specialized care given in intensive care premature nurseries, some of these infants do well, but it takes them a while to "catch up" to full term babies.

Working with Children

Home care aides will have some experiences with children throughout their career in health care. There may be children or grandchildren in the home of a client, or at some time you may be assigned to care for a sick or disabled child.

Whatever the case, you will need some understanding of children in order to work with them. Begin by reviewing the material on normal growth and development in Chapter 3. Additional information follows.

gestation
period of time between conception and birth.

prognosis
educated guess about the probable outcome of an illness.

Always consult with your supervisor regarding questions and concerns when working with children.

Need for Service

Home care agencies may provide care for children in many situations including:

- **respite care** for developmentally disabled children
- when a parent requires supervision and assistance, for example a teenage mother with a sick or disabled infant
- when ordered by the court in cases of real or suspected child abuse
- in group homes for children and mothers with AIDS
- when a child is recovering from an illness
- when a parent is ill and unable to provide child care
- when a parent has died, and the family needs temporary assistance until satisfactory child care plans can be made.

Indications of Stress in Children

Reactions of families to illness are covered in Chapter 5. However, children react deeply to any threat to their security. When a primary caregiver (parents or other) is ill or absent from the home, children and adolescents may display signs of fear and anxiety. This is shown in a variety of behaviors, including:

- nightmares and fear of going to bed or going to sleep
- being afraid of the dark
- crying and sobbing
- hiding and withdrawing from others
- aggressive acting out, may be directed toward the sick or disabled person or sibling (hitting, punching, swearing, cursing)
- regression in toilet training, a return to soiling and wetting (this is more common in toddlers and preschoolers)
- jealousy and anger toward a sick or disabled sibling
- trying to be "perfect," to please everyone
- playing one parent (or another important adult) against another
- testing the limits of rules, regulations, and routines in a family/household

Often children are unable to verbally express their fears, anxieties, and other feelings. The younger the child, the more difficulty he/she will have in asking questions and in telling "how they are feeling." Teenagers may keep their feelings to themselves and be unable to verbally communicate their emotions. Anxiety and fear are often communicated through some of the behaviors listed above.

Discipline Versus Punishment

Discipline

When supervising or caring for children, you probably will have the opportunity to reinforce the rules of acceptable behavior in the home. This system of rules that governs the way we act is known as **discipline.**

respite care
short-term care provided so that main caregivers in the family can have a break from their responsibilities.

discipline
system of rules that governs the way we act

Discipline is a positive way of teaching responsible behavior. It sets limits and provides guidelines so that children can learn how to behave in an appropriate way when the parent or caregiver is not present. Discipline should be:

- Known—the child knows the rules and what will happen if a rule is broken
- Consistent—each time a rule is broken, the consequence is the same

Recognizing the child's attempts to comply with the rules of the household and praising these efforts help to encourage acceptable behavior.

Your role as the home care aide in disciplining the child is to:

- know the rules of acceptable behavior in each family situation
- ask the family member to clarify the rules, if you are unsure
- reinforce the existing rules
- be consistent, when using discipline
- praise the child's efforts to comply with the rules

Sometimes, you may be in a home where there are very few rules of discipline. Or, you are not able to follow the existing rules because they appear to be too harsh or too loose. In such cases, contact your supervisor for assistance in handling these situation. New rules may need to be set up. Do not set up new rules of discipline without the help of your supervisor.

Punishment

Punishment is a harsh response that occurs when the discipline or rule is broken. Punishing a child for failing to follow the rules of the household is **not** a responsibility of the home care aide. If a family member tells you to do so, explain that it is not your agency's policy to carry out punishment. Ask the family member to contact your supervisor, if they have further questions. Record this information on the care record and notify your supervisor concerning the situation.

Role of the Home Care Aide

The goal is to provide a stable, secure, and safe atmosphere for the family. This is very important for sick children and for those who are experiencing stress because of illness of a family member. Recognizing each family member's needs (Chapter 3) and the family's reaction to illness (Chapter 5) can help the home care aide to provide personalized care to meet these needs and concerns. While the home care aide's responsibilities will vary in each family situation, the following are usually included:

- opening and maintaining lines of communication among all members of the family
- providing a safe, secure, and stable environment
- developing positive relationships with all family members
- maintaining the existing rules of behavior
- maintaining the daily routines as much as possible
- being alert to situations that may add stress or cause harm to the family (Box 19-8)
- reporting situations that threaten the well-being of the family

Box 19-8

Changes or Events in the Home

Report the following to your supervisor immediately:

- Violent behavior of family member (physical or verbal)
- Frequent visits by "strangers"
- Suspected drug abuse
- Excessive drinking
- Electricity, heat, or water turned off due to failure to pay bills
- Severe shortage of food or clothing
- Failure of child (children) to go to school
- Illness of child
- Sudden departure of caregiver
- Unexpected return of family member

Guidelines for Caring for Children in the Home

The following guidelines should be used when interacting with children:

Communication

- Use active listening skills—
  maintain eye contact, concentrate on what is being said
- Watch for non-verbal communication cues—
  frown, lack of eye contact, smile, hands on hips
- Answer questions simply, honestly, and clearly
- Provide non-verbal communication—a hug, touch on shoulder or arm (according to acceptable custom and culture) to comfort child
- Offer praise for something well done
- Give encouragement when the child attempts to improve behavior, even though there is only slight progress
- Use **positive** suggestions rather than negative words; avoid "Don't do…" and "No"

Rest, Sleep, Play, and Exercise

- Reinforce rituals of bedtime, nap time
- Recognize individual child's need for sleep—varies with age
- Supervise playtime—encourage active exercise, if allowed
- Avoid taking sides when disagreement occurs
- Avoid playing one child against another
- Ignore tattling, if used to get attention
- Treat each child as an individual of worth
- Do not give more attention to one child and ignore others

Mealtime

- Prepare foods that child will eat
- Do not force child to eat

Child Abuse and Neglect

The home should be a place where children can be secure, happy, and safe. However, each year, more than 2.9 million children are victims of physical, emotional, or sexual abuse or neglect, usually in their own homes. Most abusers are known and trusted by the child. This includes family members, relatives, friends of the family, or babysitters.

Causes of Abuse and Neglect

The causes of child abuse and neglect are very complex. The following factors place some people at greater risk for becoming child abusers:

- being raised by abusive parents
- being a substance abuser (alcohol, drugs)
- being a single or adolescent parent
- being isolated—no one to rely on or to assist with child care
- living in poverty

According to the National Committee to Prevent Child Abuse, there are several types of child abuse: physical, sexual, emotional, and neglect. Box 19-9 defines each type of abuse and gives some signs. It is not unusual for more than one type of abuse to occur. For example, physical and emotional abuse often occur together.

Box 19-9

Child Abuse and Neglect

Type

Physical

Injury not caused by an accident

Signs

- Unexplained bodily injury
    Bruises or welts
    Burns
    Cuts or sores
- Patterns on skin that suggest objects used
    Belt
    Cord
    Cigarette
    Iron
- Human bites

Sexual

Using child for sex: this includes rape, incest, fondling genitals

- Bruises, bleeding, irritation of genitals, anus, mouth, throat
- Difficulty walking or sitting
- Stained, torn, and bloody underwear
- Discharge of vagina or penis
- Painful urination

Emotional

Behavior that hurts the child's feelings and damages sense of self-worth

Abuser:
- Constantly belittles or criticizes child
- Uses insulting language
- Ignores child; gives no love, support, or guidance
- Screams at child
- Uses threatening language

Neglect

Failure to provide child with basic needs of food, clothing, shelter, medical care, or proper supervision

- Weight loss
- Dirty clothes, hair, body
- Urine and feces in bed
- Child left unsupervised in home
- Child wanders outside home unsupervised
- Child always hungry
- No food in refrigerator

Reporting Child Abuse

The same rules apply to reporting child abuse as reporting Elder Abuse (Chapter 18). Follow your agency's policies and procedures when you suspect or observe child abuse in the client's home. Be sure to notify your supervisor immediately. Include the following information when reporting and recording on the care record:

- the name of the abused
- the date and time the abuse occurred, if known
- how the abuse occurred, if known
- when you discovered the abuse (date, time)
- what you
  - observed
  - heard
  - were told
- where you
  - observed it
  - heard it
  - were told about it

Your agency will take steps to protect the child from further harm. It is your agency's responsibility to notify the appropriate local and state agencies.

CHAPTER SUMMARY

- Mothers experience many changes during the postpartum period.
- Home care aide's responsibilities in caring for new mothers include:
  - promoting rest and sleep
  - observing lochia
  - assisting with personal hygiene
  - observing elimination
  - encouraging proper diet
  - assisting with breast care
- Home care aides should be aware of abnormal findings to report to the supervisor.
- Infants are completely dependent on adults for their basic human needs. Always protect the infant from harm and injury.
- Signs of infant illness include:
  - elevated temperature
  - unusually quiet or limp
  - skin or diaper rash
  - vomiting and/or diarrhea
  - yellow coloring of skin
  - constant crying
- Children react to stress in the home in a variety of ways. Often, this is expressed through non-verbal communication.
- Discipline is a system of rules that governs the way we act. It is **not** the responsibility of a home care aide to punish a child who does not follow the rules of the household.

- The home care aide forms a positive relationship with children by using the following guidelines:
  - use positive suggestions
  - answer questions simply and honestly
  - offer praise for something well done
  - reinforce rituals of bedtime
  - treat each child as an individual of worth
- Child abuse is a serious problem that *must* be reported to your agency. *Suspicions* of abuse must also be reported.

STUDY QUESTIONS

1. Describe the changes that occur in the new mother's
   a. breasts
   b. uterus
   c. vaginal discharge
   d. weight
   e. emotions

2. List six responsibilities of the home care aide when caring for a new mother.

3. List seven abnormal conditions of the mother to be reported to your supervisor.

4. List five ways to keep infants safe in the home.

5. Which of the following conditions of the infant would you report to your supervisor?
   a. blue hands and feet
   b. whites of eyes are yellow
   c. spits up with burping
   d. no hair on the head
   e. limp body and very quiet
   f. skin rash

6. What is the difference between discipline and punishment?

7. List four signs of stress in children.

8. You are caring for Grandma Fink, a 93-year-old, who lives with her granddaughter and three great grandchildren. They are two, four, and six years old. List four guidelines to follow when forming a positive relationship with each of Mrs. Fink's great grandchildren.

9. List two signs of child abuse in the following categories:
   a. physical
   b. sexual
   c. emotional
   d. neglect

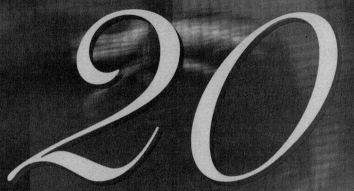

20 Mental Health/ Mental Illness

Objectives

After you read this chapter, you will be able to:

1. List five characteristics of a well-adjusted individual.

2. Define mental illness and list three effects on a person's life.

3. Define and describe three defense mechanisms.

4. Describe five abnormal behavior patterns that are common in mental illness.

5. Discuss the role of the home care aide in caring for clients with mental illness.

6. Discuss the problem of substance abuse and how it may affect the abuser and family members.

Often we say that a person with mental health is one who exhibits **normal** behavior. The dictionary defines normal as: "conforming to a standard," that is, according to the rule. So "normal" people are pretty much alike in the way they dress (warm clothing for cold weather, lighter clothing in hot or warm climates), in their behavior, and their communication. Of course, there are great variations within the definitions of normal (Fig. 20-1). Adolescents follow the "latest" dress code for their age group. Often adults may comment and complain about the bizarre appearance of some teenagers. Most are perfectly normal and are following the rule for their group.

But there are other indicators of mental health that are much broader than what we say and how we look. These have to do with a person's ability to cope with day-to-day living.

Mental Health

What is Mental Health?

What is mental health? Basically, it is a person's overall state of mind. It is how one feels emotionally rather than physically. People with good mental health are usually able to face and handle the stresses that come in everyday life (See Box 20-1). They can control their thoughts, emotions, and behavior as they do their usual day-to-day routines.

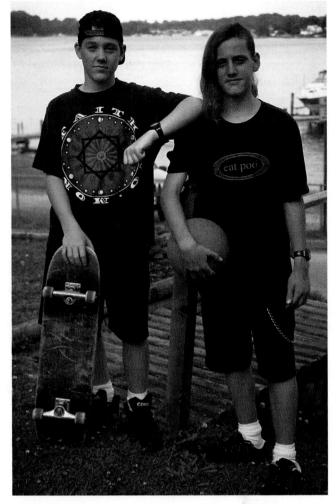

20-1 Adolescents have their own "dress code."

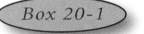

Life Stresses

Predictable

- Parenthood
- Marriage
- Death/bereavement
- Children leave home
- Retirement
- Education/testing
- Employment
- Responsibility for aging persons

Unpredictable

- Illness and/or disability
- Hospitalization
- Loss of home/job
- Accident
- Death of a child
- Divorce
- Separation
- Natural disaster
- Murder
- Suicide

normal
conforming to a standard or following the rule.

impulse(s)

a sudden, uncontrollable urge.

mental illness

a brain disorder that affects thoughts, emotions, and behavior.

defense mechanism

unconscious reactions that protect a person from real or perceived threats.

Each person responds to life's stresses differently, though. Some people can handle more stress than others—some situations will be more serious. Generally, however, people who are mentally healthy share certain characteristics. They seem to be content with their life situations, well-adjusted—normal. Some characteristics of a well-adjusted person include:

- the ability to give and receive love and affection
- knowing one's needs and how to meet them
- the ability to control one's desires and **impulses** until they can be appropriately fulfilled
- the ability to learn from experience and to let go of the past
- having a system of values and beliefs that guide behavior (a sense of right and wrong appropriate for the individual's culture)
- the ability to view oneself and one's limitations realistically
- the ability to express and control emotions in an appropriate way
- being in contact with reality

Factors That Influence One's Mental Health

Many factors can also affect a person's overall mental health. They include:

- having a strong emotional support system of family and friends (and/or community agencies)—people who can be turned to when problems arise (Fig. 20-2).

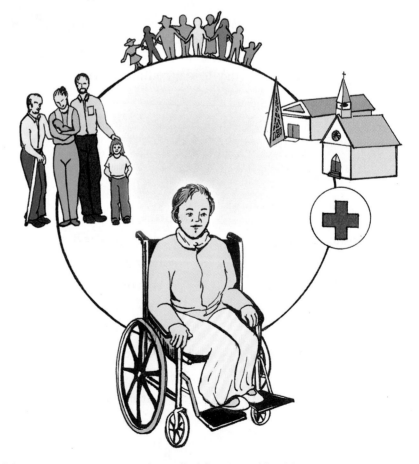

20-2 A strong support system is needed for mental health.

- physical health, disabilities, or physical limitations
- alcohol or drug use
- family history of mental illness

Mental Illness

What is Mental Illness?

Mental illness can be defined as a brain disorder that affects thoughts, emotions, and behavior. People who are mentally ill have difficulties doing the normal activities of everyday life. They may develop strange behaviors or lose touch with reality. A person who is mentally ill may show some of the following behaviors:

- Unable to carry on the normal daily activities: cannot sleep; does not get out of bed, dress, or prepare and eat meals
- Unable to function socially: withdraws from others; may have violent thoughts/behavior; may get into trouble with the law
- Becomes excessively worried, anxious, or fearful
- Loses touch with reality: may not recognize self or friends or family; doesn't know seasons, date; unable to tell correct time
- Relieves personal discomfort or troubles with increased use of drugs and/or alcohol
- Uses **defense mechanisms** all the time as a way to cope with stressful or unpleasant situations.

Mental illness is considered an illness like any other and may be accompanied by physical symptoms as well. Clients may have headaches or other pains, anorexia, a rapid heart beat, and sweat heavily. Sometimes these physical symptoms mask (hide) the emotional symptoms, and this can make mental illness hard to diagnose. See Box 20-2 for warning signs of mental illness.

Box 20-2

Warning Signs of Mental Illness

- Noticeable personality change
- Confused behavior or thinking
- Depression that will not go away
- Excessive fear, anxiety, worry
- Withdrawal from others
- Thinking or talking about suicide
- Violent thoughts or behavior
- Severe change in eating and/or sleeping patterns
- Increased use of drugs or alcohol
- Inability to cope with daily life

Mental illness can affect the quality of life of adults and children alike. Serious mental illness keeps people from leading normal lives. It can make it difficult to do life's major physical activities: eating, sleeping, dressing, and working or going to school.

Defense Mechanisms Defense mechanisms are unconscious reactions that protect a person from real or perceived threats. They help block out some of the uncomfortable and threatening feelings. This makes the situation a little easier to cope with. We all use defense mechanisms from time to time to cope with pressures and stresses of everyday life. This is normal. However, many people with mental illness use defense mechanisms constantly to postpone dealing with unpleasant feelings and thoughts.

One defense mechanism that has been discussed throughout the text is denial, which can be a normal reaction to illness. When denial becomes a pattern of behavior, it can delay, postpone, or even block treatment and may lead to serious results, even death. Some other more common defense mechanisms include:

- *Rationalization*—giving socially acceptable reasons to explain and justify one's unacceptable behavior, impulses, or feelings. For example: Your friend says, "I had to buy that dress because it was such a great bargain," although she is two months behind in her rent.
- *Projection*—attributing characteristics to others when they are actually his/her own, such as blaming others for problems rather than taking the responsibility. For example: A student fails a test and says, "That test wasn't fair. The instructor did not teach us the information that was in the test."
- *Repression*—barring painful, unacceptable thoughts, experiences, and/or impulses from our conscious mind. For example: A person who was sexually abused as a child cannot remember the abuse as an adult.
- *Regression*—returning to behavior, thoughts, or feelings used at an earlier stage of development. By acting less than one's age, the person can handle the stressful situation—or get others to take care of it. For example: An adult who is ill may show childlike behaviors and enjoy the care and attention given.

Remember that we all use defense mechanisms from time to time to help us cope with problems and painful situations. However, many mentally ill people use defense mechanisms all the time as a way of coping with life.

Causes of Mental Illness

While the exact causes of mental illness are unknown, we do know that there are many factors that play a role in its development, including:

- biochemical imbalances in the brain
- heredity
- chronic severe stress
- isolation
- alcohol and drug abuse

psychotherapy

method of treating mental disorders, primarily by "talk therapy."

- family and interpersonal relationships
- accidents
- untreated sexually transmitted disease
- diseases that impair circulation to the brain

Other long-term diseases, such as Alzheimer's disease or AIDS, do affect behavior because they affect the physical structure of the brain. However, they are classified as physical illnesses.

Myths and Realities

There are many myths and realities about mental illness, including:

Myths	Realities
People with mental illness never get well.	With treatment, people recover from mental illness. Others may develop a chronic illness that lasts for a lifetime.
The mentally ill are dangerous to themselves and others.	Mentally ill persons rarely harm themselves or others
The mentally ill are unable to work.	If the mental illness is not severe, work is possible. In some cases, a change to a less stressful job may be necessary.
Mentally ill persons can turn symptoms on and off at will.	Mentally ill persons cannot turn symptoms "on and off." Their behaviors are part of the illness and cannot be controlled.

Mental Illness Treatment and Care

In the past, mentally ill persons were confined to large psychiatric hospitals that focused primarily on meeting the patient's physical needs. Private psychiatric hospitals offered care, but only the very wealthy could afford them. Today, treatment for mental disorders is available to anyone who seeks it. Besides hospitals, treatment is offered at community mental health centers, outpatient clinics, halfway houses, and group homes. There are several health care professionals who specialize in treating mental disorders (See Box 20-3). The treatments for mental illness include **psychotherapy** (Fig. 20-3) and medication.

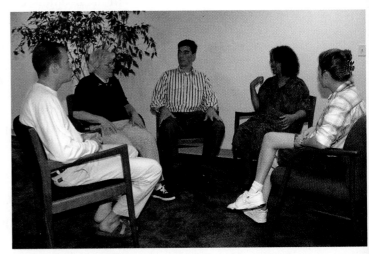

20-3 Group therapy is one way that people can learn to cope with their conditions.

Box 20-3

Mental Health Practitioners

1. PSYCHIATRIST—a physician who specializes in diagnosing, and treating chemical dependencies, emotional problems, and mental illness.

2. PSYCHOLOGIST—a person who holds a Ph.D. degree and specializes in evaluating and treating emotional illnesses. Does not prescribe or give medications.

3. PSYCHIATRIC SOCIAL WORKER—a person with a master's degree in social work (MSW) and specialized training in treating emotional illness.

4. PSYCHIATRIC NURSE PRACTITIONER—a registered nurse with a master's degree in psychiatric nursing and specializes in treating emotional illness.

Some Psychiatric Therapies

1. PSYCHOTHERAPY—method of treating mental disorders primarily by "talk therapy." This may be in an individual or group therapy session.

2. BEHAVIORAL THERAPY—attempts to solve emotional problems by changing behaviors. For example, the anxious person may learn special relaxation and breathing techniques in order to cope during periods of anxiety.

3. DRUG THERAPY—use of medications to relieve symptoms (anxiety and depression) that occur in mentally ill persons. Some drugs used to treat severe mental illness may affect behavior patterns. Drugs are prescribed by the psychiatrist and are used in combination with other psychotherapies.

Care of the Mentally Ill Client

Clients who are mentally ill may be unable to control their thoughts, emotions, and behavior. Their strange behavior may make friends, relatives, and neighbors avoid them. Family members may be ashamed of their loved one's illness. This may leave your client feeling lonely and isolated from the world around them. Your caring attitude can go a long way to provide support and acceptance for the client and family. See Box 20-4 for guidelines when caring when mentally ill clients.

Your client may be recovering from a severe illness that required a stay in the hospital. Or, your client may suffer from a chronic illness that can be treated at home. Either way, you will have several responsibilities as part of the mental health care team:

- Follow the care plan as closely as possible to provide a consistent routine of daily activities.
- Assist client to meet basic human needs, such as bathing, dressing, activity, and nutrition.
- Observe client's progress or condition and report significant changes in appearance, behavior, and communication.
- Assist client to follow medication schedule, if part of the care plan.

Abnormal Behavior Patterns

Because mental illness affects the way a person thinks and behaves, your client may act quite strangely. However, the behavior is a sign of the illness and cannot be controlled. The following lists some of the more common abnormal behaviors that mentally ill clients may have.

Box 20-4

Guidelines When Caring for the Mentally Ill Client

- Inform client about time of day, day of week, month, place, and person, as needed
- Provide safe, secure environment
- Present reality—do not go along with client's delusions or hallucinations
- Accept the person, not the behavior
- Promote behavior appropriate to age and condition
- Recognize substance abuse as a disease and not a lack of willpower or moral failure
- Record and report changes to your supervisor:
  - increase or decrease in abnormal behavior
  - increase or decrease in performing ADL
  - ease or difficulty in making decisions

- increase or decrease in ability to communicate
- change in personal appearance and grooming
- Recognize that mental illness affects everyone close to the client; listen carefully to them—offer support
- Assist with management of the home
- Avoid giving advice
- Understand your feelings and how they affect your actions
- Have an even disposition and a positive outlook
- Follow guidelines for listening, communicating (Chapter 2), and accurate recording (Chapter 10)

Confusion A mental state in which the client is disoriented about time, place or person and also may be unable to have an orderly train of thought.

Behaviors:
- Cannot give correct information about the time of day, month, season, or year.
- Cannot give correct information about where they are (at home, at the doctor's), where or with whom they live.
- Cannot recognize family, friends, others and may mistake one person for another.
- Acts bewildered and forgetful.
- Cannot remember how to perform activities of daily living correctly.
- Cannot think through a situation or problem clearly.
- Cannot remember recent events.
- Cannot remember location of bathroom, bedroom, or other parts of home.
- Wanders about the house and appears lost—particularly in the evening and at night.

Your Role:
- Communicate correct information about time, place, or person.
- Provide clues in surroundings that will help to inform client about time of day (clock), month and season (calendar) (Fig. 20-4).
- Explain events or procedures in simple, short sentences.

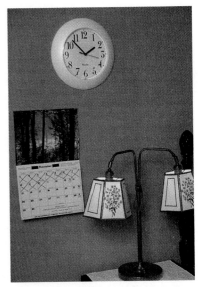

20-4 Clocks and calendars help to inform the client about time, month, and season.

- Keep a set routine—avoid making changes.
- Encourage client to perform familiar, simple tasks and assist as needed (washing hands, face, brushing teeth).
- Provide safe, secure environment—remove potentially harmful objects (see Box 20-5).

Anxiety and Panic Anxiety is an uneasy, fearful feeling about real or imagined threats to a person's well-being. Panic is a sudden feeling of extreme fear. A person may be "frozen with fear" (paralyzed) or become completely hysterical. Panic attacks come without warning and may last for minutes to hours. Their frequency varies, depending upon the severity of the condition.

Behaviors (vary according to the severity of the condition):
- Worries constantly about everything, even small things, with no real reason.
- Speaks abnormally and may be difficult to understand.
- Speaks of impending doom or danger.
- Difficulty sleeping; fatigued.
- Paces back and forth, very restless.
- Neglects personal grooming and hygiene, or is overly concerned about cleanliness or appearance.
- Frequently complains of physical discomfort.
- Poor appetite.
- Difficulty concentrating on tasks or activities.

Box 20-5

Providing a Safe, Secure Environment for Clients

- Place the following items out of sight and reach:
  - Matches and lighters
  - Sharp objects (scissors, knives, razors, breakable objects)
  - Personal care items (nail polish remover, perfumes, after-shave lotion, mouthwash)
  - Car and house keys
- Store in locked cabinets:
  - Prescription and OTC medications
  - Laundry and household cleaning agents
  - Gardening materials and fertilizers
- Reduce clutter
- Put bells on doors to signal that the client is trying to leave the area
- Place protective gate at entrance to steps and stairs
- Follow guidelines listed in Chapter 6

Your Role:

- Encourage routine periods of rest and activity as appropriate.
- Encourage client to do ADL and assist when necessary.
- Be a good listener.
- Provide a calm, safe environment.
- Speak in a calm tone of voice and use short sentences.
- Avoid discussions about client's physical complaints.
- Offer foods that are easy to eat (sandwiches, finger foods) when client is pacing.
- Encourage client to make decisions, but limit choices to make it easier.
- Offer reassurance using non-verbal behavior (sit quietly with client, touch shoulder, hand, if appropriate and culturally acceptable).
- Stay with client during panic attacks.
- Explain procedures you will perform, as needed.
- Perform tasks according to client's care plan.
- Record and report any changes in behavior to your supervisor.

Delusions and Hallucinations Delusions are false beliefs that a mentally ill person believes to be true. For example, the client may believe that the world is going to blow up at any minute. Hallucinations are sensory perceptions (things seen, heard, felt, smelled) that aren't actually there. For example, the client may "see" or "feel" bugs that aren't there.

Behaviors:

- Is suspicious of others and thinks they want to do him/her harm.
- Looks around a lot to see who is watching.
- Believes that he/she is a king, queen, president of the United States, or other well-known person.
- Mumbles to self.
- Talks about unseen objects, such as animals, space ships.
- Smiles, nods, and appears to be communicating to an unseen person.

Your Role:

- Provide a safe, secure environment.
- Leave a light on in bedroom at night if added feeling of security is desired.
- Do not go along with client's delusions or hallucinations or pretend to see or hear what the client is seeing or hearing.
- Do not argue with client about what client claims to see, hear, or feel.
- Give client correct information regarding time, place, person, as needed.
- Perform tasks according to client's care plan.
- Describe delusions or hallucinations in care record and report any changes in behavior to your supervisor.

Depression This disorder, sometimes called "clinical depression," is characterized by feelings of extreme sadness and hopelessness. Depression can also be accompanied by symptoms of physical illness, such as headaches and stomach upset. It is an illness that, for most people, can be treated effectively.

Behaviors:
- Feels very unhappy, sad most of the time.
- Cries a lot.
- Shows no interest in almost all ordinary activities (job, family, hobbies, relatives, sex).
- May overeat, or show no interest in food at all.
- May be constipated.
- Puts on or loses large amounts of weight rapidly.
- Changes in sleep patterns, such as can't sleep or sleeps all the time.
- Has no energy, feels exhausted all the time.
- Feels worthless, angry, and irritable.
- Cannot concentrate, remember things, or make decisions.
- Speaks about committing suicide or actually attempts suicide.

Your Role:
- Encourage routine periods of rest and activity, as appropriate.
- Encourage client to perform ADL and assist when necessary.
- Be a good listener.
- Provide a safe, secure environment.
- Give information, explanations, and directions to client in terms that the client can understand.
- Follow care plan to be sure that basic needs for food, fluids, and toileting are met.
- Assist client to take medications, as required.
- Be alert for signs of suicide (see Box 18-8) and report these *immediately* to your supervisor.
- Record and report any changes in behavior or problems with medications to your supervisor.

Aggression The use of violent or abusive behavior to cope with anxiety.

Behaviors:
- Is irritable and angry.
- Paces back and forth, sometimes with fists clenched.
- Appears hostile and agitated.
- Expresses rage and threats of physical abuse.
- Punches, kicks, or throws things in the environment.
- Is suspicious of others.
- Has delusions or hallucinations.

Your Role:
- Assist client to take medications as required.
- Observe client for any signs of increasing aggression and report them to supervisor immediately.
- Encourage client to perform ADL (assist as directed in care plan, if your safety is not at risk).
- Do not try to give physical comfort, such as touching or hugging, as client may try to hit or kick you.

- Be a good listener, as this may be calming to an angry client.
- Provide calm, safe environment.
- Speak in calm tone of voice and make eye contact.
- Remain calm and try to control your facial expressions—do not show anger or fear.
- Do not wake client by touching, as client may lash out—softly call out to person by name.
- Do not turn your back on an aggressive client or put yourself in a position where client could hurt you.
- If client is threatening you or does hit you, leave the home, if necessary, and call for help.
- Contact supervisor immediately if you have been forced to leave the client alone.

Suspicion (Paranoia) A pattern of behavior characterized by thoughts of persecution (that others are "out to get" him/her), secretiveness, and inability to maintain contact with reality.

Behaviors:

- Secretive; fearful of others.
- Cannot maintain contact with reality.
- Worries that someone or something is listening in on personal thoughts and watching his/her every move.
- Believes that someone or something is trying to control him/her, such as the "government" through the TV, the phone, or by computer.
- Cannot relate to others.
- Refuses to eat or drink, for fear that the food has been poisoned.
- May become aggressive under stressful situations.
- Cannot perform personal care or ADL.

Your Role:

- Do not ask client to make decisions, as this may cause confusion and increase stress levels.
- Serve foods and fluids in packages that have not been opened or that could not be easily tampered with, such as:
  - Hard cooked eggs that do not have cracked shells
  - Juice, water, or soda in individual cans, bottles, or other single-serving containers
  - Fruit cups, puddings, and yogurts in single-serving containers
  - Meals that are packaged or ready to eat (client may be suspicious of the use of a microwave oven for food preparation, as client may believe the microwave can control or hear client's thoughts)
- Do not go along with client's delusions or hallucinations.
- Do not argue with the client about what client claims to see, hear, or feel.
- Assist client to take medications, as required.
- Record and report any changes in behavior or problems with medications to your supervisor immediately.

Overactivity (Mania) A mood disorder often characterized by extreme happiness or excitement accompanied by restlessness and overactivity.

Behaviors:

- Extreme feelings of confidence or power, the ability to do anything, even fly.
- Irritable and restless—unable to sit still and relax.
- Speaks quickly in urgent tones and jumps from one topic to the next and may be difficult to understand.
- Is too busy or preoccupied with thoughts to eat, drink, or perform ADL.
- May wear bright clothes, lots of makeup and jewelry.

Your Role:

- Provide calm, safe environment.
- Provide foods and fluids that can be easily held and consumed if client is pacing the floor.
- Encourage routine periods for rest, activity, toileting, and grooming.
- Do not argue with client, as this will increase irritability and may cause aggression.
- Assist client to take medications, as required.
- Record and report any changes in behavior, especially an increase in aggression or signs of depression, to your supervisor immediately.

Sexual Acting Out Inability to control sexual desires and acts out sexual urges and fantasies in order to relieve the anxiety.

Behaviors:

- Removes clothing and insists on being nude in inappropriate settings.
- Frequently fondles, touches self.
- Masturbates frequently regardless of setting.
- Makes frequent sexually suggestive remarks or is sexually aggressive to others.

Your Role:

- Try to keep client dressed—use layers of loose, comfortable clothing appropriate to the climate.
- Keep a robe nearby for client to use in case client disrobes.
- Redress client as often as necessary.
- Try to occupy client with activities (hobbies, writing) that will keep client's hands busy and help to release the stress and anxiety.
- Provide privacy for the client who needs to masturbate.
- Observe client for signs of injury and infection that may occur with continuous masturbation:
  - vaginal drainage
  - red and irritated perineal area
  - foul odor from perineal area
  - drainage from penis
  - red and irritated skin on penis

- Try not to judge client—remember this is part of your client's mental illness.
- Maintain professional attitude, as client may mistake your friendliness for acceptance of sexual advances.
- Do not accept or ignore suggestive remarks or sexual advances—tell your client in a firm tone of voice that the behavior is not acceptable and that you do not want to be spoken to or touched in that manner.
- Record and report to your supervisor any sexual advances made by your client.

Substance Abuse

Substance abuse is the misuse of chemical substances (usually alcohol or drugs) that leads to an emotional and/or physical dependence. It is a serious problem that affects millions of Americans and their families. Unfortunately, health care workers may become substance abusers, as they often have easy access to their clients' prescription medications.

Substance abuse can alter a person's mood, consciousness, and thinking. It can cause physical changes that lead to illness—and even death. As a person becomes addicted, the body gets used to having the drugs or alcohol in the system. Then the body begins to need more and more of the substance to get the desired feeling. Soon the body becomes dependent on the substance in order to function. If the person tries to stop taking the substance, severe physical and mental distress will occur. Drug and alcohol addiction is very hard to overcome, but, with proper treatment, it can be done.

Commonly Abused Substances

The most commonly abused substances are alcohol and drugs:

Alcohol   Alcohol is a legal drug that can be obtained by anyone of legal drinking age, according to state law. It is estimated that over 15 million Americans are alcohol abusers. Alcoholism is not only a problem of older adults, it is a serious problem for adolescents—even young children. Alcohol abuse can lead to other substance abuse, too. Reasons for alcohol abuse include to help one sleep, to reduce anxiety, to lift one's spirits, or to make socializing easier. See Chapter 18 for some of the signs and problems caused by alcohol abuse in older adults.

Prescription Medications   Medications are prescribed by the doctor to treat illness and the client's symptoms, such as pain, sleeplessness, or anxiety. Some clients continue to use these medications after the initial prescription has expired. This may be done by: changing doctors frequently to get new prescriptions; changing the drug store where the prescription is filled; or obtaining prescription drugs illegally.

Illicit (Illegal) Drugs   There are many illegal drugs used in the United States. Recent reports estimate that between $49 billion and $64 billion are spent on their purchase each year. The illicit drug market tries to increase its financial profits by coming up with new drugs with exciting names to catch the interest of drug users and "hook" their victims.

Signs of Substance Abuse

The following is a partial list of signs of substance abuse:

Physical

- Changes in appearance, such as weight loss or gain, lack of attention to personal hygiene and clean clothing
- Changes in eating habits or sleep patterns
- Hides dilated or constricted pupils of eyes by wearing sunglasses
- Wears long-sleeved shirts to hide needle marks on arms
- Slurred speech; difficulty with balance
- Unusual odor to breath; unusual smell on clothing

Work or School Habits

- Difficulty concentrating on tasks to be done
- Changes in work habits, such as being late for work, calling in sick frequently, cannot perform work efficiently
- Changes in school habits, such as poor grades, lack of interest in school activities, frequently late or absent
- Disinterested in activities at work or school

Other

- Changes in personality or mood swings
- Disinterested in family activities, events
- Sudden appearance of "new" friends
- Presence of large amounts of pills, alcohol, beer (may be out of sight)
- Presence of supplies such as syringes, needles, pipes, or other drug supplies

Your Role

When You Suspect Substance Abuse

If you suspect that a co-worker, client, or client's family member may be a substance abuser, notify your supervisor. Do not discuss your suspicions with anyone other than your supervisor. This information should be kept confidential. Be sure to report accurately what you observed or heard that led you to suspect substance abuse. This is a serious responsibility, and accurate reporting is necessary so that further investigation can be made. Do not attempt to give advice to the suspected substance abuser. Your agency has resources available to handle the situation and help the abuser with this serious problem.

When You Suspect a Substance Abuser is in Your Client's Home

Some substance abusers may have bizarre behavior and can cause harm to themselves and others. Safety for yourself and your client should be your first concern. If you believe that you are in immediate physical danger, get out of the home and notify your supervisor. He/she will advise you concerning the next steps to take. If you or your client are not in any present danger, follow the directions above for reporting possible substance abuse.

When Your Client Is Presently Being Treated for Substance Abuse

Be observant for any signs that your client is returning to previous habits of abuse. Record and report your observations to your supervisor immediately so that additional help can be provided to assist your client to recover. Follow the care plan carefully. Your role includes providing support and encouragement to your client and family members during this difficult time. Recovering from substance abuse is hard work. It is important that your behavior and communication show a positive concern during this period of recovery.

CHAPTER SUMMARY

- Persons with good mental health are usually able to cope with and adjust to the predictable and unpredictable stresses of living in an acceptable way. Well-adjusted individuals are able to:
  - give and accept love and affection
  - adapt and adjust to change
  - deal with problems in a realistic way
  - accept responsibility for their own decisions, feelings, and actions
  - know their needs and how to meet them

- Mental illness is defined as a brain disorder that affects thoughts, emotions, and behavior.

- Mental illness is considered to be an illness like any other and may be accompanied by physical symptoms.

- Serious mental illness keeps people from leading normal lives.

- Defense mechanisms are behaviors that help people cope with anxiety. They protect the person from real or perceived threats. Examples of defense mechanisms are: denial, rationalization, regression, repression, and projection.

- Many people with mental illness use defense mechanisms constantly to postpone dealing with unpleasant feelings and thoughts.

- Abnormal behavior patterns seen in persons who are mentally ill include: confusion, anxiety and panic, delusions and hallucinations, depression, aggression, suspicion (paranoia), overactivity (mania), and sexual acting out.

- The home care aide's role includes:
  - following the care plan carefully
  - providing daily assistance to help the client meet basic human needs
  - observing the client's progress and reporting significant changes in appearance, behavior, and communication
  - assisting the client to follow the medication schedule
  - providing emotional support and acceptance for client and family
- Substance abuse is a serious problem that affects millions of Americans and their families. If you suspect that a co-worker, client, or client's family member may be a substance abuser, notify your supervisor.

STUDY QUESTIONS

1. List five characteristics of a well-adjusted individual.
2. Define mental illness. List three ways that it affects a person's life.
3. List three defense mechanisms and define each.
4. Describe five abnormal behavior patterns that are common in mental illness.
5. List five responsibilities of the home care aide when caring for clients with mental illness.
6. What is meant by substance abuse? How can this problem affect the abuser and family members?

Typical Clients Requiring Home Care Services

21

Objectives

After you read this chapter, you will be able to:

1. Describe the role of the home care aide when caring for clients who have the following conditions:

   Cardiovascular diseases

   Cancer

   Stroke

   Chronic obstructive pulmonary disease (COPD)

   Diabetes

   Alzheimer's disease

   Multiple sclerosis

   Parkinson's disease

   Arthritis

   Fractures

   AIDS

   Amputation/prosthesis

2. Discuss the role of the home care aide when caring for clients who are recovering from surgery.

3. Identify three purposes of support groups in helping clients and family members to cope with the illness.

4. Discuss the role of the home care aide in providing emotional support for clients and family members who are coping with illnesses identified in this chapter.

5. Apply principles of universal precautions and infection control when caring for clients.

The illnesses described in this chapter have been selected because they are typical of the types of clients you will probably care for. But, it is not possible to describe all the illnesses your clients may have. If you are not familiar with the illness and what to watch for when caring for your client, be sure to ask for help from your supervisor. Do not care for a client when you do not know your responsibilities; it can be dangerous for your client and for you, also.

For some clients, you will observe that their condition is improving with each visit that you make; this can be very satisfying for you and your client. For others, who have chronic illnesses, you may see little or no improvement. But remember, your care allows them to remain at home, in familiar surroundings, rather than in an institution. You will also care for those clients who are at or approaching the last stage of living. Basic principles of care for these clients are discussed in the next chapter.

When reading this chapter, you will be referred to material already covered in the book. It is important to refresh your memory by re-reading this information.

Cardiovascular Diseases

Definition

Cardiovascular diseases affect the normal functioning of the heart and blood vessels. A very common disorder found among home care clients is congestive heart failure. It is due to the gradual weakening of the heart's ability to adequately pump blood to all parts of the body.

The Facts

Cardiovascular disease is the leading cause of death in the United States. About 66 million Americans have some form of cardiovascular disease.

Symptoms

Clients who have congestive heart failure may have the following symptoms:

- **Edema,** especially in the feet and ankles—may also have a feeling of tightness in the fingers
- Cough due to fluid in the lungs—may or may not expel sputum
- Difficulty breathing with or without activity—needs two or more pillows to sleep
- Constantly fatigued
- Chest pain caused by lack of blood supply to heart muscle
- Anxious due to chest pains—may have symptoms of depression as disease progresses

Your Role

Communicating

- Use techniques listed in Chapter 20 for clients who are anxious.
- Clients may not want to talk a lot—it takes much energy, especially when breathing is difficult.

edema
abnormal amount of fluid in the tissues (swelling).

Maintaining a Safe Environment

- Use precautions learned for clients receiving oxygen—the client may use oxygen only when needed or all the time.
- Dispose of used tissues according to universal precautions.
- Take precautions to reduce chance of possible infectious illness—clients with congestive heart failure are at great risk for infections.
- Assist to bathroom or commode carefully—client may be receiving medications to increase urinary output.

Performing ADL

- Follow guidelines in Box 21-1, ADL for Clients with Low Energy Levels.
- Follow activity schedule—some clients may be severely limited in activity.
- Keep legs and feet elevated when sitting in chair—support area from knees to feet (Fig. 21-1A and B).
- Raise head of bed to Fowler's position, if hospital bed is used, so client can breathe more easily; if regular bed is used, provide pillows.

Maintaining Good Nutrition

- Follow care plan's directions for special diet restrictions—client may be on a sodium restricted diet to help reduce the amount of fluids in the tissues; see Chapter 8 for review of foods to avoid.
- Follow guidelines listed in Table 8-14 for ways to conserve client's energy when eating.
- Encourage fluids as indicated in the care plan.

Box 21-1

ADL for Clients with Low Energy Levels

- Do not rush the client; allow extra time to perform activities.
- Encourage self-care and assist client, as needed.
- Provide rest periods during bathing, dressing, or when you notice client is tiring during a procedure.
- Encourage client to wear non-constricting clothing that is easy to put on and take off (elastic waist bands, suspenders [not belts] for men, slip-on shoes).
- Use techniques that will save client's energy when performing ADL (chair in bathroom for bathing, toilet articles within easy reach).
- Schedule activities requiring a lot of energy (bath) for time of day when energy reserves are high, if possible.

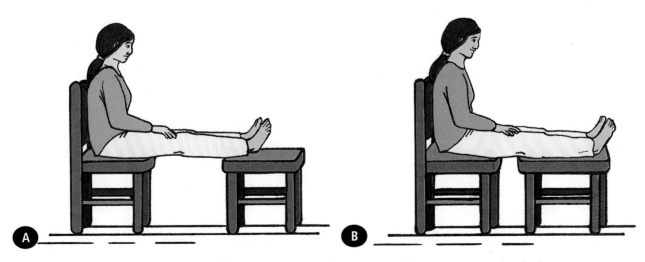

21-1 A, Incorrect position. The legs and feet are not properly elevated with no support under the knees.
B, Correct position. The legs and feet are properly elevated and knees are fully supported.

Assisting with Special Procedures

- The care plan may include the following procedures:
- Apply elastic stockings (see Chapter 17, Procedure 17-14)
- Measure intake and output (see Chapter 14, Procedure 14-3)
- Weigh daily or when listed; weigh at the same time of day; client wears similar type of clothing
- Assist client to take oral medications
- Assist client to take medication to relieve chest pain
- Take vital signs according to the care plan

Watch for... and Report

- Shallow, rapid respirations
- Coughing up blood-tinged, frothy sputum
- Wheezing or "rattling" breathing
- Cyanosis of lips and nails
- Sweating
- Weak, thready, rapid pulse
- Small amount of voiding
- Large amount of weight gain from previous time

Cancer

Definition

Cancer is a term used to describe over 100 diseases that result from the uncontrolled growth and spread of **malignant** cells. They may travel from the original site to other locations in the body.

The Facts

Cancer is the second leading cause of death in the United States. The American Cancer Society estimates that three of every four families are affected by this disease. As we age, the risk of developing cancer increases. The earlier the cancer is discovered, the greater the chance for successful treatment and recovery.

Symptoms

There are no typical symptoms shown by clients with cancer. Symptoms depend on where the cancer is located; how much of the body is affected; and the type of treatment the client has received or is currently receiving.

You may care for a client who is receiving treatment to help destroy cancer cells and prevent them from spreading. Two methods are: radiation—the use of x-rays, and chemotherapy—the use of strong chemicals in the form of medication. Unfortunately, these methods can also destroy healthy cells. Both types of treatments are usually given in hospitals or medical centers by health professionals. Sometimes, clients return home following each treatment. Your client may show the following side effects of radiation or chemotherapy:

- fatigue, exhaustion
- nausea and/or vomiting

malignant
abnormal cells causing cancer.

- anorexia
- loss of taste or smell
- skin irritation or burns in the area receiving radiation
- loss of hair
- sores in the mouth, around the lips and tongue
- bleeding gums
- upper respiratory infections—client's immune system is not functioning well

Other symptoms may include:

- pain
- constipation, due to medications given to relieve pain

Your Role

The information that follows is only a partial list of ways to assist the client with cancer. Be sure to review the care plan thoroughly before beginning care. It is important to know when the client has received the last treatment or the last medication for pain so that you can better understand the client's needs.

Communicating

- Listen to what the client tells you.
- Use non-verbal communication; it is just as important as verbal; show that you care by a touch of the hand and your presence; when a person is in pain, a lot of talking may not be welcome.
- Do not say anything that is untrue, such as "I know you will get better—don't worry."
- Encourage the client to tell you when he/she begins to be fatigued so that you can adjust the care routine, if possible.

Maintaining a Safe Environment

- Discourage visits from persons with colds or other infections—clients are at high risk for infections (see Box 21-2).
- Practice universal precautions and infection control when handling body fluids and waste.

Performing ADL

- Practice techniques to conserve client's energy described in Box 21-1.
- Provide frequent oral hygiene according to the care plan—use a very soft bristled toothbrush or foam Toothette to avoid further injury to mucous membranes—be gentle; avoid alcohol-based mouth washes—use normal saline.
- Do not remove colored lines on skin that indicate the site for radiation treatments— do not wash skin within these lines.

Box 21-2

Preventing Infection

- Use universal precautions to protect your client and yourself.
- Dispose of body wastes properly.
- Discourage visitors who have colds or other infections.
- Use disinfectants properly.
- Keep client's area clean and free of dust.
- Prepare and store foods properly.
- Wash your hands before and after giving client care.
- Wash your hands before and after handling food.
- Wash your hands before and after gloving.
- Observe skin for redness or skin breakdown.

Maintaining Good Nutrition

- Encourage fluids that client can drink.
- Prepare foods that client likes, can eat and swallow.
- Avoid foods with strong odors and high acid content, which can irritate mouth tissues.
- Prepare frequent small meals—they are usually better tolerated.

Helping Client to Cope with Pain

- Encourage client to take medication before the pain becomes severe—bring medication to client on time, according to the care plan; some pain medications cause constipation; record bowel movements accurately.
- Use techniques to help client to tolerate pain as listed in care plan (back rub, warm or cool applications to area, playing soothing music, etc.).
- Attend to client's request for spiritual aids, such as prayer or spiritual readings.
- Record type, location, and frequency of pain (see Chapter 10) on the care record, according to agency procedure.
- Assist client to record pain information (Fig. 21-2), if requested.
- Accept client's changed behavior due to pain—do not judge this behavior.

Watch for...and Report

- White or yellow patches in the mouth
- Other signs of infection
- Problems or changes in
    - swallowing, eating, or drinking
    - bowel habits—constipation or diarrhea
- Changes in type or frequency of pain
- Bruising or bleeding

Cerebral Vascular Accident

Definition

A cerebral vascular accident (CVA) is an injury to the brain caused by lack of blood to the tissues.

The Facts

Cerebral vascular accident, also known as a stroke, is the third leading cause of death in the United States. Each year about 500,000 Americans have a stroke: that's one stroke every minute, according to the American Heart Association.

Symptoms

This is a very serious illness. On admission to the medical center, the patient is very ill and requires expert care during the acute phase. Some people will not survive. Of those who do, many will be treated in a rehabilitation center before coming home. Symptoms depend on the extent

Client's Daily Pain Journal

Name: Sol Weinstein

Date: Tuesday, October 10

Location of Pain: Lower back

Medication(s): Morphine sulfate 30mg. by mouth every four hours

Pain Scale

0	1	2	3	4	5
No Pain	Mild	Discomforting	Distressing	Severe	Unbearable

TIME	LEVEL OF PAIN	MED TAKEN	ACTIVITIES AND COMMENTS
1:00 a.m	3	✓	Awake and restless
2:00	2		Awake to bathroom
3:00			
4:00			
5:00	3	✓	Awake
6:00			
7:00	2		Resting in bed
8:00	2		Breakfast in kitchen
9:00	2	✓	Shower and dress
10:00	2		Read paper, watch T.V.
11:00			
12:00 noon			
1:00 p.m.			
2:00			
3:00			
4:00			
5:00			
6:00			
7:00			
8:00			
9:00			
10:00			
11:00			
12:00			

Directions: 1. Using a Pain Scale, select the number that most closely describes your level of pain and record.

2. Record medication taken.

3. Decribe activity and any comments in column provided.

21-2 The client pain record. *(Courtesy Olsten Kimberly QualityCare, Melville, N.Y.)*

of the brain injury and the area involved. Symptoms may include problems with:

- *Communication*—due to difficulty receiving, understanding, and expressing speech and language. **Aphasia** is caused by injury to the speech center of the brain. Short attention span is also caused by brain damage. Clients may have slurred speech and problems finding the "right" word they want to say. This is very frustrating, and clients may cry or become angry because they are unable to clearly express their needs and feelings. Sometimes, they will not understand what you are asking or telling them.
- *Safety*—due to poor balance, **hemiplegia,** and **hemianopsia.** The client is at great risk for falls.
- *Activities of daily living*—due to limited mobility, weakness, and **perception** problems. There may be severe problems with performing ADL, and clients usually require a great deal of assistance with grooming and hygiene.
- *Mobility*—due to hemiplegia and enforced bed rest.
- *Pain in affected shoulder and/or arm*—due to weight of paralyzed arm pulling on joints.
- *Elimination*—due to incontinence, urinary retention, and constipation.
- *Nutrition*—due to difficulty in swallowing, self-feeding, and perception problems.
- *Depression*—due to effects of serious illness, problems with mobility, and prolonged rehabilitation. Clients may have low self-esteem because of the many losses they have experienced and the need to depend on others for so much care. Emotions change so quickly that the client and family may not understand what is happening. These rapid mood swings are a result of damage to the brain tissue and are not an indication of true feelings.

Your Role

Home care aides provide support to client and family during the long road to recovery following a stroke.

Communicating

- Follow the guidelines in Chapter 2 for communicating with persons who are hearing impaired; clients may not be hard of hearing but usually have difficulty understanding and responding to speech.
- Ask questions that can be answered with a simple "yes" or "no".
- Use non-verbal communication—gestures, pictures (Fig. 21-3 A and B), chalkboards, flash cards, typewriters, and computers.
- Try to anticipate your client's need before he/she has to ask for something.
- Follow the instructions given by the speech therapist.

Maintaining a Safe Environment

- Follow the principles of safety in Chapter 6.
- Protect from infection.
- Discourage visitors with respiratory infections.

aphasia
absence of speech.

hemiplegia
paralysis of one side of the body.

hemianopsia
blindness or defective vision in one half of the field of vision.

perception
ability to recognize sensations through the senses.

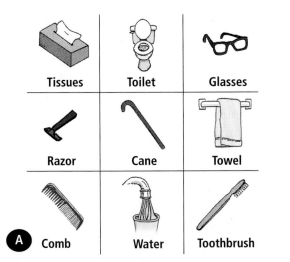

A	B	C	D	E
F	G	H	I	J
K	L	M	N	O
P	Q	R	S	T
U	V	W	X	Y
Z	END OF WORD	PERIOD .	YES	NO
1	2	3	4	5
6	7	8	9	0

21-3 Communications charts. **A,** A picture communication chart.
B, An alphabet communication chart.

Performing ADL

- Follow the care plan; encourage the client to become as independent as possible.
- Use assistive devices, for example, special toothbrushes, combs, soap-on-a-rope, as directed by occupational and physical therapists.
- Promote mobility through range of motion exercises and ambulation, if possible.
- Change position every two hours and check skin for injury; client should not lie on affected side any longer than one hour.
- Do not pull on or use affected limb when lifting or moving client.
- Apply sling or elevate paralyzed arm according to care plan and directions of physical therapist.
- Watch for swelling, discoloration, and pain in affected limb.
- Schedule rest periods between activities; these clients tire easily.
- Take to bathroom for elimination, if possible; a raised seat will make it easier for the client to use the toilet; a commode may also be used; clothing that is easy to get off will help to prevent accidents; see Chapter 14 for additional information on elimination.

Maintaining Good Nutrition

- Remind client to follow speech therapist's instructions about proper swallowing techniques.
- Feed client from the unaffected side; see Procedure 8-1, Feeding the Client.
- Check the paralyzed side of the mouth to make sure no food is "pocketed" inside the cheek.
- Encourage client to self-feed when possible.
- Use assistive devices when needed.

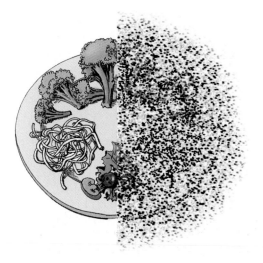

21-4 The client may only see half of the plate.

- Rotate plate so client can see and eat all of the food; clients with perception problems may only see half the food on the plate. (Fig. 21-4)
- Feed slowly and watch for aspiration of food and choking; know how to perform abdominal thrusts (Heimlich maneuver); see Chapter 23.
- Follow suggestions in Table 8-13 for clients with difficulty chewing and swallowing.

Handling Behaviors

- Be patient with your client; follow the suggestions found in Chapter 5, Working with the Ill and Disabled.

Assisting with Special Procedures

- Follow the care plan for special procedures to improve mobility, including: turning, positioning, range of motion exercises, and ambulation with or without assistive devices.
- Assist client to take medications according to schedule.
- Take blood pressure and pulse according to care plan.

Watch for...and Report

- Problems eating and swallowing
- Incontinence
- Constipation
- Skin changes
- Complaints of pain
- Depression
- Signs of infection

Chronic Obstructive Pulmonary Disease (COPD)

Definition

COPD is a term used to describe a group of chronic diseases (adult asthma, chronic bronchitis and emphysema) that causes the client to have difficulty inhaling and/or exhaling air from the lungs. Usually there are permanent physical changes in the lungs and alveoli.

The Facts

COPD affects about one in 14 persons over the age of 45. Smoking, lengthy exposure to air pollutants, and chronic irritation from dust and fumes in the workplace are factors that contribute to COPD.

Symptoms

Home care clients may show the following symptoms:

- difficulty breathing when performing ADL and even when resting (in the later stages of the illness)
- breathes through the mouth

pursed lips
lips positioned for whistling.

- inhaling is not as difficult as exhaling; may have **pursed lips** (Fig. 21-5) in an effort to force out air that is trapped in the lungs
- bluish color of lips, nail beds, and skin
- cough due to thick hard plugs of mucus in lungs that are difficult to expel
- "barrel chest" because of an enlarged rib cage
- fatigue—most of the energy is taken just to breathe
- wheezing

Your Role
Communicating

- Use calm, reassuring approach.
- Follow guidelines listed in Chapter 2 if client is hearing or visually impaired.
- Be patient; do not cut off conversation if client has difficulty talking and breathing, too; practice your active listening skills.

Maintaining a Safe Environment

- Use safety precautions when clients receive oxygen; follow safety guidelines listed in Chapter 17.
- Reduce the amount of dust in the air by damp dusting, especially in the client's bedroom; keep this room as dust-free as possible.
- Eliminate household odors from cleaning products by opening window after use, when possible; environment should be free of aerosol sprays, perfume sprays, etc.
- Teach client proper way to dispose of used tissues containing sputum.
- Use universal precautions when handling used tissues.
- Protect client from visitors who have respiratory infections.

Performing ADL

- Assist client to perform ADL according to instructions given by occupational therapist or care plan.
- Help client to maintain comfortable sleeping or resting position (Fig. 21-6).
- Follow guidelines in Box 21-1 for assisting clients with low energy levels.

Maintaining Good Nutrition

- Encourage increased fluid intake to help in coughing up sputum, according to care plan.
- Provide small, frequent meals—eating takes energy!
- Avoid gas-forming foods.
- Avoid milk—it tends to thicken mucous secretions and makes coughing up sputum even more difficult.
- Follow guidelines in Boxes 8-6, 8-7, and 8-8 for ways to help your client maintain good nutrition.

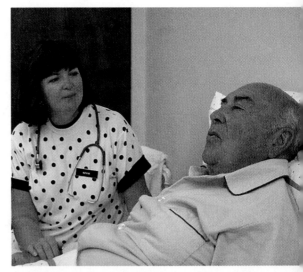

21-5 The client exhales through pursed lips.

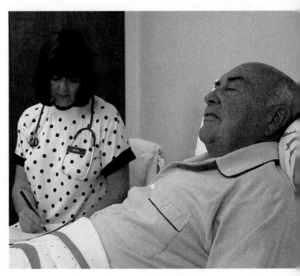

21-6 The client sleeps best in an upright position.

Assisting with Special Procedures

- Help client to practice techniques to control the feeling of panic during coughing episodes; these techniques have been taught by the professional nurse or respiratory therapist and may be listed in the care plan.
- Support and encourage the client to use correct breathing and coughing techniques as taught by the respiratory therapist; if unsure of the technique, notify your supervisor for help.
- Assist client, as needed, to take medications orally or by means of metered dose inhalers (see Procedure 17-5).

Watch for... and Report

- Signs of infection
- Increase in panic attacks
- Severe difficulties in performing ADL
- Signs of depression

Diabetes

Definition

Diabetes mellitus is a chronic illness in which the pancreas is unable to produce enough (or any) insulin to meet the body's needs for carbohydrate, fat, and protein metabolism. There are two types of diabetes:

- Insulin-dependent diabetes mellitus (IDDM)—clients take insulin daily.
- Non-insulin-dependent diabetes mellitus (NIDDM)—clients do not take insulin but control the diabetes with a proper diet and oral medications; this type of diabetes usually occurs after age 40.

The Facts

About 14 million Americans have diabetes. They are two to six times more likely to have a heart attack or stroke than those who are not diabetics. More than 50% of diabetics have high blood pressure, and they are prone to many other problems, such as: nerve damage (especially in hands and feet), blindness, leg and foot ulcers, kidney failure, impotence, infection, and poor healing. The disease is more common in Native Americans, African Americans, Hispanics, and Asian Americans than whites.

Symptoms

The symptoms vary according to the type of diabetes. Those who are already diagnosed and receiving treatment should have few disease symptoms. However, long-term effects of the disease may lead to serious problems, such as stroke, heart disease, leg ulcers, or amputation.

Your Role

Many times you will be caring for the client because of another condition—stroke, fracture, amputation. But, he/she is also a diabetic and requires special care.

Maintaining a Safe Environment

- Protect the client from injury; sense of touch may be missing in hands and feet; burns or injuries may not be felt.
- Shoes or hard-soled slippers should be worn when walking; inspect ankles and feet (between and under toes) for changes in the appearance of the skin; report abnormal findings; prompt treatment is essential to prevent infection and permanent damage to the tissues.
- Be alert for signs and symptoms of infection (see Box 9-1).
- Dispose of used insulin syringes properly (see Chapter 9).

Performing ADL

- Assist client to perform activities of daily living according to the care plan.

Maintaining Good Nutrition

- The proper diabetic diet is prescribed for each client (see Chapter 8).
- Be sure the client eats the entire meal, no more and no less; if the client does not eat the entire meal, notify your supervisor.

Assisting With Special Procedures

- Assist client to take blood sugar level and record in daily diary (see Chapter 17).
- Weigh client according to care plan.
- Assist client to take medications according to care plan.
- Be alert for signs of low blood sugar (Box 21-3)—THIS IS AN EMERGENCY SITUATION—if client is able to swallow, give 4 ounces (120 ml) of orange juice and notify your supervisor immediately; follow instructions; client should feel better within a short amount of time; if no improvement, call supervisor; if client is unable to swallow, phone 9-1-1 or your local emergency number immediately; then call your supervisor.

Watch for…and Report

- Nausea and vomiting
- Excessive thirst
- Fruity odor to breath
- Rapid breathing
- Confusion
- Diarrhea
- Extreme fatigue
- Signs of low blood sugar
- Not eating meals
- Sores on skin

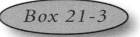

Box 21-3

Signs of Low Blood Sugar
(Sometimes called "insulin reaction")

Early signs include:

- Faintness
- Sudden weakness
- Excessive perspiration
- Irritability
- Hunger—"empty feeling" in stomach
- Palpitations
- Trembling
- Headache

Other signs:

- Confusion
- Slurred speech
- Blurred vision
- Difficulty walking

If untreated, may progress to loss of consciousness and seizures.

Treatment:

- If client can swallow, give 4 oz (120 ml) of orange juice; notify supervisor.
- If unable to swallow, notify Emergency Medical Services.

Alzheimer's Disease

Definition

Alzheimer's disease is a progressive, currently not treatable, and fatal disease that results from the gradual destruction of brain cells.

The Facts

It is the fourth leading cause of death in older adults. More than four million Americans are affected. It is <u>not</u> a normal result of aging.

Client Behaviors

There is no "typical" client with Alzheimer's disease. Symptoms and behaviors vary. As the disease progresses through various stages, the client loses more and more control over the ability to function mentally and physically. Families will often tell you how difficult it is to see their loved one change in personality and in ability to care for himself/herself and be helpless to reverse the changes. Some health care professionals say that the family is the real victim of the disease; the client may not be aware of the devastating mental and physical changes that are occurring.

The following are behaviors you may observe in your client:

- *Speech*—slow, hesitant; difficulty completing a sentence; loses train of thought; struggles to use simple words; uses inappropriate words
- Confused about time and place
- *Changes in mood*—may have rapid mood swings; for example, may be calm, then have outbursts of anger, for no apparent reason
- Personality changes—may be anxious, agitated, aggressive, abusive, or be in a depressed state, suspicious, or show inappropriate or annoying behavior
- Difficulty thinking through a situation or reasoning; unable to make decisions
- *Difficulty in performing ADL*—forgets how to dress, toilet, and groom self
- Difficulty remembering family members and location of key areas of the home (bathroom, kitchen, bedroom)
- *Wandering*—particularly in late afternoon and evening

Your Role

The needs of each client will vary according to how the disease is advancing and the types of behaviors the client shows. Follow the care plan carefully and note any changes in the client's physical and mental condition. The following are some general rules when caring for your client:

Communicating

- Speak slowly.
- Use simple words in short sentences.
- Repeat instructions as often as needed.
- Do not change topics suddenly.

- Follow information in Chapter 2 on communicating with hearing-impaired clients (while the client may not be hearing impaired, the same principles apply).
- Place signs on doors to identify the bedroom, bathroom, and other rooms frequently used; a drawing on the signs may help (Fig. 21-7).
- Wear name tag with title to help client remember; family members may also wish to wear name tags such as "Betty—Daughter" or "Bob—Husband."
- Client should wear a bracelet engraved with the words **Memory Impaired** that includes client's name, address, and phone number (Fig. 21-8); this will help to identify the client who may wander from the home.

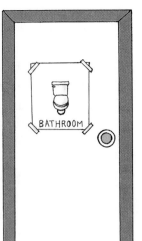

21-7 Labels help Alzheimer's clients to identify rooms.

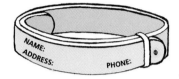

21-8 Wandering clients should wear identification bracelets.

Maintaining a Safe Environment

- Follow guidelines on safety for confused clients in Chapter 20.
- Lock doors to unsafe areas (garage, basement, etc.).
- Keep doors to outside locked.
- Do not rearrange furniture; it may cause more anxiety and possible injury from tripping or falls.
- Place plastic bags out of reach—may cause choking or suffocation.
- Remove artificial fruits, vegetables, or food-shaped kitchen magnets—client may try to eat them (Fig. 21-9); also, remove items such as coins, safety pins, and other small objects—the client may confuse them with things to eat.
- Cover thermostat so client cannot reach the controls to raise or lower the temperature of the home.
- Remove control knobs from the stove.
- Unplug appliances when not in use.

Performing ADL

- Be alert for signs that client needs help to perform ADL.
- Assist client only when needed or when client shows signs of frustration.
- Do not rush—provide ample time for the activity.
- Divide an activity into steps that are easy to follow.
- Take one step at a time and talk the client through each step.
  Example:
  1. Pick up the spoon.
  2. Put pudding on the spoon.
  3. Bring the spoon up to your mouth.
  4. Open your mouth.

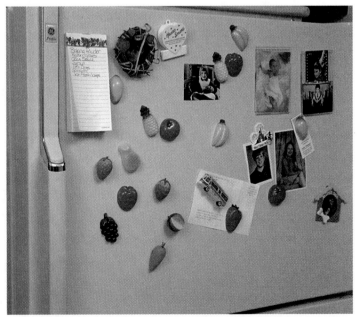

21-9 Artificial "food magnets" may be confusing to the Alzheimer's client.

- Encourage and praise accomplishments.
- Do not force client to perform the activity; if resistive, complete task yourself, if possible; you may need to return later to perform the activity when the client is calmer.
- Be alert for signs that client needs to use the bathroom (restlessness); the care plan may include a toileting routine.
- Lay out clothes in the order they are to be put on; clothing should be easy to put on and remove.

Maintaining Good Nutrition

- Provide extra time for eating.
- Encourage self-feeding—provide finger foods that client can handle easily.
- Offer foods high in protein and complex carbohydrates for between-meal snacks, as indicated on the care plan.
- Give reminders on how to use utensils, if needed.
- Remind client to chew food slowly.
- Remind client to swallow food.
- Serve foods and liquids that are not too hot or too cold to avoid burns.
- Avoid possible confusion and frustration by:
  - reducing the number of food choices
  - placing one utensil and one food in front of the client at a time
  - using unbreakable plates and cups, if available.
- Do not be concerned about poor table manners—give praise for attempts to feed self.

Handling Behaviors

- See Chapter 20 for ways of handling behaviors such as aggression, sexual acting out, anxiety, delusions, and hallucinations.

Wandering

- Approach calmly, walk with client and gradually guide back, if client is found wandering outside the home.
- Distract client by offering a favorite snack or drink.
- Remain calm—do not use physical force or startle client.

Hiding Objects/Suspiciousness

- Determine favorite hiding places (under bed, between chair cushions, under pillows); the care plan may provide this information.
- Ask caregiver to remove valuables and lock them securely.
- Offer to help find missing item (check favorite hiding places first).
- Do not argue with client.
- Do not whisper; it just reinforces the client's suspicions.

Watch for...and Report

- Changes in confusion or wandering
- Changes in ability to perform ADL and to communicate
- Signs of infection
- Refusal to take medications

remission(s)
partial or complete disappearance of symptoms of illness or disease.

exacerbation(s)
return of symptoms of illness or disease following a remission.

Needs of the Informal Caregiver

The day-to-day responsibilities of caring for the person with Alzheimer's disease can affect the caregiver in a variety of ways. It is not unusual for him/her to experience feelings of helplessness, frustration, and anger. For many caregivers, the home care aide's visits may be the only contact with someone they can talk to and express these emotions. Take the time to listen to your client's caregiver and to express your understanding of the difficult situation they are handling each day. Caregivers also appreciate words of praise for doing a good job!

Multiple Sclerosis

Definition

Multiple sclerosis is a chronic, slowly progressing disease of the central nervous system causing changes in the brain and spinal cord.

The Facts

Multiple sclerosis is a major cause of chronic disability in young adults.

Symptoms

The symptoms of multiple sclerosis vary widely and may change almost daily. The disease is characterized by **remissions** and **exacerbations** of the symptoms, which include:

- weakness, paralysis, poor coordination
- stiffness or fatigue of a limb
- walking problems: staggering, falling, inability to walk
- visual disturbances: blurred vision, double vision, dark spots in front of the eyes
- incontinence of bowels and bladder
- mood swings, depression, irritability

Your Role

Activities of daily living present the most problems and challenges for the client. Some clients will be able to perform self-care within the limits of the disease, while others may be totally disabled and unable to perform any self-care.

Communicating

- Use large print written materials for clients with visual problems.
- Follow the suggestions for communication with hearing impaired in Chapter 2 when ringing in the ears may interfere with hearing.

Maintaining a Safe Environment

- Encourage client to use assistive devices when walking.
- Remove any hazards in the home.
- Be alert for signs of infection; the risk of infection is always present.

Performing ADL

- Help the client as needed.
- Do not allow him/her to become tired.
- Schedule rest periods.
- Change positions every two hours; range of motion, ambulation, and other exercises will be used to ease stiff muscles.
- Observe output; record intake and output as ordered.
- Watch for constipation; watch for signs of a urinary tract infection—cloudy, foul-smelling urine, fever, pain when voiding.
- Keep skin clean and dry; watch for any sign of skin breakdown.

Maintaining Good Nutrition

- Buy food or prepare meals as indicated in the care plan.
- Offer foods from the entire Food Guide Pyramid; plenty of fluids (3000 ml) and high-fiber foods will help to prevent constipation.

Providing Emotional Support

- Help to maintain independence as much as possible. Mood swings are common and are often produced by fatigue, infection, or physical or emotional stress.
- Understand that clients and their families may grieve the losses caused by this disease. Many clients have low self-image. They may be angry and depressed about what is happening. Counseling services and support groups may be helpful. Some clients will find great comfort from spiritual support.

Assisting With Special Procedures

- Assist client to take medications according to care plan.
- Applications of heat or ice may be ordered to relieve muscle spasm before exercising.
- Use wheelchair and other assistive devices as needed.

Watch for...and Report

- Signs of infection
- Increasing problems with the symptoms
- Severe behavioral and emotional changes
- Elimination problems—urinary retention, constipation, incontinence
- Skin breakdown

Parkinson's Disease

Definition

Parkinson's disease is a chronic, slowly progressing degenerative disease of the central nervous system characterized by stiffness, slowed movements, and **tremors.**

The Facts

Parkinson's disease usually occurs after the age of 50. The total disability that occurs from this disease may take years to develop. Eventually, most clients will require care in a nursing home.

tremors
purposeless, continuous, quick movements of skeletal muscles, especially in the hands.

Symptoms

- Fine tremors of hands
- Rigid muscles
- Slow movements
- Slow speech with a monotonous tone
- Slow, shuffling gait
- Expressionless face
- Drooling

Your Role

Self-care presents the biggest problem for client and family. As the disease progresses, ability to perform ADL is lost, and the client needs more care. An effort is made to help the client maintain the abilities that are present for as long as possible.

Communicating

- Allow plenty of time for clients to answer your questions. Do not rely on their facial expressions to indicate understanding. While it may not appear that your client understands what you are saying, do not be fooled. They do understand but may be very slow in responding. This is due to problems with muscle movement, not with intelligence or brain function.
- Encourage client to perform exercises to strengthen speech and facial muscles as taught by the speech therapist.

Maintaining a Safe Environment

- Remove clutter and hazards that may cause the client to fall.

Performing ADL

- Help the client as needed.
- Use assistive devices for grooming, bathing, and ambulation; clothing should be easy to put on and take off.
- Offer plenty of fluids and fiber in the diet, if possible; this is not always realistic because of chewing problems.
- Observe for constipation.

Maintaining Good Nutrition

- Remember that self-feeding, chewing, and swallowing are complex tasks involving the nerves and muscles (see Box 8-7).
- Offer foods from all levels of the pyramid.
- Use a spoon with a built up handle and a plate guard on the plate, if available; clients with tremors will have great difficulty using a fork or spoon.
- Serve foods that are easy to get to the mouth; avoid peas or other similar foods that are difficult to balance; spilling is common; protect the client's clothing from stains (Fig. 21-10); clients are easily frustrated by spilling and the length of time it takes to eat, chew, and swallow.

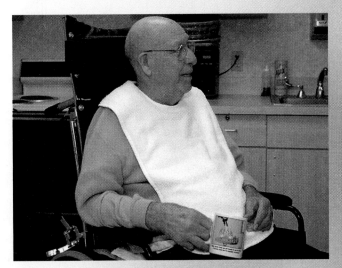

21-10 Protect the client's clothing from spills.

- Provide small, frequent meals, instead of three large meals; they may be easier for the client to eat.
- Give abundant amounts of fluids, as much as 3000 ml a day.
- Encourage client to practice exercises to strengthen muscles used in chewing and swallowing as taught by the speech therapist.
- Use adaptive equipment as ordered by the occupational therapist.

Providing Emotional Support

- Listen to the client and allow him/her to express feelings. Clients express many feelings because of the enormous losses caused by this disease. Anger, frustration, low self-image, hopelessness, and worthlessness are common emotions associated with Parkinson's disease.
- Work with the family and agency staff to find ways to help client cope with problems. Prayer and spiritual support can be uplifting for many of these clients. Regular visits from clergy or church members are welcomed by clients who have participated in religious activities. Support groups and counseling are also beneficial.

Assisting With Special Procedures

- Assist clients to take medications at the proper time; Parkinson's disease is treated with many medications; these do not stop the progress of the illness but do relieve the symptoms.
- Apply heat to reduce rigidity of the muscles, according to the care plan.
- Weigh client according to the care plan.

Watch for...and Report

- Increasing problems with mobility
- Changes in behavior—severe anxiety, depression, withdrawal
- Signs of infection
- Problems with elimination
- Increasing difficulty with eating
- Weight loss

Arthritis

Definition

Arthritis is a group of conditions that damages the joints, cartilage, and connective tissue causing limitation in movement. About 100 different diseases are listed under the category of arthritis. Two common types are:

- *Osteoarthritis (OA)*—a localized, degenerative disease, involving the weight-bearing joints
- *Rheumatoid arthritis (RA)*—a progressive, chronic inflammatory disease that causes joint changes; this is the more serious of the two diseases because other organs (heart, lungs, muscles, eyes) can also be affected.

The Facts

More than 50 million Americans have some type of arthritis; four million are completely dependent. They are unable to work, go to school, play, or carry out many activities of daily living.

Symptoms

Symptoms depend on the degree and the type of arthritis. Some common symptoms include:

- Swelling, redness, tenderness, and chronic pain in the affected area
- Stiffness, especially after being in the same position for a length of time, for example, 30 minutes
- Inability to move the involved joints
- Weight loss
- Difficulty sleeping, moving, and performing ADL
- Chronic fatigue

Your Role

Maintaining a Safe Environment

- Prevent falls and injury.
- Use assistive devices, if needed, for safe ambulation.
- Protect client from infection.

Performing ADL

- Allow client to be as independent as possible. Grooming and hygiene activities may take a long time. Be patient; assist the client only when necessary. Stiffness occurs in the early morning and may take an hour or two to subside. A shower will ease the stiffness and helps to "get the client going."
- Encourage use of assistive devices. Clothing should be easy to put on and take off (Fig. 21-11).
- Assist with range of motion (ROM) exercises to prevent stiffening of joints. Some clients will have painful joints, so be careful when performing ROM exercises. Do not hurt the client.

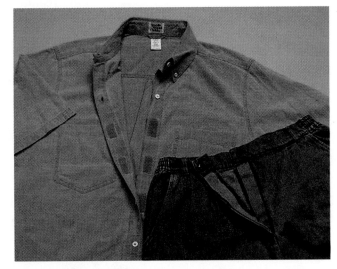

21-11 Clothing with Velcro or snaps makes dressing easier for the client.

Maintaining Good Nutrition

- Use assistive devices for self-feeding.
- Use light-weight cups and glasses; fill to only $1/2$; clients may not be able to lift cups and glasses that are full of liquid.
- Follow instructions from the occupational therapist regarding assistive feeding devices.
- Offer foods from all levels of the pyramid; the client should remain at normal weight.

Providing Emotional Support

- Use listening skills to help client express feelings; clients can become discouraged and disgusted with their condition; it is hard to adjust to the lifestyle changes brought about by arthritis
  NOTE: Clients will say they have "good days" and "bad days." On a good day, a person may do too much because he/she feels good—and pays for that overactivity for many days after. Learning to pace oneself is an important approach to coping with this disease.

Assisting with Special Procedures

- Assist client to take medications as ordered; they are used to relieve inflammation and pain.
- Apply heat and cold, according to the care plan, to relieve pain and stiffness.
- Use positioning devices, such as splints and slings according to the care plan.
- Lift, move, and position client carefully to avoid pain in the joints; it is always best to have the client move himself/herself, even if it takes a long time.

Watch for…and Report

- Increasing pain and immobility
- Signs of infection
- Skin breakdown
- Swelling, redness, and tenderness in a joint
- Severe anxiety and depression

Fractures

Definition

Fractures mean broken bones caused by injury, such as falls, or diseases that weaken bones.

The Facts

Each year, over 200,000 hip fractures occur in older adults, primarily due to falls in the home. Fractures are the leading cause of injury-related disability and death in older adults.

Symptoms

The location of the fracture(s) and the method used to treat the fracture determine the type of symptoms your client may have. For example, the client with a fractured wrist will probably have a cast from the hand and extending to the upper arm. If the cast is on the dominant hand (right hand for right-handed person), the client may have great difficulty feeding himself/herself with the other hand. But, the client who has had surgery to replace a fractured hip will not have difficulty eating because of the injury. However, learning to use a walker and exercising to strengthen the muscles of the injured leg are activities for this type of client.

Sometimes, you may care for a client who has both a fractured wrist and a fractured hip. Sometimes, the client may not return home until he/she is able to bear weight on the wrist and use a walker for support.

Your Role

Caring for a Client with a Cast

Casts, made of fiberglass, are applied by the doctor to a part of the body to keep it immobile. The cast keeps the bones in proper position while healing takes place. The following are important points when caring for your client:

- Keep the cast clean and dry; wash with soap and water, if necessary; do not soak the cast.
- Be careful to avoid wetting the inside edges of the cast; they are difficult to dry and can cause irritation of surrounding skin.
- Cover the cast completely with plastic before assisting client to take a shower, if permitted.
- Discourage client from putting objects into the cast (coat hanger, "back scratcher") to relieve itching of the skin; notify supervisor if client complains of severe itching.
- Observe limb for signs of problems affecting the circulation and nerves (see Box 21-4).

Follow instructions in care plan for:

- Assisting with ADL
- Assisting with exercises or instructing client about exercises to strengthen limb or maintain range of motion, according to physical therapist's directions
- Observing client's ability to use walker correctly (see Chapter 11)
- Assisting with toileting, if needed
- Assisting at mealtime (cut food, butter bread, if wrist is casted)

Caring for a Client Following Surgical Repair of a Fracture

Another way to repair the fracture is by placing pins in the bones to keep them in proper position for healing. Sometimes, the bone is so damaged that it must be replaced with an artificial part. Both procedures require surgery. After the initial postoperative period in the hospital, the client may be transferred to a rehabilitation center or other nursing facility to strengthen injured muscles and learn to perform various activities correctly, such as walking, transfer techniques, and ADL. Before returning home, the home care team may visit the primary caregiver and assess the home environment (see Chapter 1).

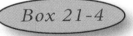

Box 21-4

Check Limb with Cast for...and Report to your Supervisor

- Skin color—white or bluish
- Skin temperature—cool or cold to the touch
- Size—swollen fingers, toes compared with the non-casted limb
- Movement—difficulty or inability to move fingers, toes
- Also report client complaints of
  - pain under the cast
  - pain when moving fingers, toes
  - numbness or tingling in the area

Follow the care plan, which may include:

- Assisting with mobility excercises as instructed by the physical therapist
- Assisting with ADL as instructed by the occupational therapist
- Encouraging client toward independence—assist only when needed
- Observing that client uses correct technique for
  - walker
  - crutches
  - transfers (see Chapter 11)
- Encouraging rest periods so client does not become fatigued, resulting in further injury

AIDS

Definition

AIDS (acquired immunodeficiency syndrome) is an infectious, currently incurable disease caused by the HIV (human immunodeficiency virus). It breaks down the body's immune system and, therefore, destroys the body's ability to fight infection and illness. Not all persons with HIV will develop AIDS, but all AIDS victims have the HIV.

The Facts

About 1.5 million people in the United States are infected with HIV. HIV is transmitted in several ways: having sex (homosexual or heterosexual) with someone who has HIV; sharing needles or syringes with an illicit drug user who has HIV; passing HIV from infected mother to her infant during pregnancy and/or breast-feeding; coming in contact with infected blood. Unfortunately, there is no vaccine to prevent the HIV infection.

Transmission of HIV

HIV **IS** transmitted from the client's body when the virus, (contained in blood, vaginal secretions, breast milk, bloody urine, feces, or vomitus and other body substances, such as draining wounds), enters the caregiver's body through a break in the skin (open sore, cut).

HIV is **NOT** transmitted from client to the caregiver during routine contact, such as touching, hugging, talking, transporting, bathing, or feeding. See Box 21-5 for myths and realities of AIDS.

When caring for the client with AIDS, it is very important that universal precautions and infection control procedures are followed. See Chapter 9 to review this information.

The Effects of HIV on the Immune System

Clients infected with HIV may have no symptoms for a long period of time. However, the virus is multiplying and begins to affect the body's ability to fight infections and other diseases. The client may eventually show signs of infection, such as fever, fatigue, night sweats, diarrhea, and weight loss. These symptoms show that the body's natural defenses are no longer able to destroy the pathogenic organisms. Blood tests and

Box 21-5

Myths and Realities of AIDS

The following are some myths and realities of the disease:

The Myth	The Reality
1. *Only homosexuals and drug users get AIDS.*	1. Anyone exposed to the HIV is at risk of contracting AIDS; HIV passes from the infected person into the other's bloodstream.
2. *AIDS can be spread by touching, hugging, or being near a person with AIDS.*	2. AIDS is not transmitted through casual contact.
3. *Using public toilets and swimming pools are sources of the virus causing AIDS.*	3. HIV is very fragile and does not survive for long outside the body.
4. *Men are most prone to getting AIDS.*	4. AIDS is the sixth leading cause of death in women age 15–44, and these numbers are rising; 34% of all HIV-infected women contracted HIV through heterosexual contact; the number of HIV-infected infants is rising rapidly.

a physical examination help the doctor to diagnose the client as having AIDS. AIDS is the last stage of this chronic illness.

Your client may have a variety of types of infections that affect many body systems. This is because the damaged immune system is no longer able to fight disease. As a result both common and rare diseases may occur.

Caring for the client with AIDS means:

- using universal precautions to protect him/her from further infection
- using universal precautions to protect yourself from the virus

The Client as a Person

Sometimes, health care workers are so concerned with the proper procedures to take that they lose sight of the client as a person. Regardless of how HIV was acquired, the client is a human being who is living his/her life as fully as possible.

Since AIDS is a chronic illness, clients and their families may have times when they are discouraged and frustrated. Since AIDS is a fatal illness, they may express many emotions, such as fear, anger, and sorrow. AIDS is an illness of many losses, and all concerned are deeply affected.

You can help both client and family to cope with the effects of AIDS by showing, through action and communication, that you:

- accept the client as a person of worth
- accept the family as they are—"family" may be the client's lover or friends
- encourage both client and family to express feelings and emotions
- maintain a positive outlook.

Families may be fearful of touching the loved one, fearing that AIDS is transmitted in this manner. Touching, caressing, and hugging are all ways of expressing tenderness and love. Encourage family members to have contact with the client through these means, if appropriate for their culture.

Sometimes, there may be conflicts between the client and other family members. Each may turn to you to express concerns. Your role includes listening and providing comfort and support. Use your active listening skills. Share with your supervisor your own feelings and concerns about what they tell you.

Some clients will tell you how lonely it is to be homebound. Friends and family may not visit, fearing they will also become infected. Your visit may be the only contact the client has with another person.

Symptoms

There are no "standard" symptoms for the AIDS client. The types of symptoms vary according to the progress of the illness and the types of infection present. Some clients spend most of the day out of bed and may need some help with bathing and dressing. Others are so ill that they are in bed most of the time and require complete care.

Your Role

The client is at high risk for infection. Therefore, every action you take must be toward preventing possible infection. Listed below are some basic principles to follow. Your client's care plan will provide specific tasks to perform.

Communicating

- Follow the guidelines in Chapter 2 if your client is hearing or visually impaired.
- Use non-verbal communication to express your support; touch communicates just as well as words in many situations.
- Contact your supervisor if you believe that the client and/or the family may need more assistance than you are able to give in handling the day-to day problems of coping with AIDS.

Maintaining a Safe Environment

Safety includes using universal precautions when needed; disposing of client's waste according to policy and procedures of your agency; eliminating chances for infection; and maintaining home safety. Some tasks include:

- Keeping living area well ventilated, but avoiding drafts
- Damp dusting client area and keeping it as dust free as possible
- Instructing client about proper technique for coughing into tissues and disposing of them; many clients have pneumonia and cough up a lot of sputum.
- Discouraging persons who have colds or other infections from visiting the client
- Following directions in Chapters 6 and 7 for maintaining a safe, clean environment
- Discouraging client from cleaning birdcages, cat litter boxes, or fish tanks; organisms that live in these areas can easily travel to the client.
- Washing all fruits and vegetables thoroughly
- Washing client's dishes with HOT, soapy water, using gloves; dishes do not have to be separated, unless indicated in the care plan.
- Following rules for universal precautions listed in Box 21-6

Box 21-6

Basic Rules for Universal Precautions

- Wear gloves when there is a chance of being in contact with client's blood, semen, vaginal secretions, mucous membranes or other body fluids.

- Wear gloves when the skin of your hands is broken or irritated.

- Wash hands before applying gloves and immediately after removing gloves.

- Wash hands immediately after being contaminated with blood or other body fluids.

- Clean up blood or body fluid spills immediately with bleach and water solution (1:10); remember to prepare solution daily.

- Do not handle used "sharps," such as needles.

- Ask client to place used "sharps" in puncture-resistant container or Biohazard Needle Box container provided by your agency or community.

- Wear personal protective equipment as required by your agency.

- Avoid splashing when disposing of contents of bedpan, urinal, or commode; if splashing occurs, clean area immediately.

- Wear gloves when disposing of soiled sanitary napkins or tampons.

- Do not eat, drink, apply cosmetics, or handle contact lenses in areas where exposure to blood or other potentially infectious materials is possible.

Performing ADL

The amount of assistance required depends on the condition of the client. Fatigue is usually a common complaint. Follow directions previously given in Box 21-1. Other tasks include:

- Using special care when performing oral hygiene, if the client has sores in the mouth, on the tongue or lips, or bleeding gums; be gentle, wear gloves, and follow directions given for cancer clients who have similar problems; the care plan may require the use of special medicated mouthwashes.
- Observing the skin for reddened areas or signs of skin breakdown—record and report.
- Encouraging good personal hygiene and grooming—assist as necessary
- Following directions in the care plan for handling episodes of diarrhea, a common problem; wear gloves when washing anal area; when removing fecal material from clothing, bed linen; and when washing soiled materials.

Maintaining Proper Nutrition

One of the major symptoms of AIDS is loss of weight. As the illness progresses, clients lose a lot of weight. This is called wasting. Serving nutritious meals that the client will eat is a real challenge for the home care aide. Serving high-calorie supplements between meals may be ordered by the doctor. Listed below are some additional guidelines to follow:

- Avoid serving foods with high acid content (citrus, pineapple, tomatoes) for clients with sore mouths.
- Avoid serving foods containing raw eggs because of risk for infection.
- Encourage fluids, especially during episodes of diarrhea, to prevent dehydration.
- Boil tap water, according to directions in the care plan.
- Follow directions in Chapter 8 for clients who have nutrition problems caused by fatigue, difficulty swallowing, etc.
- Prepare and store food properly—wash fresh fruits and vegetables thoroughly—refrigerate leftovers immediately; see Chapter 8 for other directions to reduce the chance of infection from foods.
- Follow guidelines in Box 8-6 and 8-8.

Other Procedures

Your client may be receiving other treatments to handle a variety of problems, such as:

- oxygen—for difficulty breathing
- intravenous fluids—for dehydration
- intravenous medications—for infections
- intravenous nutrition—for problems with nutrition

Follow the directions listed in Chapter 17 for caring for clients receiving these treatments.

surgical incision(s)
a cut produced during surgery that creates an opening into an organ or space in the body.

wound
physical injury causing a break in the skin during surgery or an accident.

Caring for clients with AIDS requires the home care aide to use all the knowledge learned in this program to give proper care. The care plan will give specific information to help you to give appropriate care to meet the client's needs. Unfortunately, the client will eventually develop an infection or disease that he/she can no longer fight. During this end stage of the illness, follow the information in the next chapter about caring for the client who is dying.

Watch for...and Report

- Reddened areas on skin or skin breakdown
- Signs of infection
- Coughing, difficulty breathing
- Inability or failure to drink fluids or eat meals
- Unusual vaginal discharge
- Severe diarrhea
- Skin changes—sores, draining wounds
- Decreased urinary output
- Confusion, changes in vision and hearing

The Postoperative Client

Definition

The term **postoperative** refers to the time following surgery.

The Facts

Some clients come home the day of surgery or the next day. Depending upon the type of operation, some people may be hospitalized for several days or weeks.

Your Role

Home care aides may care for postoperative clients. Your role depends on:

- type of operation
- condition of client
- type of care needed

Always follow the care plan.

Maintaining a Safe Environment

- Protect client from falls.
- Support client when ambulating.
- The **surgical incision** is an opening in the skin, the body's first line of defense against infection; nursing staff will change dressings and empty surgical drainage devices.
- Protect client from **wound** infection.
- Report fever, pain in incision, and foul-smelling drainage on dressings.
- Practice universal precautions; do not handle anything stained with body drainage without wearing gloves.
- Wash hands according to principles in Chapter 9.

incentive spirometer
instrument that is used to encourage the client to breathe deeply and correctly.

- Teach client to wash hands at appropriate times.
- Protect from infections of the respiratory tract by encouraging deep breathing, coughing (see Procedure 21-1), moving, turning, and ambulation.
- Encourage client to use **incentive spirometer** (Fig. 21-13) according to the care plan.
- Discourage visitors with respiratory infections.

Procedure 21-1

Assisting Postoperative Clients to Deep Breathe and Cough

Deep breathing

1. Explain what you are going to do.
2. Provide privacy.
3. Assist client into sitting position.
4. Have client place hands over lower end of rib cage with tips of third fingers just touching each other.
5. Instruct client to deep breathe by:
   a. Exhaling until the ribs move down as far as possible.
   b. Breathe in through the nose as deeply as possible. Client will be able to feel fingers separate during inhalation.
   c. Hold the breath for a count of three.
   d. Exhale slowly through pursed lips until the ribs move as far down as possible.
6. Repeat according to care plan, usually every one to two hours while awake.

NOTE: An incentive spirometer is often used to assist clients with deep breathing. Follow instructions from your supervisor.

Coughing

1. Explain what you are going to do.
2. Ask client to place interlaced fingers or a small pillow over the incision (chest or abdomen) (Fig. 21-12A and B).
3. Have client take two deep breaths (as above).
4. Tell client to take another deep breath, hold it for a count of three, and then cough twice with the mouth open.
5. Repeat according to care plan, usually two or three coughs per hour.

CAUTION: Stand away from client. Do not let client cough on you. If client's hands are free, mouth should be covered with a tissue. Any sputum produced is coughed into tissue and discarded by client into waste container. If you are handling soiled tissues, wear gloves. If client is coughing on you, wear a mask.

Record what you have done. Report any abnormal observations.

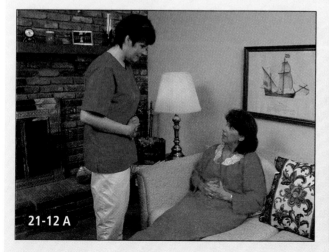

21-12 A

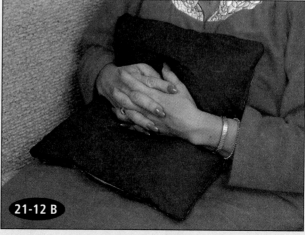

21-12 B

Performing ADL

- Assist as necessary; encourage movement and independence as permitted; most clients will be permitted to ambulate.
- Change position every two hours and carry out range of motion exercises, if bed rest is ordered; leg exercises help to prevent formation of blood clots.
- Check output; be alert for constipation.

Maintaining Good Nutrition

- Offer fluids regularly.
- Follow special diet according to care plan.
- Use suggestions in Box 8-6 for loss of appetite, which is a common postoperative problem.

Providing Emotional Support

- Encourage clients to try to move and become more independent.
- Follow suggestions in Chapter 5, Working with the Ill and Disabled.

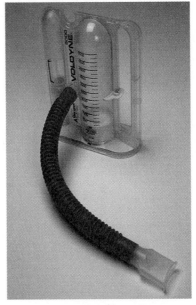

21-13 An incentive spirometer.

Special Procedures

- Assist with medications at the correct time.
- Reinforce dressings as necessary.
- Apply elastic stockings or bandages as directed.

Watch for...and Report

- Signs of infection
  - fever
  - foul-smelling drainage
  - coughing up sputum
- Fresh blood on dressings
- Nausea and vomiting
- Constipation
- Pain in chest and/or difficulty breathing
- Leg pain—especially in calf muscles

Caring for a Client with a Prosthesis

Definition

A prosthesis is a mechanical device used to replace a part of the body that has been surgically removed (amputated) because of disease or injury. Sometimes a prosthesis replaces a part that is deformed due to a birth defect. Prostheses are specially made to fit the client by a specialist, called a prosthetist. Plastic, metal, and wood are some materials used to make a prosthesis.

The Facts

Prostheses are very expensive. One that replaces an upper and lower leg may cost over $15,000. Cardiovascular problems and diabetes are two of the most frequent causes of amputation. More than 75% of lower-limb amputees are over 60 years of age.

Symptoms

Your client returns home after an initial period of time in the hospital recovering from surgery that may have been followed by a stay in a rehabilitation center. Learning to adjust physically and emotionally to the loss of a limb can be a long, difficult process. Clients may mourn their loss in silence or express their feelings verbally or non-verbally. It is not unusual for them to be sad during this period of adjustment.

Some clients will tell you about pain, tingling, or numbness in the missing limb. This is called "phantom limb pain" and is due to changes in the region of the brain that once controlled the function of the now-missing limb. These feelings are real and should not be viewed by others as "silly" or "crazy." Medical researchers are experimenting with ways to eliminate these symptoms.

Your Role

While at the rehabilitation center, the client learns to apply and remove the prosthesis. If a part of the arm or leg is amputated, the prosthesis fits over the stump. A stockinette covers the stump to protect the skin. Learning the proper care and maintenance of the prosthesis is very important for both client and caregiver. The physical therapist instructs the client about exercises to perform so that the remaining muscles of the limb remain strong. The occupational therapist teaches the client to perform ADL using the prosthesis.

Your role in assisting the client may include:

- placing the prosthesis near the client so that it can be reached
- assisting the client to put on or remove the prosthesis, if necessary; check the condition of the stump; note any signs of pressure, such as redness, bluish color, bruising, or skin breakdown.
- storing the prosthesis properly after the client has removed it
- washing and drying the stockinette, if the client is unable to perform this activity; wash with mild soap and water; rinse well before drying; store stockinette in the proper location
- noting any complaints, such as pain or discomfort in the stump or other areas.
- recording and reporting complaints and signs of pressure to your supervisor

Support Groups

Many communities sponsor support groups to assist clients and caregivers to cope with the day-to-day aspects of living with the illnesses described in this chapter. These groups, usually led by a health professional and/or counselor, provide the chance for members to share their experiences; discuss ways to handle typical problems; and express feelings and concerns. Through participating in support groups, clients and caregivers say that they receive encouragement and renewed strength to cope with the limitations of the illness.

Sponsors of support groups include local hospitals and medical and rehabilitation centers. Local chapters of national organizations, such as the Alzheimer's Association, American Lung Association, American Heart Association, and the American Cancer Society, also sponsor support groups. Information about where and when the groups meet can be obtained by telephoning the sponsoring agency or association.

CHAPTER SUMMARY

The home care aide cares for clients with many conditions.

- Frequently seen conditions are:
  - cardiovascular diseases
  - cancer
  - stroke (CVA)
  - chronic obstructive pulmonary disease (COPD)
  - diabetes
  - Alzheimer's disease
  - multiple sclerosis
  - Parkinson's disease
  - arthritis
  - fractures
  - AIDS
  - amputation with prosthesis
- Your role includes:
  - communicating with client and family
  - maintaining a safe environment
  - performing ADL
  - maintaining good nutrition
  - assisting with special procedures
- Clients returning after surgery require special care. The home care aide watches for and reports abnormal signs and symptoms.
- Support groups provide caregivers and clients with the opportunity to:
  - share experiences
  - express feelings and concerns
  - discuss ways to cope with the day-to-day aspects of living with the illness
- Home care aides provide emotional support to clients and family members coping with illness.
- Universal precautions and infection control practices are essential in the care of all clients.

STUDY QUESTIONS

1. Select six conditions described in this chapter and give two ways in which you will:
   a. communicate with the client
   b. maintain a safe environment
   c. perform ADL
   d. maintain good nutrition
   Also, list three observations to report to your supervisor (Watch for...and Report).

2. Describe the care of a postoperative client. What will you watch for and report to your supervisor?

3. Identify a support group in your community. Where does it meet? How often? What are its purposes?

4. List two ways the home care aide can provide emotional support for the client (or family) with:
   a. AIDS
   b. Alzheimer's disease
   c. stroke
   d. cancer
   e. multiple sclerosis
   f. amputation
   e. cardiovascular disease

5. Discuss how you will use the principles of universal precautions and infection control when caring for clients with:
   a. COPD
   b. AIDS
   c. diabetes
   d. cancer
   e. Parkinson's disease
   f. arthritis
   g. surgical wounds

Caring for the Dying Client

22

Objectives

After you read this chapter, you will be able to:

1. Recognize your own feelings about death and dying.

2. Discuss the emotional reactions of clients and their families to a terminal illness.

3. Define the terms: living will, durable power of attorney, DNR (do not resuscitate).

4. Understand the hospice approach to caring for clients who have a terminal illness.

5. Explain how the home care aide meets the physical, emotional, social, and spiritual needs of the dying client.

6. Identify the signs of approaching death and the signs of death.

7. Give postmortem care.

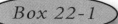

Attitudes About Death

- When did you first learn about death?
- Who died?
- Who told you about death?
- What feelings do you remember?
- What did you do about those feelings?
- Did you attend the funeral/memorial service/burial?
- What are some fears that a dying person may have?

At some time during your career as a home care aide, you may be assigned the care of a client who will not recover from his/her illness. This client is said to have a **terminal illness** or **end-stage disease.** No matter which term is used, the client is expected to die from this particular disease process.

You may feel uncomfortable being around a person who is dying. You may not know what to say or do for this client. Because of your own attitudes about death and dying, you may avoid being with your client. This behavior, of course, causes the client to feel abandoned, rejected, and isolated. It is important for you to examine and understand your own feelings about death (See Box 22-1). These are attitudes that we learned from family members and may change as we grow older. Religious and cultural influences affect our attitudes about death. Some people believe that death is the end of everything; others believe in an eternal afterlife, where the good are rewarded and the evil are punished; some others may believe in reincarnation into a new life or life form. Whatever your attitudes or beliefs, the fact remains that we all will die. Humans do not live forever.

Most clients are told that they are dying. This is done by the physician or a family member. Sometimes, the family does <u>not</u> want the client to know that the illness is terminal. In this case, you must follow their wishes. This can be very difficult for you because you may feel as if you are lying to your client. Discuss these feelings and your concerns with your supervisor. Other times, clients find their diagnosis/prognosis by:

- reading their medical records when no one is looking
- overhearing conversations about their condition
- realizing that they are becoming sicker—not better
- recognizing that the treatment is no longer effective and may be stopped.

Emotional Reactions to Death and Dying

The news that one has a fatal illness is overwhelming for the client and family. Dr. Elisabeth Kübler-Ross, a psychiatrist, spent many years working with dying persons. She has described the emotional stages experienced by the dying person (Fig. 22-1). It is important to remember that:

- the stages may overlap
- people may go from one stage to another and then back again
- everyone is different, and not all people will go through each stage
- clients and their families will also experience these stages

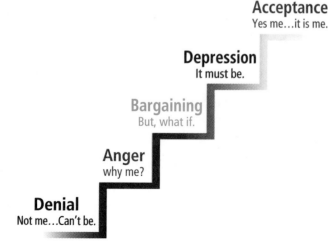

Acceptance
Yes me...it is me.

Depression
It must be.

Bargaining
But, what if.

Anger
why me?

Denial
Not me...Can't be.

22-1 Stages of dying.

Stage 1—Denial

Denial is a defense mechanism that protects the client from unpleasant reality. Understand the client's need to deny what is happening. Partial acceptance may follow. Sometimes, the denial will continue. In this case, do not argue with your client or try to change his/her thinking. Accept the client's behavior and understand the reasons for it.

Stage 2—Anger

The client is angry with everyone, everything—his/her family, you, God. They take their anger out on family, friends, and caregivers. Do not take it personally. They are angry because they are dying; they are not angry at you. Be kind and patient. **Empathy** is important. Use your listening skills.

Stage 3—Bargaining

Bargaining is an attempt to postpone the unavoidable. This mechanism is effective only for a brief period and is often associated with unexpressed guilt. For example, the person may promise God that he/she will do some wonderful thing if God will cause a miracle cure. This is unrealistic and can cause some guilt because the client may feel that he/she could have been a better person.

Stage 4—Depression

The client becomes very sad for many reasons—including the loss of all they love, the loss of self, the loss of opportunity to change, loss of the future. Do not try to cheer up the client. Allow him/her to be sad—it's "OK" to feel this way. It is a part of the preparation for death and final separation from all the client loves.

Stage 5—Acceptance

The client is neither depressed nor angry. The client is just there and seems to have almost no feelings. At this time, the family needs support because the client begins to withdraw from them. Many times family members cannot understand why the client is "giving up" and will not fight the disease any longer. There comes a time when the body is no longer able to fight, no matter what the family wants. Of course, not all clients quietly accept death, close their eyes, and die. Some will fight the illness and continue treatment for as long as possible.

Advance Medical Directives

Advance directives are documents in which a person states choices for medical treatment (or appoints others to make treatment choices) if he/she should lose decision-making ability.

Advance medical directives are:

Living Will
- Written instructions
- Called a living will because it takes effect while the person is still alive

terminal illness
an illness that causes the end of life.

end-stage disease
terminal or final illness.

empathy
understanding the feelings of another.

living will
an advance medical directive that specifies treatment to be given or withheld if a person becomes terminally ill or incapable of making decisions himself/herself.

DNR
an abbreviation for "do not resuscitate," meaning do not artificially restart the heartbeat.

durable power of attorney
an advance medical directive that names another to make health care decisions if a person becomes unable to do so.

hospice
a program of care that helps dying persons live until they die and helps the family live with them.

bereaved
those who mourn the death of a loved one.

- Specifies treatment to be provided or withheld if a person becomes terminally ill and/or incapable of making decisions himself/herself; for example, the document may specify:
  - Organ donation after death—which organs
  - **DNR**—Do Not Resuscitate

Durable Power of Attorney

- Written instructions
- Names another person (called a "proxy") to make health care decisions if the person is unable to do so himself/herself

An advance medical directive can be changed or canceled at any time. It does not go into effect until the time when the client can no longer make or communicate decisions for himself/herself. Loved ones should be included in advance directives discussion and decision making.

The home care agency provides all adult clients with information about their rights under state and federal laws to make health care decisions, including the right to refuse or accept treatment and the right to execute advance directives. This is clearly explained in the Client's Bill of Rights. If you or your client (and family) have any questions concerning advance medical directives, notify your supervisor.

Hospice

Many people who are at home with end-stage disease will be in a **hospice** program. These programs provide physical, emotional, and spiritual care given by a medically supervised team of professionals and volunteers. One of the main goals of hospice care is to help clients live comfortably until they die and to help the family live with them as they are dying. The focus is on caring rather than on curing. All services are provided through the hospice program. As death approaches, there are no calls to 9-1-1 for EMS (Emergency Medical Services). All calls are directed to the hospice. You will direct calls and questions to your supervisor.

Principles of hospice care include:

- providing comfort when cure is no longer possible
- giving care to the whole person and whole family
- placing the client at the CENTER of the team of caregivers (Fig. 22-2)
- offering education, preparation, and support about the natural process of dying
- having a system of care that supports the client and family 24 hours a day, 7 days a week
- supporting the **bereaved** for one year following the client's death

To work in a hospice program is a commitment to be there for the client and family—for the "long haul." They rely on the hospice team, especially

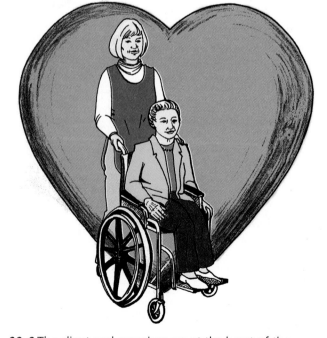

22-2 The client and caregiver are at the heart of the hospice system.

the home care aide, to provide personal care and hygiene for the client. It is almost as if you become a family member; you are "in it" with them. Clients have a great fear of being deserted; don't abandon them. If you will be late for work or absent, notify your supervisor so the family will not worry about you and a substitute can be sent.

Caring for the Dying Client

The following principles are important to remember when caring for clients with end-stage disease.

Help Clients Live Until They Die

- Encourage socialization (Fig. 22-3).
- Use listening skills. Always be honest; you will be asked many questions that you will be unable to answer. Say, "I don't know, but I'll ask my supervisor."
- Help client to finish any unfinished business. For example, Mr. Schmidt wanted to make a quilt for each one of his children. His home care aide gathered all the materials and placing them within his reach so he could complete his work. The aide arranged Mr. Schmidt's schedule so that he would have the energy to do what was important to him.
- Offer your clients some control over their lives. Give them choices regarding routines, foods, activities, etc.
- Promote independence—encourage your client to do as much as possible within his/her ability and energy level.
- Offer comfort and support.

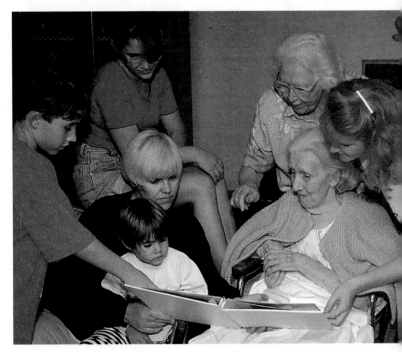

22-3 Encourage socialization for dying clients.

Encourage Hope

- Hope is present throughout all the emotional stages of death and dying.
- Hope keeps the client going through months of suffering; it maintains the spirit and helps people go on.
- Hope changes. Clients hope for a better day tomorrow, a good sleep tonight, less pain.
- All hope for the "miracle" of a complete cure. We all hope for this along with the client and family. While this is not realistic, it is always in the "back of one's mind." Do not discourage the client's hope and demand that he/she be realistic. Research has revealed that people with hope live longer and have a better quality of life than those who are hopeless. If and when acceptance comes, and hope seems to be gone, just listen to your clients and care for their needs. Hope may not be appropriate at this time.

Relieve Pain

rite(s)
formal ritual(s) used in religious or solemn practices.

- Assist clients to take medications as ordered. These are usually taken every four hours (q4h) around the clock, instead of when needed.
- When pain medication is to be taken as needed (prn), clients should take it when the pain begins and not wait until the pain becomes intolerable.
  - Notify your supervisor, if the:
    - medication is not effective in relieving the pain
    - client wants to take more medication than what is prescribed
    - client wants to take the medication more frequently
  - Many prescribed pain medications cause constipation. Observe the bowel movements and report any problems.
  - Keep client's environment as quiet and calm as possible to promote rest and sleep. Music may be soothing and comforting.
  - Good hygiene, a back rub, and clean bed linens also promote comfort and will enhance the effect of the pain-relieving medications (Fig. 22-4).
  - If activity causes pain, provide personal care about an hour after the client takes his/her medication.

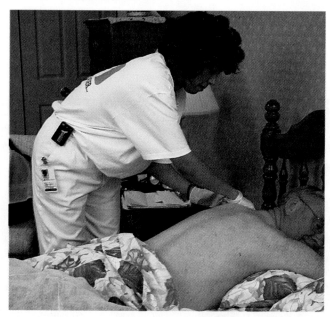

22-4 A back rub can help clients to rest and relax.

Assist with Religious Consolation

- Some clients will find their own relationship with God a strong source of strength at this time. Clients may want you to read scriptures or other religious books to them. Do so.
- Allow time for visits from clergy, chaplain, or others from the client's religious community or from the hospice (Fig. 22-5). Have the client ready for the visit. Whenever possible, schedule personal care and hygiene activities before the visit so the client feels and looks as good as possible.
  - Catholic clients who wish to receive the Sacrament of Reconciliation will need private time alone with the priest. For Sacrament of the Sick, the priest anoints the client with blessed oils and prays for healing. Family members may be present and pray with the priest. For those clients who are receiving Holy Communion (Eucharist), have a glass of water nearby.
  - When a client's religious belief is unfamiliar to you, ask the family or your supervisor to explain the belief and its **rites** to you.
  - If your client does not belong to any specific faith tradition and wants to see a clergyperson, the hospice team will be able to help. Notify your supervisor about your client's need.

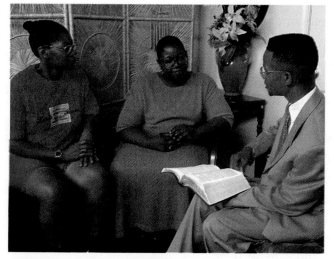

22-5 The chaplain attends to the client's spiritual needs.

- Some clients will not find religion to be a source of help. Recognize that each person has his/her own needs and beliefs that are to be respected.

Provide Good Physical Care

- Meet client needs for grooming, hygiene, and toileting.
- Keep skin clean and dry; change positions and perform range of motion exercises; skin breaks down very quickly; report any skin changes to your supervisor immediately.
- Give mouth care before meals.
- Offer foods from all levels of the pyramid; offer fluids between meals.
- Do not force the client to eat.
- Follow the care plan regarding protein supplements and special preparation of food.
- Feed client as necessary. (See Chapter 8 for further information on feeding clients.)
- As body systems fail, increasing physical care is needed.
- Try to anticipate your client's needs.

Needs of Caregivers

This is a difficult and stressful time for caregivers. Accept their feelings; listen to them; and demonstrate your concern for them. Acknowledge their problems. However, realize that you can't solve all of them. Notify your supervisor when necessary. The hospice will provide assistance when possible.

Needs of the Home Care Aide

Caring for dying people is hard work, both physically and emotionally. You will have many feelings about working with hospice clients. Do not withdraw from your client and caregiver. Discuss your feelings with your supervisor. You may participate in hospice team meetings. Don't be afraid to discuss your feelings and observations with team members. Perhaps you just need to express what you are feeling and know that it's "OK" to feel this way. Perhaps you need some time off or a different assignment. The most important thing is to remember that you have needs, too—so take care of yourself, as well as your client.

Signs of Approaching Death

As death approaches, physical changes can be seen as each system shuts down. Many clients slip into death very much like the way they have fallen asleep during life. Seizures, hemorrhages, and a "death agony" are quite uncommon, although these may happen. If family members are present, let them stay with the client and assist with personal care, if they are able.

The last sense to leave the dying person is hearing. Remember, the client may be able to hear what is going on, even if he/she is unable to respond. Everyone should speak with the client knowing he/she understands and needs to know who is there and what is happening. Holding

expire
die.

postmortem
after death.

the loved one's hand, saying "I'm here," is very comforting. This, too, may be the time to say any last words and good-byes to the dying person.

Common physical changes in the near-to-death client include:

- Circulation is slowed. The pulse becomes rapid and weak, almost impossible to count. The skin becomes cold, especially the arms, legs, hands, feet, and nose. Cover the client with a light blanket and elevate the limbs to return the flow of blood to the heart. A heavy blanket will make the client too warm, and restless from trying to remove the covers. Lips and nail beds may be cyanotic. Oxygen may be given.
- Respirations are slow and shallow until breathing stops. Clients breathe through the mouth. Give oral hygiene frequently. Be careful the client does not aspirate liquids. Moisten and lubricate lips and tissues of the mouth frequently. Breathing may become noisy from mucus in the throat—the so-called "death rattle."
- Incontinence may occur. Keep client clean and dry. Provide good skin care to prevent additional discomfort from skin breakdown.
- Clients become very still. Movement is almost absent. Sensations gradually disappear.
- Appetite and thirst are lost, although some clients awaken from an unconscious state and take tiny sips of fluids.
- Client is usually unconscious.

Death may come quickly, over a period of hours, but, for some persons, the process of active dying may take several days. This is emotionally and physically draining for family and caregivers. You will know that death has occurred when your client has stopped breathing for a few minutes and you cannot feel a pulse. Note the time and call your supervisor.

You may feel very sad that your client has died. You may even cry along with the family and loved ones (Fig. 22-6). This is normal. Home care agencies and hospices hold "support sessions" for staff members whose clients have died. It helps, and it is important to discuss your feelings and experiences when your client **expires.**

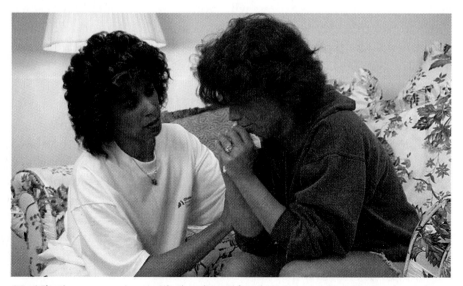

22-6 Sharing your sorrow with the client's family is a normal and natural reaction.

Care After Death

Care of the body after death is called **postmortem** care. Once you have notified your supervisor of the client's death, the doctor and funeral director are notified. Before the funeral director can remove the body, the client must be legally/officially pronounced dead. The procedure for this pronouncement varies from state to state. Your agency will know what to do.

The body is prepared for removal from the home. The caregiver may need some time alone with the client to say the final good-byes. Some specific religious or cultural practices may be followed at this time. Special preparation of the body may be done by the caregiver or others according to religious rites. These should be done only after the legal pronouncement of death. Check with your supervisor concerning religious and cultural practices.

When appropriate, and according to the agency policies, prepare the body in the following manner:

- Place one pillow under the head.
- Bathe the body, if necessary; clean genital area if there has been any incontinence.
- Reinforce dressings if needed (don't forget to wear gloves).
- Close eyes, put dentures in mouth, if possible.
- Keep body flat on back, legs straight, arms folded over the abdomen.
- Follow agency policy regarding jewelry; if taken by family members, be sure to document who took what off the body.
- Do not try to straighten limbs if there are contractures.

After the body is removed from the room, strip the bed and wash the linens, if there is sufficient time. Equipment is removed; rented equipment is returned to the providers. The hospice program arranges to have equipment returned.

You may wish to attend the viewing and funeral of your client. This will give you a chance to say good-bye and to let the family know that you really did care for the client. This is your decision; there is no right or wrong. You must do what is best for you.

CHAPTER SUMMARY

- The home care aide's feelings about death and dying will influence his/her ability to care for dying clients. You may feel uncomfortable caring for dying persons—this is normal.
- Both client and family react to a terminal illness. Typical reactions include:
  - denial
  - anger
  - bargaining
  - depression
  - acceptance
- Advance medical directives are documents in which a person states choices for medical treatment if he/she should lose decision-making ability.
- Hospice is a program that provides total care for dying clients.
- Guidelines for caring for dying persons include:
  - Help client live until he/she dies.
  - Encourage hope.
  - Relieve pain.
  - Assist with religious consolation.
  - Provide good physical care.
- Caring for dying persons is hard work, both emotionally and physically. If you have concerns, questions, and uncomfortable feelings, you are not unusual. Discuss these feelings with your supervisor.
- The home care aide recognizes the signs of approaching death and offers comfort to both client and family.
- Follow agency policy and procedures when the client has died.

STUDY QUESTIONS

1. What are two factors that influence our attitudes about death?
2. How do people find out they have a terminal illness? What are the "typical" emotional reactions?
3. Define the following terms:
   - advance medical directives
   - living will
   - durable power of attorney
   - DNR
   - hospice
4. List five principles to remember when caring for clients with end-stage disease. Explain three ways the home care aide can implement each.
5. List five signs of approaching death.
6. What are the home care aide's responsibilities when the client has died?
7. Discuss appropriate behavior for the home care aide whose client has expired.

Emergencies

Objectives

After you read this chapter, you will be able to:

1. Define the term "emergency."

2. Describe three ways to prepare for medical emergencies.

3. Discuss five rules to follow when there is an emergency.

4. List the information needed to report an emergency by telephone.

5. Describe first aid procedures to follow for four common medical emergencies.

6. Discuss the importance of recording and reporting your actions in an emergency to your employer.

7. Demonstrate the use of universal precautions when giving first aid.

Roger, the home care aide, has just entered the front door of his client's (Marjorie), apartment house when her daughter runs from the elevator screaming and crying. She pulls his arm and leads him into the kitchen of the apartment. Roger finds Marjorie sitting at the table, unable to speak or breathe, with her hands around her neck. Her face is turning blue, but she is conscious. The daughter says that her mother started to choke while eating a piece of meat and then stopped breathing. Roger tells the daughter to call 9-1-1 for help. He immediately performs abdominal thrusts (Heimlich maneuver) to help Marjorie to expel the meat from the trachea and begin to breathe again. The piece of meat is expelled after the second thrust. "You are a miracle worker," says Marjorie. "I thought I would die—you came just in time."

Recognizing an emergency, calling for help, and giving first aid calmly and skillfully are responsibilities of the home care aide.

What is an Emergency?

The term **emergency** is used when the following are present:
- serious situation
- arises suddenly
- threatens the life or welfare of a person or group of persons

Emergencies may be due to accidents (injury to leg due to falling from a ladder), a **medical crisis** (chest pain), or natural disasters (injuries due to a hurricane or tornado).

Each emergency situation requires immediate action. This is called "**first aid.**" It is the immediate care given to the person before treatment by trained medical personnel.

Preparing for Emergencies

Because emergencies arise suddenly, using time wisely is critical. For example, taking time to search for emergency phone numbers so help can be called is not wise. So, planning for emergencies in advance is very important.

Emergency Telephone Numbers

In Chapter 6, Box 6-8 lists telephone numbers to use in case of a household emergency. These numbers also can be used in medical emergencies. Many communities have a 9-1-1 number to contact Emergency Medical Services (EMS). The person answering the phone is called an "emergency dispatcher" who has special training in handling crisis situations over the phone. The dispatcher will ask questions to find out what type of help is needed (police, fire, or medical services). Answer the questions as completely and clearly as possible. The dispatcher will also give directions about what to do while waiting for emergency medical personnel to arrive. **DO NOT HANG UP THE PHONE UNLESS TOLD TO DO SO.** See Box 23-1 for the types of questions you should be prepared to answer.

emergency
a serious situation arising suddenly that threatens the life or welfare of a person(s).

medical crisis
event requiring immediate attention.

first aid
immediate care given before treatment by trained medical personnel.

Box 23-1

Reporting an Emergency

Answer the questions that the dispatcher asks. Typical questions are:

1. What is the exact location or address of the emergency?
   - Give name of town, city, or area, and address
   - Give landmarks, nearest cross streets
   - Give building name, floor, room, or apartment number
   - Give other information that will help in finding the location
2. Where are you calling from?
   - Provide phone number
3. Who are you?
   - Give your name and title
4. What happened? How many people are involved?
   - Give as much information as possible, as briefly as possible
5. What is the condition of the victim(s)?
   - Provide information as requested
6. What first aid is being given?
   - Tell what you are doing

Stay on the phone until you are told to hang up or the dispatcher hangs up.

Knowing What to Do

This chapter gives some common medical emergencies that may occur in the home and other places. However, it does not include all possible emergency situations. You are encouraged to take a first aid course and be certified to perform cardiopulmonary resuscitation (CPR). This is a procedure used to help start breathing and restore the heartbeat. Agencies in your community offer such courses, including the local rescue squad, local chapter of the American Red Cross, or your own home care agency. Being trained in first aid and using these skills in an emergency can mean the difference between life and death for the victim. Being prepared helps to reduce fears and panic that many feel when an emergency occurs. Panic can make a person immobile. The worst thing to do in an emergency is nothing.

Calling for Help

When in doubt, call for help. The following situations require an immediate call for help.

The victim:

- is unconscious
- has no pulse
- is not breathing or has difficulty breathing
- is bleeding severely (Fig. 23-1 on page 436)

Sometimes, the victim may not want you to call for help. But, you must use your judgment. When in doubt about calling for help, **CALL.** In many situations, minutes, even seconds, count in getting the proper care for the person.

When a telephone is not available, you should know where the nearest phone is located. If another person is in the home, ask him/her to make

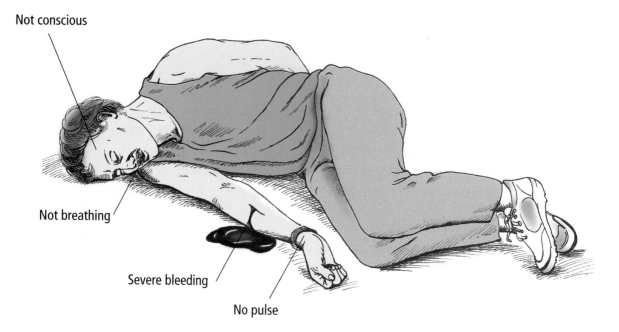

Not conscious

Not breathing

Severe bleeding

No pulse

23-1 Four signs of a life-threatening emergency.

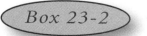

Box 23-2

Important Parts of the First Aid Kit

- Adhesive tape
- Gauze pads and roller gauze
- Scissors and tweezer
- Band-Aids (assorted sizes)
- Antiseptic ointment
- Triangular bandage
- Hand cleaner
- Latex gloves

the call for help. Prepare the person to answer questions about the victim. In this case, your role is to stay with the victim until help arrives. If you are alone and there are neighbors nearby, shout for help.

The First Aid Kit

Having a first aid kit available is another way to prepare for an emergency. A kit should be available to use in the home, automobile, workplace, and other locations (restaurants, boats, etc.). First aid kits may be purchased or assembled. Box 23-2 gives the essential supplies needed.

Guidelines for Handling Emergencies

While each emergency situation is different, listed below are general guidelines to follow (Box 23-3).

- Do not put yourself in danger—check the scene for hazards (live electrical wires, broken stairs).
- Protect yourself from the victim's body fluids (Box 23-4).
- Remain calm and in control; it helps you, and it helps the victim to feel more secure.
- Observe the victim—is he/she conscious? is there a pulse? is there severe bleeding?
- Observe the area—try to find out what happened, what caused the emergency, and how the victim was injured.
- Talk to the victim; reassure him/her and try to find out what happened; bystanders may be able to provide additional information; try to get as much information as possible from the victim and others.
- Explain to the victim what you are doing and that help is being called.

- Call 9-1-1 or your local emergency number.
- Give first aid as needed.
  - Cover victim with blanket, coat, or sweater to maintain body temperature.
  - Do not move a seriously injured victim unless there is an immediate danger (strong odor of gas, fire, flooding); then, move carefully according to the procedures you learned while taking the first aid course; ask the victim not to move—moving can cause additional injury and pain.
  - Do not give any food or fluid.

Bystanders may provide some help to you (according to the situation), such as comforting the victim or other persons involved.

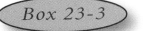

Box 23-3

The Four Cs of Emergency Care

CAUTION   never put yourself in danger.

CHECK   the victim's condition and area where found.

CALL   9-1-1 or your local emergency number; if in doubt, dial 0 for the operator.

CHECK   for the victim until help arrives, using the first aid skills you have learned.

Box 23-4

First Aid Situations that Increase the Home Care Aide's Risk for Infection

Victim is

- bleeding
- vomiting
- coughing up sputum
- incontinent

The Wound is

- bleeding
- weeping fluid
- caused by a bite (animal or insect)
- caused by chemicals

TAKE PRECAUTIONS

- Create a barrier between yourself and any body fluids and/or mucous membranes.
  - use latex or rubber gloves, if available

  or

  - use plastic bag, plastic wrap to cover your hands, if available

  or

  - use sterile dressing, clean dry pad, or clean, dry clothing to cover a wound
- Wash hands thoroughly after giving first aid.

When EMS Personnel Arrive

Your role in caring for the victim ends when emergency personnel arrive. They may ask more questions about the victim or about the first aid you have been giving. Answer the questions accurately and quickly. Time is very important. If they need your assistance, they will ask for help. Otherwise, do not interfere. Remain with other family members to provide comfort and support.

Some home care aides have said that EMS personnel ignored them and did not give them credit for giving first aid. In many cases, this is true. EMS personnel are highly trained to handle all types of emergencies. Their focus is on the victim; giving the necessary emergency care; and transporting him/her to the hospital as quickly as possible. There is usually not much time for them to recognize your contributions to helping the victim.

Reporting to Your Agency

As soon as possible following the emergency, contact your agency and report the following:

- Your name
- Your client's name or name of victim
- The emergency
- Where and when it happened
- What you did (first aid given; called 9-1-1)
- What happened when EMS arrived
- Results (client or victim to hospital?)

Your agency will give you further directions to follow. Remember to record the information listed above in the client's record. Some agencies will ask you to complete and sign an Incident Report. This is a special form used when unusual situations occur, such as emergencies. Your agency will provide you with the form and give you special directions for its completion.

Common Emergencies

The following is a discussion of a few of the more common emergencies you may encounter as a home care aide.

Choking

The airway is blocked by a piece of food or other object (candy, marbles, small pieces of plastic). While common in infants and children, more adults die from choking than children. Choking can result from such activities as trying to swallow large pieces of poorly chewed food; eating too fast; eating while laughing; or running with food or other objects in the mouth.

Partially Blocked Airway The victim is getting enough air in and out of the lungs to cough, make wheezing noises, and may even be able to talk. Encourage the person to continue coughing. If the object is not expelled, call 9-1-1 for help.

Totally Blocked Airway No air can get in or out of the lungs. The victim cannot speak, cough, or breathe, and may turn blue (cyanosis). Sometimes, the person may make high-pitched sounds or cough weakly. He/she usually puts his hand around the throat—a universal sign of choking (Fig. 23-2). This is a very frightening experience for the victim and a life-threatening emergency. ACT AT ONCE.

Action

Have someone call 9-1-1, while you begin to give abdominal thrusts (Heimlich maneuver). This is a series of thrusts to the upper abdomen above the navel and below the ribcage. These thrusts force air out of the lungs and the object is pushed out—like a cork from a champagne bottle. Follow these directions for giving abdominal thrusts:

Directions for Abdominal Thrusts

Victim is Standing or Sitting

1. Stand behind victim and wrap your arms around the victim's waist (Fig. 23-3).
2. Make a fist with one hand and place the thumb side against the middle of the victim's abdomen, just above the navel and below the ribcage (Fig. 23-4).
3. Grab your fist with your other hand and give quick, inward and upward thrusts into the abdomen (Fig. 23-5).
4. Repeat these thrusts until the object is forced out.
   NOTE: If victim is noticeably pregnant or extremely overweight, give chest thrusts. Place your fist against the center of the breastbone. Grab it with your other hand and give quick thrusts into the chest.

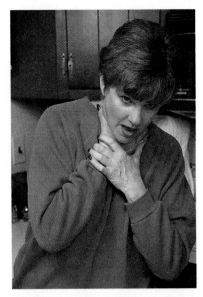

23-2 The universal sign of choking.

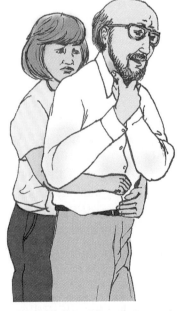

23-3 Stand behind the victim and wrap your arms around the victim's waist.

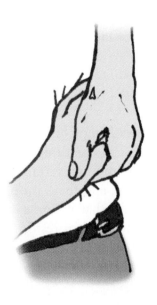

23-4 Make a fist with one hand and place the thumb side against the middle of the victim's abdomen, just above the navel and below the ribcage.

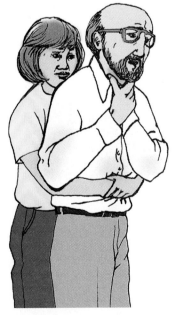

23-5 Grab your fist with your other hand and give quick inward and upward thrusts into the abdomen.

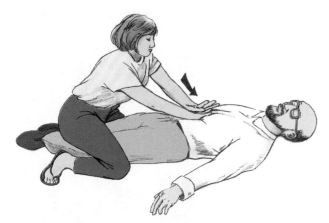

23-6 Straddle the victim's hips.

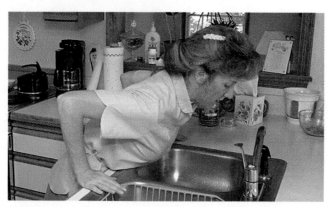

23-7 To give yourself abdominal thrusts, press your abdomen into a firm object, such as a kitchen counter-top.

Victim is Lying Down

1. Position victim on his/her back.
2. Straddle victim's hips, if possible (Fig. 23-6).
3. Place heel of one hand against the middle of the victim's abdomen, between the ribcage and the navel, with fingers pointing toward the victim's chest.
4. Put your other hand on top of the fist.
5. Press into the victim's abdomen with quick upward thrusts until object is expelled.

When You Are Alone and Choking

1. Lean over and press abdomen against a firm object, such as the back of a chair, kitchen sink. Avoid using an object with sharp edges or corners that can cause further injury (Fig. 23-7).
2. Use your hands to give abdominal thrusts as listed above.

No Breathing

When breathing stops, the person will lose consciousness very shortly. If breathing is not restored, the heart stops beating, and blood does not circulate throughout the body. Lack of oxygen to the tissues causes other body systems to fail, leading to death. Breathing must be restored for the person to stay alive.

Action

Rescue breathing is the only way of supplying needed oxygen to the person. Rescue breathing means that another person is breathing air into the victim's lungs to maintain a supply of oxygen. If the victim is not breathing and there is no pulse, CPR must be started. It is highly recommended that all home care aides take a course in CPR to learn the proper techniques for restoring breathing and the heartbeat. If you are certified to give CPR, it is important to keep your skills current.

Bleeding

Bleeding occurs when capillaries and blood vessels are injured. Severe bleeding (hemorrhage) is caused when one or more large blood vessels are involved. If untreated, the victim may die within a short period of time.

rescue breathing
another person breathes air into the victim's lungs to maintain supply of oxygen.

There are two types of bleeding:

- *External*—bleeding is visible and comes from an open wound.
- *Internal*—bleeding occurs inside the body. The location of the bleeding cannot be seen, but the victim's symptoms show that the injury is internal. For example, the victim vomits bright red blood. Sometimes, the vomitus appears like coffee grounds. This means that the gastric juices of the stomach have acted on the blood, making it appear like ground coffee.

When severe bleeding occurs, the person may also show the following signs:

- rapid, weak pulse
- moist, cool skin
- pale or bluish skin
- very thirsty
- swollen, tender, hard areas of the body, such as the abdomen
- confusion, drowsy, or unconscious

Action

Severe bleeding is a medical emergency. Assist the victim to a comfortable position—usually lying down and keep him/her from getting chilled or overheated.

For External Bleeding From an Open Wound

- Put on disposable latex gloves, if available. If not available, place a barrier (dressing, cloth, plastic bag, plastic wrap) between you and the blood.
- Place a clean dressing over the wound and apply direct pressure. If a sterile dressing is not available, use anything that is clean and dry (clean towel, face cloth, shirt, blouse, sock). If dressing becomes soaked with blood, apply another dressing over it and continue to apply pressure. Do not remove the original dressing or peek under the dressing(s) to see if the bleeding has stopped. This could cause blood clots to be dislodged and cause more bleeding.
- If victim can help, ask him/her to apply pressure to the wound.
- Raise the injured area above the level of the heart, if possible. If you suspect that the wound involves a fracture, <u>do not</u> move.
- Apply a bandage snugly over the dressing to keep it in place.
- Wash your hands immediately after giving care.
- Call 9-1-1 for help.
- Do not give food or fluids.

For Signs of Internal Bleeding

- Save specimen containing blood (vomitus, feces, urine, sanitary pad, or other specimen containing blood).
- Wear gloves, if possible, when handling blood. If not available, wash hands immediately after care.
- Call 9-1-1 for help for signs of severe bleeding.
- Do not give food or fluids.

Shock

Shock is a condition where the circulatory system is not able to transport adequate amounts of blood to all parts of the body. Some causes of shock include: severe bleeding, electrical shock (victim is in contact with live electrical wires), serious body injury, severe burn, allergic reaction, and emotional reaction to sudden illness. Shock can also be caused by an insulin reaction (see Chapter 21).

Signs of shock include:

- weak, rapid pulse
- shallow, irregular, labored breathing
- cold, clammy skin
- paleness in light-skinned persons; grayish in dark-skinned persons
- restlessness
- dazed look—eyes dull and pupils wide
- may be confused

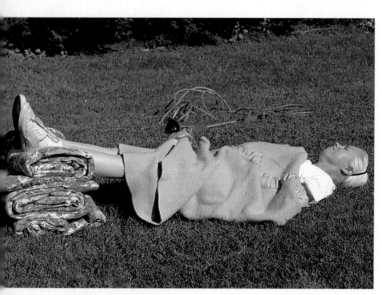

23-8 Elevate the victim's legs approximately 12 inches.

Action

- Do not touch the victim until the source of electrical current is turned off, if electrical shock is suspected.
- Assist victim into position with head lower than the legs—this helps to keep the blood flowing to the brain (Fig. 23-8); if you suspect head, neck, or back injuries, keep victim flat.
- Loosen any tight clothing to make breathing easier.
- Maintain body temperature.
- Remain with victim until help arrives—have someone call 9-1-1.
- Reassure victim that help is coming.

Stroke

Care of the client with a stroke was discussed in Chapter 21. However, first aid for the victim who has signs that a stroke has occurred is very different. Signs may include:

- Weakness or paralysis on one side of the body
  - drooping of eyelid, mouth, facial muscles
  - loss of movement of arms, fingers, legs, toes
  - tingling sensations in weakened areas
  - lack of ability to grasp objects, poor grip in hand
- Slurred speech or aphasia
- Staggering gait
- Conscious, may be confused
- Unconscious

shock
a condition in which the circulatory system is not able to transport adequate amounts of blood to all parts of the body.

Action

- Place victim in comfortable position; if lying down, keep head and shoulders raised; if unconscious, place victim on the affected side to allow saliva to drain from the mouth.
- Keep victim calm; reassure.
- Maintain body temperature.
- Have someone call 9-1-1.
- Remain with the victim until help arrives.

Falls and Fractures

Throughout this textbook, safety for both client and home care aide have been discussed. However, many people are not safety conscious. Falls are a common medical emergency for all ages. Most falls happen in or around the home because of carelessness or physical conditions of the victim that cause dizziness or unsteady gait. The risk of fractures is always present when falls occur. Listed below are some general signs of fractures.

- Pain or tenderness in the area of the fracture
- Deformity of the affected limb
- Loss of function; the victim cannot move or has difficulty moving
- Swelling in the area; bruising of the skin
- Victim may say that he/she felt or heard the bone snap or pop.

Action

- **DO NOT** move the victim unless he/she is in danger; if the victim <u>must</u> be moved, try to get help; if no help is available, move gently to safe area; protect injured area from further damage; the first aid course will give instruction on the proper ways to keep the part immobile.
- Do not attempt to straighten the limb or have the victim try to move it.
- Maintain body temperature and keep the victim as comfortable as possible.
- Have someone call 9-1-1 for help.
- Remain with the victim; provide reassurance.

Burns

Burns are injuries to tissues of the body caused by heat, electricity, chemicals, radiation, or gases. Burns are classified according to the amount of damage caused to the skin—epidermis, dermis, and structures beneath the skin (muscles, nerves, bones). They are described by degrees, as follows:

- *First degree*—involves the epidermis. The skin appears red and dry. Swelling may be present. The area is painful.
- *Second degree*—involves the epidermis and the upper part of the dermis. The skin is red with blisters. Blisters may open and weep clear fluid making the skin appear wet. Swelling may be present. The area is painful.

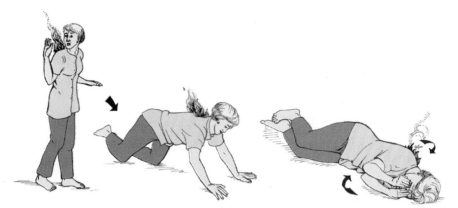

23-9 Stop, drop, and roll to smother flames and stop the burning process.

- *Third degree*—involves the epidermis, dermis, and any or all structures beneath the skin. The skin appears to be charred. Structures underneath may appear to be white. There may be an odor of burned flesh. The area may be painful or not, depending on the amount of injury to the nerve endings.

A first-degree burn of the finger can be painful, but it is not life threatening. Third-degree burns are very serious and can be life threatening when they cover large amounts of skin surface.

Action

When the victim is burned, take the following action:

- Remove the victim from the source of the burn, such as put out flames (smother with blanket, roll victim on floor to put out flames) (Fig. 23-9).
- Pour large amounts of cool water over the burned area or soak towels, sheets with cool water and apply to the area; this helps to cool the burned area and reduce the burning process; for chemical burns to the skin or eyes, flush with large amounts of cool running water until EMS arrives; Do not use ice or ice water—too much body heat is lost when ice is used (Box 23-5).

Box 23-5

Burn Care Cautions

- Do not try to clean up the burned area by
  - removing pieces of clothing or jewelry that stick to the burn
  - washing the area with soap and water
- Do not apply ointments, butter, cooking oil, burn creams, or other substances to severely burned areas.
- Do not break blisters; they protect the injured skin below.
- Do not apply ice directly to a burn unless it is very minor.

- Remove any clothing surrounding the burn that has not stuck to the burn area.
- Cover the burn using a dry, sterile dressing (if available) or dry, clean cloths to prevent infection; loosely bandage to keep them in place.
- Call 9-1-1 for help if there are severe burns.

Seizures

A seizure (convulsion) occurs when the normal functioning of the brain is disrupted by injury, infection, or disease. Seizures may occur because the victim has epilepsy, a chronic condition usually controlled by medication. Seizures may be mild blackouts or a sudden, uncontrolled series of muscle contractions that the victim cannot control. They may last for several minutes.

Action

- Protect the victim by:
  - placing him/her on the floor, if possible
  - removing furniture or other objects that the victim might strike against during uncontrolled body movements
  - placing a folded towel or clothing under the head
  - remaining with the victim during the entire seizure
- If there is saliva, blood, or vomitus in the mouth, roll the victim on his/her side to allow fluid to drain from the mouth.
- Do not place anything in the victim's mouth.
- Do not restrict the victim's movements during the seizure; this could cause more injury.
- Have family member call 9-1-1 for help.

Poisoning

A poison is a substance that, when taken into the body, causes injury or illness. There are four ways poisons enter the body:

1. *Respiratory System*
   Examples: breathing in carbon monoxide gas or fumes from paints or from drugs (crack cocaine)

2. *Digestive System*
   Examples: eating foods containing poisons; drinking household cleaning products; abusing or misusing drugs

3. *The Skin*
   Examples: handling fertilizers or pesticides improperly; contact with certain poisonous plants

4. *Circulatory System*
   Examples: injecting poisons into the body through bites or stings of insects, animals; drugs injected by needle and syringe

Action

Signs of poisoning vary according to the type of poison and how it entered the body. If you suspect that poisoning has occurred, take the following action:

- Call the Poison Control Center immediately; the phone number should be included on your Emergency Phone Number List; if the number is not known, call 9-1-1 or the local emergency number.
- Follow the directions that the Center staff will give; they will also tell you whether to call for an ambulance.
- See Box 23-6 for additional guidelines.

Chest Pain

Chest pain is the major symptom of a heart attack. A heart attack is a condition where the heart muscle is not receiving enough blood due to damage of the blood vessels in the area. The only way to know if the victim is having a heart attack is by medical examination and tests. Therefore, getting medical help as quickly as possible is very important. While chest pain can be a symptom of other problems, the person who is having chest pain should be treated as if he/she is having a heart attack. Signs of heart attack include:

- Squeezing, uncomfortable pressure, fullness or dull pain in the center of the chest that lasts for more than two minutes
- Pain that radiates to shoulders, arm, neck, or jaw (Fig. 23-10)
- Symptoms of shock (see page 442)

Box 23-6

Do's and Don'ts When Caring for a Suspected Poisoning Victim

DO

- Call the Poison Control Center or local emergency number.
- Try to find out what caused the poisoning (empty bottle of pills, etc.) and when it happened; give this information to the Poison Control Center.
- Listen for directions about caring for the victim until help arrives.
- If fumes were inhaled, get the victim to fresh air, if possible (open windows).

DON'T

- Cause victim to vomit, if poison has been swallowed.
- Follow directions on the container's label; they may not be correct.

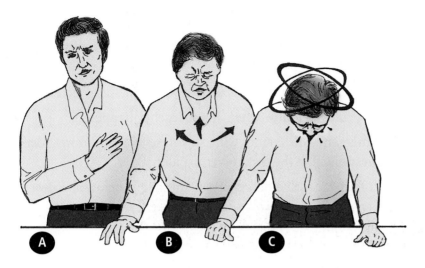

23-10 Signs of a heart attack. **A,** The feeling of pressure in the chest. **B,** Pain that spreads from the chest, up the neck, and down the left arm. **C,** Dizziness and sudden sweating.

Action

- Help victim into comfortable position, usually sitting.
- Loosen tight clothing.
- Encourage victim to remain quiet.
- Take pulse and respirations.
- Have someone call 9-1-1 for help.
- Remain with victim until help arrives.
- Comfort and reassure victim; chest pain is very frightening.

CHAPTER SUMMARY

- "Emergency" is a term used to describe a serious situation that arises suddenly and threatens the life or welfare of a person or group of persons. The immediate action taken is called "first aid."

- Preparing in advance for an emergency is very important. This includes knowing: the local emergency telephone number to call; the types of questions the dispatcher may ask; and how to care for common medical emergencies until help arrives.

- Taking a first aid course is highly recommended.

- There are several general guidelines to follow when emergencies occur.

- Reporting to your agency following the emergency is very important. Do not forget to record in the client's care record what happened and what first aid care you gave.

- Medical emergencies, such as choking, difficult or no breathing, severe bleeding, lack of a pulse, and unconsciousness require immediate action and an immediate call for help.

- The Poison Control Center must be contacted immediately if you suspect that the victim has been poisoned.

- Shock is a condition that can result from severe bleeding, serious body injuries, severe burns, allergic reactions, and emotional reaction to sudden illness. Prompt treatment is important.

STUDY QUESTIONS

1. What does the term *emergency* mean? Give four examples of medical emergencies.

2. Give three ways you will prepare for medical emergencies.

3. List five rules to follow when an emergency happens.

4. The emergency dispatcher will ask you several questions. Identify six questions that the dispatcher usually asks.

5. Select four medical emergencies from the list below and describe the first aid you will give for each emergency.
   a. Choking
   b. Shock
   c. Chest pain
   d. Poisoning
   e. Fracture
   f. Severe external bleeding
   g. Third-degree burns
   h. Seizures
   i. Stroke

6. Why is it important to record your actions on the care plan (if the victim is your client) and prepare an Incident Report for your employer?

Getting a Job and Keeping It

24

Objectives

After you read this chapter, you will be able to:

1. Discuss two resources available to obtain information about job openings.

2. Complete a job application correctly.

3. Discuss four basic principles to follow when preparing for a job interview.

4. Identify five "do's and don'ts" to follow during an interview.

5. Explain the meaning of certification and how it is obtained and maintained in your state.

6. List six rights of employees.

7. List six rights of employers.

8. Understand why the employer evaluates employee performance and how the evaluation is useful to the employee.

9. Discuss the importance of continuing education for the home care aide.

10. Give notice of resignation correctly.

> Janet and LeRoy sing in the same choir. They both have successfully finished a training program for home care aides. Janet was hired and trained by her agency, so she already has a job. LeRoy took the home care aide course at a local vocational school, and he needs to find a job. Phyllis has just moved here from another state. She is a certified home care aide with five years of experience. She, too, needs to find a job.

Just as training to become a home care aide takes time and energy, so does finding the right job. There is preparation and thought involved, including:

- locating job openings
- completing the **job application form**
- preparing for an interview
- participating in the interview
- deciding to take the job (or not)

This chapter presents the guidelines to follow in your job search. Remember that looking for the right job should be done in an organized and orderly manner. Job-seeking, job-getting, and job-keeping skills are important to develop.

Locating Job Openings

Sources of information that can help you identify job openings in your area are:

1. *Networking*
    This is an informal way to find out about job openings. Networking takes place when you let other people (those who work in home care and those who don't) know that you are looking for a job. For example, Janet may be able to tell LeRoy if her employer is looking for more home care aides. If Phyllis worked for an agency with offices in other states, her previous employer may have some job leads. Also, other persons in your community, church, PTA, or other groups might know of job openings. If you have a computer, don't forget to check the on-line bulletin boards.

2. *Newspaper*
    Newspaper advertisements give a general listing of the jobs open in your community. Look in the special section that lists medical/health care jobs. Also, check for the listing, home care aides, in the general Help Wanted ads. There is an art to reading want ads—a basic understanding of abbreviations used and reading "between the lines" will help you to understand the ads (Table 24-1).

3. *Employment agencies*
    There are two types of employment agencies, public and private. Both match job seekers with potential employers. Public employment agencies are free. Private employment agencies charge a fee for service to the employer and often to the job seeker, YOU. Fees are based on your earnings and the amount of services provided to you. A private employment agency will ask you to sign a con-

job application form
a form to be filled out when applying for a job.

networking
informal method of exchanging information about job openings.

employment agencies
private or governmental agencies that match job seekers and potential employers.

job placement counselors
persons in a school who help students to find part-time employment while in school. (Services may also be available to graduates seeking full-time jobs.)

reference
person who will speak in another's behalf.

Table 24-1

Want Ad Abbreviations and Meanings

Abbreviation	Meaning	Abbreviation	Meaning
Cert.	Certification	F/T	Full time
CHHA	Certified Home Health Aide	HHA	Home health aide
Comp.	Companion	Lic.	License
Eve.	Evenings	M-F	Monday through Friday
Excel.	Excellent	Wknd	Weekend
Exp. Pref'd	Experience Preferred	Reim.	Reimbursed
		Req.	Required

tract that outlines fees to be paid and other information about the rights and responsibilities of both parties. IF YOU DON'T UNDERSTAND THE CONTRACT, DON'T SIGN IT.

4. *School **job placement counselors***
   Some schools have job placement counselors. They help students find part-time employment while still in school. Sometimes, schools offer job placement services to their graduates.
5. *Your instructors*
   Your teachers are excellent sources of contacts in the home care field. They have had experience working with you in your program. They can often supply leads to your first job or to a new and more challenging one. Do not be afraid to ask for their help. Ask them, too, if you can use their name as a **reference.**

Completing the Job Application

When you have located a possible job opening, call the agency or visit in person to find out if this is true. Ask about the job and about filling out an application form. Some employers will send an application form in the mail, while others require you to complete it in their office. If you are going to the office, be sure to dress appropriately. Many times the application form is completed just before the interview. Bring a copy of the information you will use to fill out the form. Be sure to bring:

- Social Security card
- proof of citizenship or legal residency
- names and addresses of personal references and former employers (if applicable)
- certification
- driver's license (if applicable)
- a pen

Always completely fill out the application in ink and print all information so it is easy to read (Fig. 24-1). Be truthful. Do not give any false information.

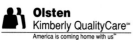

Olsten
Kimberly QualityCare℠
America is coming home with us℠

Application for Employment

Type or print clearly. This form should be completed carefully and fully. It is essential that we have complete information regarding your training and experience. Please complete all sections even if you have already provided us with your resumé. Your present employer will not be contacted for a reference without your consent. Reasonable accomodations will be made for applicants when requested.

TODAY'S DATE

NAME:	LAST	FIRST		MIDDLE

ADDRESSES FOR THE LAST FIVE YEARS (Present address first)	1. STREET	CITY	STATE	ZIP
	2. STREET	CITY	STATE	ZIP
	3. STREET	CITY	STATE	ZIP

TELEPHONE #	OTHER PHONE
( )	( )

Are you legally authorized to work in the USA? ☐ Yes ☐ No
(Should you become employed by Olsten Kimberly QualityCare, you will be required to provide documentation proving your identity and eligibility to work in the USA.)

POSITION APPLYING FOR (CLINICAL/CAREGIVER HEALTH CARE APPLICANTS—ALSO SEE SECTION BELOW)	MIN. SALARY REQUIREMENTS	DATE AVAILABLE TO BEGIN WORK

HOW WERE YOU REFERRED TO OLSTEN KIMBERLY QUALITYCARE?
☐ NEWSPAPER   ☐ TRADE PUBLICATION   ☐ EMPLOYMENT AGENCY
☐ OLSTEN CORPORATION EMPLOYEE, NAME: WORK LOCATION
☐ JOB FAIR/OPEN HOUSE; LOCATION   ☐ OTHER REFERRAL SOURCE

EDUCATION	HIGH SCHOOL NAME	LOCATION	LAST YEAR COMPLETED: ☐ 9 ☐ 10 ☐ 11 ☐ 12	DID YOU GRADUATE? ☐ YES ☐ NO	COURSE OR MAJOR	DIPLOMA OR DEGREE	GPA
	COLLEGE NAME	LOCATION	LAST YEAR COMPLETED: ☐ 1 ☐ 2 ☐ 3 ☐ 4	DID YOU GRADUATE? ☐ YES ☐ NO	COURSE OR MAJOR	DIPLOMA OR DEGREE	GPA
	GRADUATE SCHOOL NAME	LOCATION	LAST YEAR COMPLETED: ☐ 1 ☐ 2 ☐ 3 ☐ 4	DID YOU GRADUATE? ☐ YES ☐ NO	COURSE OR MAJOR	DIPLOMA OR DEGREE	GPA
	BUSINESS SCHOOL NAME	LOCATION	LAST YEAR COMPLETED: ☐ 1 ☐ 2 ☐ 3 ☐ 4	DID YOU GRADUATE? ☐ YES ☐ NO	COURSE OR MAJOR	DIPLOMA OR DEGREE	GPA
	OTHER	LOCATION	LAST YEAR COMPLETED: ☐ 1 ☐ 2 ☐ 3 ☐ 4	DID YOU GRADUATE? ☐ YES ☐ NO	COURSE OR MAJOR	DIPLOMA OR DEGREE	GPA

OLSTEN KIMBERLY QUALITYCARE PROFESSIONAL AND PARAPROFESSIONAL CLINICAL/HEALTH CARE APPLICANTS ONLY

LICENSE/ CERTIFICATION/ REGISTRATION (Use additional pages as necessary)	LICENSE TYPE	LICENSE/CERTIFICATION/REGISTRATION NO.	STATE	EXPIRATION DATE
	LICENSE TYPE	LICENSE/CERTIFICATION/REGISTRATION NO.	STATE	EXPIRATION DATE
	LICENSE TYPE	LICENSE/CERTIFICATION/REGISTRATION NO.	STATE	EXPIRATION DATE
	CPR EXPIRATION DATE	LAST PHYSICAL EXAM		LAST TB/CXR DATE

Please check the specialty area(s) that best match(es) your education, experience and interest.
☐ **Home Care**
☐ INTERMITTENT CARE   ☐ EXTENDED CARE   ☐ HOSPICE   ☐ RESIDENTIAL CARE
☐ IV THERAPY   ☐ MED/SURG   ☐ PEDIATRICS/MATERNAL CHILD   ☐ REHABILITATION
☐ **Supplemental Staffing**
☐ NURSING HOME   ☐ CLINIC (SPECIFY) _____
☐ HOSPITAL: ☐ GERIATRIC   ☐ PSYCHIATRIC   ☐ MED/SURG   ☐ PEDIATRIC/MATERNAL CHILD   ☐ ICU/CCU   ☐ LABOR/DELIVERY
☐ OTHER SPECIALTY _____
☐ **Nurse Travelers:** ASSIGNMENTS OF 8+ WEEKS IN ANOTHER CITY/STATE

Please check the shift(s) and days of the week you are available to work:
☐ FULL-TIME   ☐ PART-TIME   ☐ 7 A.M.–3 P.M.   ☐ 3 P.M.–11 P.M.   ☐ _____ VISITS ONLY
☐ MONDAY   ☐ TUESDAY   ☐ WEDNESDAY   ☐ THURSDAY   ☐ FRIDAY   ☐ SATURDAY   ☐ SUNDAY

24-1 An application form. *(Courtesy Olsten Kimberly QualityCare, Melville, N.Y.)*

Preparing for the Interview

Make an Appointment

Most employers will set up an interview when you call or after you submit a completed application form. Once the appointment time has been set, be sure to get there before the time arranged. If it is not possible to keep the appointment, notify the person *immediately* to explain why you cannot come and to set up another appointment. Otherwise the employer may decide that you are unreliable. If you don't know the exact location of the office where you will be interviewed, a practice trip may be helpful. It will give you an idea of how much time you need to get there. Remember, YOU need the job. If you miss the interview without notifying the potential employer, you may not get another chance.

Gather Information

Get to know some facts about the employer and the agency. Get the agency's brochure from the office. Is it a branch of a national agency? Is it Medicare-approved? What kind of services does it offer? What do others in your community and the health care field have to say about it?

Prepare Questions

Make a list of questions to ask during the interview that pertain to the job responsibility and the agency. For example:

- How long has the agency been open?
- What type of clients do you serve?
- How many clients do you serve?
- How many home care aides do you employ? Full-time? Part-time? How are they supervised? How often? By whom?
- What other staff do you employ?
- Do I wear a uniform?
- What geographic areas does your agency cover?
- What area(s) will I work in?
- Do I use public transportation? Drive my own car?
- Tell me about your infection control plan.

Asking questions shows that you are interested in the agency and the job. Avoid asking questions about sick time, vacations, or pay raises unless the interviewer gives no information about them. Questions that focus almost entirely on pay, vacations, and holidays give the impression that you are more interested in "off-time" benefits rather than the responsibilities of the job.

Prepare Answers

Most interviewers have a basic set of questions they ask all applicants. It is impossible to guess all the questions that might be asked, but the following are often included:

- Tell me about yourself.
- Why are you interested in working here?
- What experience have you had in home care? Have you worked in any other health field?

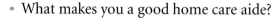

- What makes you a good home care aide?
- Why did you select this field of health care?
- What personal characteristics are necessary for success as a home care aide?
- What are your strengths? Weaknesses?
- If already employed, why do you want to change jobs?

Preparing answers to these questions (before the interview) may be helpful so you can be ready to answer if any of the topics is discussed.

There are some questions that interviewers cannot ask because they violate a person's civil rights. According to federal law, the following questions may not be asked by the employer prior to employment:

- When were you born?
- How old are you?
- How many children do you have?
- Do you have any children?
- Do you have a boyfriend/girlfriend?
- How much do you weigh?
- What type of military discharge do you have?

If any of these questions is asked during the interview, you have the right to refuse to answer the question.

Dress Appropriately

It is said that interviewers make their decisions about hiring an applicant within a few minutes after the initial contact. Therefore, first impressions are extremely important. Preparing for the interview means being well groomed and dressing professionally (Fig. 24-2). Do not show up in casual "playclothes" for an interview (Fig. 24-3). Your appearance at the interview is a preview of your grooming while "on the job." Box 24-1 lists some tips on dressing and grooming for a job interview.

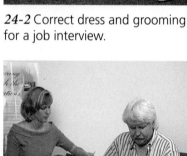

24-2 Correct dress and grooming for a job interview.

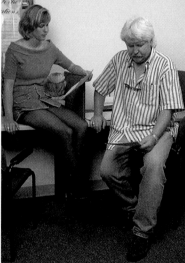

24-3 Incorrect dress and grooming for a job interview.

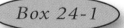

Box 24-1

Dressing and Grooming for the Interview

- Dress as you would for the first day on the job (unless the agency requires a uniform).
- Wear neat, casual clothes and comfortable shoes:
  - skirt and blouse
  - slacks and shirt
- Hair should be neatly combed; shoes and clothes clean.
- Males should be cleanly shaven; if facial hair is worn, be sure it is neatly trimmed.
- Do not wear excessive jewelry, makeup, or cologne.

Participating in the Interview

Purpose

The interview is the most important step in obtaining the job. The actual interview lets the employer:

- get to know you
- consider you as a future employee
- explain the details of the job
- tell you about the agency and the clients served

You will have the opportunity to:

- explain why you are suitable for the job
- ask specific questions about job responsibilities, working condition, benefits, etc.
- ask other questions

The interview helps to answer two basic questions:

"Is this the person for the job?" (employer)
"Is this the job for me?" (applicant)

If you have prepared ahead of time, you should feel confident and ready for the interview. Arrive about 10 minutes before the appointment. This shows your interest and reliability. It also gives you a chance to calm down and concentrate on the upcoming interview. Remember, you are prepared; you have the skills the employer needs; you are a winner. Go for it!

Guidelines

The following "do's and don'ts" will help you through the interview.

Do

- Greet the receptionist politely.
- Give your name and reason for being there.
- Remove coat (and hat) before the interview.
- Complete the job application form; read it completely before starting.
  - Use your notes.
  - Complete the entire form; print "None" or "N/A" for parts that do not apply to you.
- Take several deep breaths to relax before you enter the interview area.
- Firmly shake hands with the interviewer and greet by name when introduced; smile.
- Maintain eye contact during the interview.
- Speak clearly; use proper grammar.
- Be polite.
- Maintain good posture; sit up straight.
- Answer all questions honestly.
- Emphasize your strong points.
- Think about the question asked and how to answer it before you begin to speak.

- Give clear, short answers.
- Be honest.
- Ask questions you have prepared in advance (use notes you have made).

Don't

- Bring children or friends to the interview
- Write in spaces labeled "office use only" on application form
- Fidget, squirm, wiggle, or move nervously
- Chew gum, smoke, or eat anything during the interview
- Use slang expressions, obscene words or gestures
- Interrupt the interviewer when he/she is speaking
- Brag about yourself
- Rush when giving answers
- Talk too much or too long

At the end of the interview, thank the person for the opportunity to be interviewed. Firmly shake his/her hand and leave the room.

A positive interview may result in a job offer. Sometimes, you may be offered the position immediately. If not, the interviewer will tell you when you will hear about the job.

While you are waiting to hear about the job, keep looking for another one. After all, an interview does not guarantee a job offer. Even if you are not the successful candidate for the job, you have been through the job-seeking process and have learned what to do and what not to do. Keep trying; don't give up. There IS a job for you.

Deciding to Take the Job

Now that you have completed the application and interview, the next step is deciding if the job is for you. Some factors to consider in the decision are:

1. *Starting wages or pay (salary)*—weekly, every other week, monthly? Can I budget myself to live on the amount offered?
2. *Pay raises*—how often? how much? based on length of employment and/or performance?
3. *Benefits*—medical insurance (type of plan, insurer, cost to employee)? dental insurance? disability insurance? life insurance? pension plan? plan for prescription drugs? eyeglass plan?
4. *Paid sick leave*—how much? can it be carried over from one year to another?
5. *Vacation*—how much? based on length of employment?
6. *Holidays*—how many?
7. *Location of areas where you will work*—accessible by public transportation? fares paid? personal auto needed? amount reimbursed per mile? type and amount of automobile insurance required? safety of areas served?
8. *Uniform worn?*—paid for by agency? self? any allowance for uniform maintenance?
9. *Education*—Continuing education or in-service education available?
10. *Conference/office time*—how often? how long? paid?
11. *Hours*—work schedule?

certification
recognition by a governmental or nongovernmental agency that an individual has met certain requirements.

mandatory
required.

Making Your Decision

Put all of the information about the job(s) offered to you in writing and compare the positive aspects and the negative aspects. Also, consider these questions:

- Will the job meet my career goals?
- Will I find job satisfaction?
- Can I work comfortably and safely for this employer in this agency?
- Will I be able to give good care to clients as an employee of this agency?
- Will I be able to safely use my skills and abilities?

Once you have answered all of these questions you are ready to make your decision. It's your choice!

Certification

Certification is recognition by a governmental or nongovernmental agency that a person has met certain qualifications. The home care aide must attend a training program that is approved by the certifying group. Sometimes, a comprehensive examination is given to test the aide's knowledge and competence. You must apply and pay a fee to take this test. Your instructor can tell you how and what to do. In some states, certification is obtained when a student successfully finishes a training program. He/she applies to the appropriate state regulating body and pays a fee for certification. In some states, certification is **mandatory.**

Each state has its own requirements for certification. If you move from one state to another, you may be required to contact the appropriate regulating body in that state to apply for certification. Remember, in order for your agency to receive Medicare reimbursement for your services, you must be a certified home care aide.

In order to keep your certification active, you must meet the requirements set up by your state. This may involve participating in educational programs and/or working a specific number of days within a certain time period. For example, you must work a minimum of 14 days within 2 years. In addition, you will have to follow the rules and regulations for certified home care aides in your state. These usually govern what tasks you can legally perform, honesty, safety of clients, and substance abuse. Some states require that certification be renewed every year or every two years. A fee is charged for renewal.

Certification is very valuable to you. It demonstrates that you have met a required level of knowledge and competence. This credential gives you the opportunity to work in many agencies.

For additional information about certification:

1. Consult your instructor or agency.
2. Consult the state regulatory agency
   (State Health Department, State Board of Nursing).
3. Write to: National HomeCaring Council
   519 C Street, NE
   Washington, DC 20002

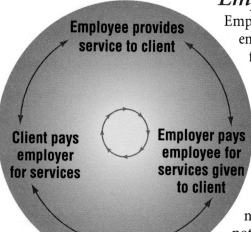

24-4 Employment is a partnership between employer and employee.

Employment—A Partnership

Employment is a partnership. If the partnership is a good one, both employer and employee benefit. The employer has agreed to pay you for the services that you will provide. You have agreed to perform these services to the best of your ability. In this way, both of you benefit. The home care agency receives monies from the client based on the services given by its employees. Because the employees perform these services accurately and skillfully, the employer is able to pay the employees from monies received from the client (Fig. 24-4).

It is this mutual agreement—employer to employee and employee to employer—that makes the real difference. Unfortunately, there are many employees, in all types of businesses, who do not understand that the employer *cannot* pay the employee unless the product or service being produced is *sold* or *used*. In the automobile industry, the product is the car. In the home care industry, the product is not as easy to see or touch. The product is the delivery of a variety of home care services to many different clients (mothers and their newborn infants, children, younger and older adults). Your ability to produce the desired services will affect your employer's ability to have enough monies to pay you. Therefore, performing your duties and responsibilities accurately and skillfully is very important.

Employer and Employee Rights

In this partnership, both parties have rights. Listed below are some of the rights of your employer and some of your rights.

Employer Rights

- Right to expect that the home care aide will perform the duties properly
  That you will:
  - practice your skills correctly
  - perform your duties and responsibilities accurately
  - know what you are **not** permitted to do
  - give care according to the care plan
  - refuse to perform skills that you are not trained to perform or not permitted to do
- Right to expect that the home care aide will keep accurate records of client care given and billable time
  That you will:
  - use the correct forms, provided by your agency, to record client care and billable time
  - use other forms, such as Incident Report forms, when necessary
  - be honest in recording time spent caring for your client and the care given to your client
- Right to expect that the home care aide will use correct safety practices to protect himself/herself and the client
  That you will:
  - practice safety awareness at all times
  - use universal precautions and infection control procedures when needed

personnel policies
a set of rules and regulations to be followed by employees; these usually pertain to employer and employee rights and responsibilities.

- report to your supervisor situations in the client's home that you believe to be unsafe
- Right to expect the home care aide to follow the agency's **personnel policies** and procedures
  That you will:
  - follow all personnel policies and procedures: looking and acting professionally (Chapter 1), and code of behavior (Chapter 2)
  - ask your employer to explain any policies or procedures you do not understand
- Right to supervise and evaluate the home care aide's job performance and to discipline him/her, if necessary
  That you will:
  - accept constructive criticism offered by your supervisor
  - follow suggestions for improving your job performance
- Right to expect that the home care aide will protect and respect the client's privacy and property
  That you will:
  - keep all information confidential about client and family (Chapter 2)
  - treat client's property with respect and consideration
- Right to expect that the home care aide will treat all agency personnel with respect
  That you will:
  - follow the agency's code of behavior

Employee Rights

- Right to be paid for the work you perform
  That your employer will:
  - provide payment according to an agreed-upon rate and according to the agency's pay schedule
  - provide the correct amount of money for the time worked
  - provide additional monies for extra time worked (overtime, holidays, etc.)
  - keep accurate records of work time and income taxes and Social Security paid
- Right to a safe working environment
  That your employer will:
  - provide the necessary equipment and supplies to protect you from possible infection (mask, gloves, etc.)
  - remove you from situations in the home where there is danger to your well-being
  - follow Federal regulations regarding exposure to blood-borne pathogens (see Chapter 9)
- Right to be supervised properly
  That your employer will:
  - supervise you on the job regularly
  - inform you of the results of the supervision—verbally or in writing
  - explain how you can improve your performance, if needed
  - respond promptly when you contact the agency to report abnormal conditions in your client

- Right to be evaluated and to be informed if your performance is not satisfactory
  That your employer will:
    - evaluate your performance on a regular basis
    - inform you of the results of the evaluations—verbally and in writing
    - inform you about ways to improve your performance
    - inform you about what will happen if your performance does not improve
- Right to receive copies of the agency's personnel policies and job description
  That your employer will:
    - give you copies of the personnel policies and job description
    - answer any questions, if you do not understand the meaning of any policy or procedure
    - honor the personnel policies as printed
- Right to attend in-service education programs provided by the employer to maintain your skills and develop new ones
  That your employer will:
    - provide in-service education programs regularly
    - keep records of your attendance
- Right to be treated with respect by all agency staff
  That your employer will:
    - treat you with respect and dignity at all times
    - recognize that you are an important part of the home care team

Supervision and Evaluation

Supervision is a process used by employers to observe employees doing their jobs. The purpose is to assist them to improve client care skills and to perform their duties and responsibilities more effectively.

Evaluation is the process employers use to find out how well the employee performs on the job and how well he/she relates to client/family and members of the home care team.

From time to time, you will be supervised and evaluated by your employer. You will be told how often supervisory visits will be made during the year. You may or may not be given advance notice. Remember that these visits are made to help you to improve your client care skills, organization, and home management abilities. Supervisory visits give you the chance to ask questions and receive helpful hints from your employer. Following each visit, your supervisor records the observations and discussions with you about your performance, including directions given for improvement.

Employee evaluations are given according to a time schedule (every six months or yearly), which your employer will explain. As a new employee, you may be evaluated more frequently. One of your rights as an employee is to know in advance what areas will be covered in the evaluation. See sample evaluation form (Fig. 24-5).

After evaluating your performance, your employer will meet with you privately to discuss the findings. He/she should discuss your strengths and those areas that need improvement. The purpose of the evaluation

supervision
process of observing employees doing their jobs.

evaluation
process of judging employee performance to determine suitability to remain in the job.

OLSTEN Health Care

RECORD OF EMPLOYEE OBSERVATION/EVALUATION

☐ **Observation**   ☐ **Evaluation**

Employee's name

Job classification

Client's name   Diagnosis

	Yes	No	N/A
Does employee prepare and/or follow the plan of care?	☐	☐	☐
Is employee's charting accurate and complete?	☐	☐	☐
Does employee use equipment properly?	☐	☐	☐
Does employee relate well to co-workers?	☐	☐	☐
Does employee relate well to client(s)?	☐	☐	☐
Does employee relate well to family members?	☐	☐	☐
Does employee show an interest in learning?	☐	☐	☐
Does employee report pertinent information to supervisor?	☐	☐	☐

RATE EMPLOYEE	Above	Average	Below
Adaptability	☐	☐	☐
Attitude	☐	☐	☐
Cooperativeness	☐	☐	☐
Coping ability	☐	☐	☐
Initiative	☐	☐	☐
Punctuality	☐	☐	☐

Quality and
Quantity of Work _____

_____

_____

Teaching _____

_____

_____

Comments and
Recommendations _____

_____

_____

_____

_____

_____

_____ _____ __/__/__ _____ _____ __/__/__
Signature of Employee   Title   Date   Signature of Observer/Evaluator   Title   Date

NOTE: An _observation_ requires the signature of the observer; an _evaluation_ requires the signature of both the observer and the Healthcare staff employee.

©1991 The Olsten Corporation. Printed in U.S.A. EOE M/F/H/V   HC 01073 (10/91)

24-5 A sample evaluation form. *(Courtesy Olsten Kimberly QualityCare, Melville, N.Y.)*

is to help you to progress on the job. It is to your employer's advantage to assist you to improve; it is to your advantage to follow your employer's recommendations.

There is space on the evaluation form for the employer and employee to give written comments. You may agree or disagree with the evaluation. Give your reasons in writing, sign, and date the form. Each evaluation is kept as a permanent, confidential part of your employee record.

Continuing Your Education

We are living in a time when approaches to health care change rapidly. New techniques and procedures are being developed to improve the care given to clients at home. Sometimes procedures we have been taught are changed; sometimes new procedures need to be learned to replace outdated ones. It is very important to keep up with these changes so that your skills remain sharp and current. One way to do this is by participating in continuing education programs offered by your employer. Ask your supervisor about the types of programs given.

Some states consider continuing education to be so important that certification renewal depends on proof of the person's participation in these activities. Your employer can give you more information about your state's requirements.

Deciding to Leave Your Job

Leaving a job can be a most frustrating, difficult, and stress-producing experience. But it need not be, if approached properly. There are many reasons for deciding to leave a job. Perhaps you are moving to another area of the state or country. Or, you are planning to continue your education full-time. Maybe there are people you work with whose behavior is causing you difficulty in performing your job effectively.

The final decision to leave should be based on careful thought. It should not be a decision made in haste—on the spur of the moment. Some employees storm the employer's door with the statement, "I quit!" This behavior shows that the person's decision is probably based on the immediate problem rather than on a review of the factors leading to the actual event. At any rate, should you decide that the only thing to do is to leave the job, it is important that you have a new job **before** leaving your old one. It is much more difficult to find a job after you have already left your employer, no matter what the reason.

Before deciding to leave, you need to think about the reasons for leaving. If a problem situation exists, have you taken the steps necessary to solve the problem? Can it be solved? Have you talked to your supervisor about it? The best approach to handling the situation may not be to leave your employer. Talking to your supervisor about the problems and possible solutions may help you to decide whether to leave or to stay.

Leaving the Job Gracefully

According to the latest statistics, the average worker in the United States will change jobs at least seven times during one's work life. Therefore, it is important to develop skills needed to leave the job gracefully. Once you have decided to leave, the following steps need to be taken:

1. Follow your agency's policy about notifying superiors about your decision. For example, your agency may request two week's notice of resignation. Make sure that you honor this policy. Let your employer know as soon as possible so that there will be time to hire a replacement.

2. Speak to your supervisor and explain why you are leaving.

3. Avoid discussing your intentions to leave with co-workers before speaking with your supervisor. It is poor practice to inform everyone but those who really need to know. Information spreads rapidly through the "grapevine," and you do not want your employer to hear about your leaving from this source.

4. Share the news with your client(s) after you have told your employer. Your client will appreciate your telling him/her yourself.

Some agencies conduct an exit interview with each employee who is leaving. This gives the employer the chance to ask you for information about the job you are leaving. Your honest answers help the employer to improve working conditions in the future. Do not take this opportunity to gripe about your supervisor or other staff members. You may, at some future time, want to return to the agency. Don't "burn your bridges"—always leave the interview on a positive note.

Take the opportunity during this exit interview to ask the employer if:

- you can use their name as a reference
- there are other offices located in the new area (if you are moving to a new location)

CHAPTER SUMMARY

- Seeking, finding, and keeping a job are important skills to develop.

- There are several resources for obtaining information about job openings, including:
  - networking
  - newspaper advertisements
  - employment agencies
  - school job placement counselors
  - your instructors

- Prepare for the job interview by:
  - making an appointment
  - gathering information
  - preparing questions and answers
  - dressing appropriately

- Certification is recognition by a governmental or nongovernmental agency that you have met specific qualifications as a home care aide.
- Both employers and employees have rights.
- Evaluation and supervision are important to the employer, employee, and client.
- Continuing education helps you learn new information and skills that will help you give better care to your client.
- Agency personnel policies regarding resignation should be followed when possible.

STUDY QUESTIONS

1. Locate a job opening using the following sources:
   a. local newspaper
   b. your instructor
   c. home care agency within your community

2. Write a list of four questions to ask during a job interview.

3. Select four questions (from this chapter) that an interviewer might ask you. Write answers for each question.

4. Prepare your own index card (or small sheet of paper) that lists the information you will need during an interview.

5. How is certification obtained in your state? Is certification mandatory? Gather the same information about another state that is the closest to your home state.

6. List two reasons for employee evaluation. How can you use the results of evaluation and supervision by your employer?

7. List six rights of employers and six rights of employees.

8. Your co-worker complains about attending the agency's continuing education programs. How would you respond?

9. Give two reasons for leaving a job and explain how you would do this.

Glossary

Abuse Mistreating or causing harm

Acute illness An illness with a rapid onset, severe symptoms, and of short length

Advance directive Documents that indicate a client's wishes about health care

Aerobic Able to live in the presence of oxygen

AIDS Abbreviation for acquired immunodeficiency syndrome

Ambulate To move the body with or without assistance, to walk

Anaerobic Able to live without air or oxygen

Analysis Determining the substances present in a specimen

Anorexia Loss of appetite

Antiembolism stockings Elastic stockings worn to prevent the formation of blood clots in the legs

Areola Colored, circular area surrounding the nipple

Aspiration Breathing in or inhaling a substance into the bronchial tubes and lungs

Assess To determine the client's needs for home care services

Assistive devices Equipment or other items to help clients perform activities of daily living more easily

Atrophy Decrease in size or a wasting away of tissue

Baby boomers Those born between 1946 and 1964

Bacteria Microorganisms causing disease

Bed cradle A device to keep the top bedding from resting on client's legs and feet

Bereaved Those who mourn the death of a loved one

Bias(es) To like or dislike someone or something without a good reason; prejudice

Blood pressure The pressure of blood in the large arteries

Blood-borne pathogens Pathogenic microorganisms that are present in human blood and can cause disease in humans

Body mechanics Proper use of muscles to move and lift objects and maintain correct posture

Body structure(s) Construction and arrangement of cells, tissues, and organs

Bond Emotional attachment between infant and parents, especially the mother

Bony prominence Part of bone that is near the skin's surface

Calculi Abnormal stones formed in the body due to accumulation of mineral salt

Carbon dioxide Gas eliminated from the lungs during exhalation

Care record A permanent written record of client's progress during illness and rehabilitation

Carrier A person or animal who spreads disease to others but does not become ill

Catheters Hollow, flexible tubes made of soft plastic or rubber that can be inserted into the body to withdraw or to insert fluids

Certification Recognition by a governmental or nongovernmental agency that an individual has met certain requirements

Cesarean birth Surgical procedure where the baby is delivered through an incision in the abdomen

Chart To record in writing information on client's record

Chronic illness A disease showing little change, slow progress and of long duration; not an acute illness

Closed bed Made when the bed will remain empty for a period of time. May be made with or without a bedspread

Combustible Capable of catching fire and burning

Communication Sharing of thoughts, information and opinions with others

Compress (compresses) Gauze, washcloths, or small towels applied to a body area. May be moistened with hot or cold solution

Confidentiality Something spoken or written in confidence; in secret

Congenital Present at birth

Constrict To narrow

Contaminated Dirty, exposed to harmful organisms, making the object unsafe for use as intended

Contamination Introduction of harmful organisms

Contract To become smaller, tighter

Contracture Shortening of muscle whereby a joint becomes permanently immovable

Crisis A critical time

Decubitus ulcer Sore on the skin caused by prolonged pressure on the part; also called bed sore or pressure sore

Defense mechanism Unconscious reactions that protect a person from real or perceived threats

Deficiency A lack of one or more essential nutrients in the diet

Dehydrated/dehydration Excessive water loss from body tissues resulting from not enough fluid intake

Denial A refusal to admit the truth

Depression, Depressed A feeling of intense sadness

Diabetes Disease resulting from lack of insulin secreted by special cells of the pancreas. Causes blood sugar to be elevated

Diagnose(d) To determine the type and cause of an illness or condition based on a variety of information

Diastole Relaxation of the heart muscle causing its chambers to fill with blood

Diastolic (blood) pressure Force of blood pushing against walls of large arteries when the heart is relaxing

Digestion Complete physical and chemical breakdown of food

Dilate Expand or open wider

Disability Physical, mental, or emotional handicap that interferes with abilities to carry out activities of daily living

Discipline System of rules that governs the way we act

Disinfect To destroy germs

Disinfectant A chemical that can be applied to objects to destroy germs

Distilled water Water that goes through a special process to remove minerals and other substances

Diuretic(s) A drug or other substance that causes urine to be produced or excreted

DNR An abbreviation for "do not resuscitate," meaning do not artificially restart the heartbeat

Document To describe in writing observations or action taken. Also called recording or charting

DRG (diagnostic related group) A listing of diagnoses used in establishing reimbursement by Medicare and Medicaid for hospitalization and medical care

Durable Power of Attorney An advance medical directive which names another to make health care decisions if a person becomes unable to do so

Dysuria Difficulty urinating

Ecologically Relating to the environment

Edema Abnormal amount of fluid in the tissues (swelling)

Elimination The process of removing waste products from the body

Embolus A blood clot that travels through the circulatory system until it lodges in a distant blood vessel

Emergency (emergencies) A serious situation that comes on suddenly and threatens life or well-being

Emesis basin A kidney shaped basin that fits against the neck to collect vomitus

Empathy Understanding the feelings of another

Employment agencies Private or governmental agencies which match job seekers and potential employers

End-stage disease Terminal or final illness

Endocrine Glands that secrete hormones directly into the bloodstream

Ethics Code of behavior or conduct

Evaluation Process of judging employee performance to determine suitability to remain in the job

Exacerbations(s) Return of symptoms of illness or dieease following a remission

Exocrine Glands that secrete substances into a duct

Expire Die

Exposure incident A specific eye, mouth, other mucous membrane non-intact skin or parenteral contact with blood or other potentially infectious material that results from the performance of an employee's duties

Fatigue Loss of strength and endurance

Feces Formed body waste discharged from the bowels

Fever An abnormal elevation of body temperature

First Aid Immediate care given before treatment by trained medical personnel

Flammable Burns easily

Flatus Air or gas in the intestine that passes through the rectum

Footboard A positioning device to keep client's feet in an upright position

Footdrop Inability to keep the foot in a normal walking position

Fracture Broken bone

Function(s) Action performed by any structure

Genetic Inherited through the genes

Genitalia (genitals) Organs of reproduction, usually external organs

Gerontologists Specialists in the study of aging

Gestation Period of time between conception and birth

Grief Physical and emotional responses associated with extreme sorrow or loss

Grievance(s) A wrong, considered as grounds for a complaint

Habit A repeated pattern of involuntary behavior or thought

Health A state of physical, mental, and social well-being

Hemorrhoids Varicose veins in the rectum or anus

Hepatitis B An infectious disease of the liver spread through contact with blood and caused by a virus

HIV Abbreviation for human immunodeficiency virus

Hormones Chemicals produced by endocrine glands

Hospice A program of care that assists the dying client to stay at home and maintain a satisfactory life style during the end stage of an illness

Hospital Discharge Planner Person who arranges for the care of a patient upon release from the hospital. May be a professional nurse or social worker

Humidifier Equipment used to increase the amount of moisture in an oxygen delivery system

Hypertension High blood pressure

Hypotension Low blood pressure

Illness The state of being sick

Impaction The presence of a large, hard mass of feces in the rectum or colon

Impulse A sudden, uncontrollable urge

Incentive spirometer Instrument that is used to encourage the client to breathe deeply and correctly

Incident An unexpected event

Incontinent The inability to control urination or bowel elimination

Infection Occurs when harmful organisms enter the body and grow, causing illness or disease

Informal caregivers Unpaid persons who care for clients on a voluntary basis

Intravenous (IV) infusions Administration of nutrients or medications through a vein or veins

Invasive Entering the body

Job application form A form to be filled out when applying for a job

Job Placement Counselors Persons in a school who help students to find part-time employment while in school. (Services may also be available to graduates seeking full-time jobs)

Lancets Short, pointed blades used to obtain blood from capillaries

Lifting or Turning sheet Folded sheet placed under client from shoulders to thighs

Living Will An advance directive which specifies treatment to be given or withheld if a person becomes terminally ill or incapable of making decisions him/herself

Lochia The discharge from the vagina after childbirth

Lubricant A fluid, ointment, or other substance for reducing friction between parts that rub together and making a surface slippery. It protects skin and prevents drying

Malignant Abnormal cells causing cancer

Malnutrition Any disorder of nutrition

Mandatory Required

Medicaid A state and federal program of hospitalization and health care for low income persons of all ages

Medical asepsis Use of techniques and practices to prevent the spread of pathogenic organisms

Medical crisis Event requiring immediate attention

Medicare A federal program of hospitalization and health care insurance for persons over 65 years. Participation is voluntary

Medications Substances used in the treatment of diseases or illness; drugs

Mental illness A brain disorder that affects thoughts, emotions, and behavior

Metabolism Burning of food to produce heat and energy in the body

Microorganisms A living plant or animal that can only be seen by a microscope

Microscope Instrument for viewing objects that cannot be seen with the naked eye

Mourn The process of grieving caused by great personal loss

Muscle atrophy Wasting of muscle

Muscle tone Readiness of muscle to work

Nasal cannula A two-pronged device that delivers oxygen. Short prongs are inserted into client's nostrils

Need Requirement for survival

Neglect Inability or failure to provide needed care

Networking Informal method of exchanging information about job openings

Nonpathogenic Usually not capable of causing or producing a disease

Nonverbal communication Communication without the use of words

Normal saline solution A solution of table salt and water in the same concentration as in the body tissue

Nutrition The process by which food is taken in and used by the body

Observe (observation) Act of watching carefully and attentively

Occupied bed Made while the client is in the bed

Open bed Made when the bed will be occupied shortly. Top linens are fan-folded to foot of bed

Output All fluids lost from the body that can be measured

Oxygen Gas essential for life

Parasites Organisms that live in or on another organism

Parenteral Piercing mucous membranes or skin through needle sticks, human bites, cuts, and scrapes

Pathogenic Capable of causing or producing a disease

Peers Persons who are one's equal

Perineal (perineum) Pertaining to the perineum, the area between the legs. In women, the area between the vagina and anus. In men, the area between the scrotum and anus

Peristalsis Rhythmic, involuntary movement that occurs in hollow tubes of the body

Personal Protective Equipment (PPE) Specialized clothing or equipment worn by an employee for protection against a hazard

Personnel policies A set of rules and regulations to be followed by employees. These usually pertain to employer and employee rights and responsibilities

Physiological Pertaining to the normal functioning of the body

Pigment Coloring matter in the body

Pneumonia Inflammation of the lung

Policy (policies) A set of rules and regulations

Postmortem After death

Postpartum period The first six weeks following the birth of a baby

Prefix The word part attached to the beginning of a word root to modify its meaning

Prejudice Having or forming a preconceived judgment or opinion without fair reasons

Primary caregiver A person who provides most of the care early in one's life

Prognosis Educated guess about the probable outcome of an illness

Prostheses Devices used by disabled persons to replace a missing body part

Psychotherapy Method of treating mental disorders, primarily by "talk therapy"

Pulse Throbbing felt over the arteries with each beat of the heart

Pursed lips Lips positioned for whistling

Reference Person who will speak in another's behalf

Reimbursement To make payment for expense incurred

Remission(s) Partial or complete disappearance of symptoms of illness or disease

Rescue breathing Another person breathes air into the victim's lungs to maintain supply of oxygen

Reservoir A place where a pathogen is stored, can live and grow

Respiration(s) Act or process of breathing

Respite care Short-term care provided so that main caregivers in the family can have a break from their responsibilities

Rite(s) Formal ritual(s) used in religious or solemn practices

Role Usual function of a person or object

Rooting reflex Normal reaction infants have that makes them begin to suck when their cheeks are stroked

Secrete (Secretion) Release of a substance that serves a special function in the body

Sedative(s) A substance, procedure, or measure that has a calming effect

Self-actualization State of reaching one's full potential and being able to cope with problems

Self-esteem Thinking and feeling good about yourself

Shearing Pressure against surface of skin and skin layers as client is being moved—one surface rubs against another surface

Shock A condition in which the circulatory system is not able to transport adequate amounts of blood to all parts of the body

Sibling A brother or sister

Sphincters Rings of voluntary and involuntary muscles that surround external and internal body openings

Sputum Material coughed up from the lungs and spit out through the mouth

Standard a gauge that is used as a basis for judgment

Stereotype A generalization about a form of behavior in an individual or group

Sterile Free from all living organisms

Suffix A word part attached to the end of the word root to modify its meaning

Supervision Process of observing employees doing their jobs

Surgical incision A cut produced surgically by a sharp instrument creating an opening into an organ or space

Surrogate One who is appointed to act for another

Systole Contraction of heart muscle causing blood to leave the heart

Systolic (blood) pressure Force of blood pushing against walls of the large arteries when the heart is contracting

Temperature The amount of heat produced by the body as it uses food for energy

Terminal illness An illness which causes the end of life

Thermometer An instrument for measuring temperature

Thrombus Blood clot

Toxic Poisonous

Traction To put under tension by means of weights and pulleys to straighten or immobilize a body part or to relieve pressure on it

Transfer Moving client from one place to another

Transmitted Passed from one person or place to another

Trauma Injury caused by external force or violence

Tremors Purposeless, continuous, quick movements of skeletal muscles, especially in the hands

Unit prices A method of pricing food

Universal Precautions An approach to infection control designed to prevent the spread of blood-borne diseases

Urinate Process of eliminating urine

Verbal communication Communication using the spoken or written word

Vital signs Essential signs of life: temperature, pulse, respirations, and blood pressure

Vomitus Material expelled from the stomach when vomiting

Word root The word part that is the core of the term, contains the basic meaning of the word

Wound Physical injury causing a break in the skin during surgery or an accident

Index

Note that page numbers in italics indicate figures and those followed by t indicate tables.